AF718685

Supplementing Dietary Nutrients

A Guide for Healthcare Professionals

THE STANDARD
ROAD MAP SERIES

Supplementing Dietary Nutrients

A Guide for Healthcare Professionals

by
Thomas G. Guilliams Ph.D.

POINT INSTITUTE
STEVENS POINT, WI

The Point Institute was founded by Thomas Guilliams, Ph.D. as an independent research organization focused on examining and disseminating information about the use of natural therapeutic options for treating and preventing chronic disease. Along with therapies generally defined as lifestyle interventions, the Point Institute specializes in the evidence and application of nutraceuticals (dietary supplements, herbs, vitamins, minerals, etc.) as therapeutic and preventative agents in clinical practice.

Disclaimer: This publication is intended only to inform and educate healthcare professionals; and combines both established and emerging nutritional information. The scope of this publication is limited and is not intended to replace the role of comprehensive textbooks on nutrition. Nothing herein is intended to replace guideline recommendations or promote specific therapies for individual patients. Healthcare providers are responsible to make their own determination of the usefulness and applicability of the information within this publication. Neither the publisher, author, nor reviewers assume any liability for any injury to persons arising from the use of the information found in this publication.

ISBN: 978-0-9856158-0-2

Dedication

This work is dedicated to those who seek the truth wherever it may be found; and follow the question wherever the answer leads; and to all those in awe of the orchestrated beauty and design of the human frame.

> *"It is highly dishonorable for a reasonable soul to live in so divinely built a mansion as the body she resides in- altogether unacquainted with the exquisite structure of it"*
>
> Robert Boyle (1627-1691)

Acknowledgements

To the many thousands of people, past and present, who have dedicated their lives to the study of nutrition and human health; your dedication to research and willingness to write down your observations have made it possible to practice today's nutritional medicine.

To those who have asked me difficult questions about the evidence and mechanisms related to nutrient supplementation; you pushed me to find the intersection between clinical research and clinical reality.

To those who helped get this manuscript ready for the world to see: to Jamie, Dave, Roni and Liz for their great help editing and proofreading; to Nathan and Sara for their dedication in making the cover and layout design under the time-crunch they were given; and for my friends and coworkers who kept me motivated through the whole project. To Lindsey Drake for helping to make tweaks for the second printing and for helping to find the little mistakes we all missed the first time around.

To the many experts I phoned or emailed throughout this project, thanks for helping me to understand the nuances that rarely get published. Special thanks to Loren Israelsen (UNPA) for his comments on the regulatory section, and to Mark Blumenthal (ABC) for his comments on the herbal section and for permission to reprint *HerbalGram* material in the appendix.

Finally, to my wife, Lori, and my children, Caleb, Naomi, Josh, Katie, Elisabeth and Matthew: If you want to take the time to read through this book, it will help answer the burning question of exactly what Dad does when he's at work all day. May God grant that you would always be blessed with health and abundance; and a generous heart to share these gifts with others.

Table of Contents

Table of Contents

Table of Contents

Preface

The purpose of this book is simple: to help guide healthcare professionals in making dietary and nutritional *supplement* recommendations for their patients. This Road map is not intended to be an exhaustive work on nutrition; there are many excellent textbooks that cover this in detail. Nor is this intended to replace the need for a nutritionist or dietitian within the clinic, though I hope they, too, will find this resource helpful. What most nutrition textbooks and many nutritional courses lack is the practical and clinically relevant relationship between the science of nutrition and the available products used in clinical practice. This book is intended to fill that gap.

I have spent over 20 years attempting to create an interface between epidemiological data, clinical research, clinical practice challenges and commercially available foods and supplements. I have had the privilege to interact and teach with some of the leading functional medicine/integrative clinicians in the country, honored to engage with some of the leading nutrient researchers in the world, and have an intimate knowledge of the raw material supply chain that provides the ingredients that make up dietary supplements. This Road map represents nearly two decades of researching answers to questions posed by clinicians on behalf of their patients, along with my own insatiable curiosity to know "why" and "how."

The scope of this Road map is limited to the principles and applications of foods or dietary supplements as nutrients, not as therapeutic agents. For instance, while we discuss detailed differences between natural and synthetic vitamin E and other tocopherols, we do not attempt to summarize the vast clinical research on the same. In addition, we cover for the clinician a host of practical aspects of using dietary supplements completely absent from nutritional textbooks, such as regulatory issues, adverse event reporting, bioavailability issues and much more. This book can function as a mini-textbook on the practical clinical application of nutrients or kept handy as a reference for its monograph information. The Point Institute publishes many monographs and white papers on the use of dietary supplements as therapeutic agents, and several Road maps outlining condition-specific lifestyle and nutritional intervention are also available (see back pages).

Some of the conclusions and recommendations here may be less sensational than the marketing claims used to sell supplements. Often what we believe to be true about a food or supplement actually turns out to be false, or at least unsubstantiated. In many cases, nutrient claims purporting to be true are simply too difficult or costly to research in humans, at least for now, and we are often left with a nutrient's potential mechanisms and the clinician's intuition. While we do not discount the benefit of this level of evidence within the clinical practice, our recommendations are mostly based on published clinical research where available.

In today's scientific world, nutritional research and guideline recommendations are constantly changing. We welcome your input. If you know of reputable scientific information that would challenge or modify our recommendations, we ask you to communicate with us at info@pointinstitute.org so we can evaluate the information and consider revising our recommendations. Before doing so, please be sure you have the most recent update of this Road map. You can check our website, www.pointinstitute.org, or the retailer of this book for updates on this or other publications.

[This copy is a second printing of the first edition that includes minor updates, mostly pertaining to changes in the labeling requirements of daily values in U.S. starting July of 2018. Other small changes to correct errors were also made prior to reprinting].

Lifestyle-based Therapy : Our Core Philosophy

Our core philosophy is simple: the human body has an amazing ability to maintain its own health when provided with appropriate amounts and types of healthy signals. When harmful signals are removed and appropriate signals are enhanced, cells and organ systems are capable of creating healthy outcomes. Lifestyle-based therapy (i.e., Lifestyle Medicine), then, provides the tools and incentives to help individuals assess and prioritize the signals in their lives that require changing and offers a bridge of support through the journey to a healthier outcome.[1]

For the clinician, implementing lifestyle medicine means understanding chronic disease prevention and intervention from a different perspective, one that fully integrates the relationship between lifestyle inputs (what we will call "signals") and the patient's ability to convert these signals into healthy outcomes. As Hippocrates understood it nearly 2,400 years ago, *"Everyone has a physician inside him or her, we just have to help it in its work. The natural healing force within each one of us is the greatest force in getting well."* Voltaire put this a bit more bluntly when he said, *"The art of medicine consists of amusing the patient while nature cures the disease."*

Lifestyle-based therapy is truly patient-centered in that it requires assessing all the signals that influence an individual's health (unlike clinical trials that view patients within a cohort), recognizing that individuals have differing capacities to translate signals and change behaviors. Clinical success is dependent, in this model, on an ongoing relationship between an engaged clinician and an empowered patient.

Physiological Resilience and Metabolic Reserve

While the name we give to chronic diseases might depend on the organ system or tissues involved, such as atherosclerosis, osteoarthritis, Alzheimer's, type 2 diabetes or cancer, the chronic dysfunction involved in each of these conditions is ultimately caused by the presence of signals that overwhelm the body's ability to heal itself, or the absence of signals that would allow tissues to recover. Our lifestyle synergy model describes two layers of resistance against poor lifestyle signals: Physiological Resilience and Metabolic Reserve.

Essentially, physiological resilience is the capacity of each cell or organ system to withstand the necessary (and immediate) changes that create the rhythm of a healthy organism. The ability of arteries to dilate when blood flow increases, the ability to quickly dispose of excess glucose after a meal, or the ability to increase (and decrease) cortisol when a stressful situation arises (and resolves) are just a few examples of physiological resilience. Each of these systems, and thousands more, are like coils or rubber bands, capable of being stretched for a particular physiological purpose, designed to snap back to their original condition. Some are stretched and snap back in an instant (nerve conductivity), others in hours (like blood glucose control). Some follow a circadian cycle (like the HPA axis) and others a monthly cycle (menstruation).

When signals begin to overwhelm our physiological resilience, the stretching of an organ system does not immediately resolve. Perhaps the best example of this is the slow progression of impaired glucose tolerance/insulin resistance, sometimes referred to as the "metabolic continuum." Note in Figure 1 the "stretching" of the post-prandial glucose affects the area under the curve (AUC) of glucose much more than the change in the eventual fasting state. By the time a patient is deemed to be a "type 2 diabetic," their ability to reach normal fasting levels is compromised by changes in peripheral insulin sensitivity and pancreatic insulin capacity—a depletion of metabolic reserve.

1. The Core Philosophy is further described in the book, *The Original Prescription: How the Latest Scientific Discoveries Can Help You Leverage the Power of Lifestyle Medicine*. Point Institute. 2012.

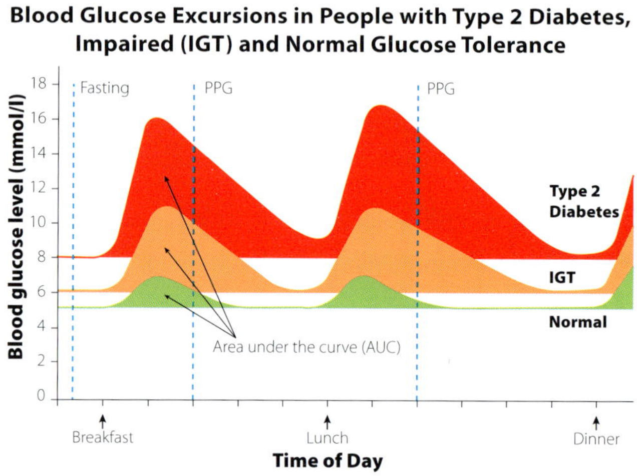

Figure 1 : Blood Glucose Excursions based on Glucose Tolerance.
These three curves show the relative blood glucose excursions in response to typical meals throughout the day for individuals with normal glucose tolerance, impaired glucose tolerance, or diagnosed type 2 diabetes. Fasting glucose is usually measured after an overnight fast, while post-prandial glucose (PPG) is typically measured 2 hours after consuming a meal. Note the large difference in the area under the curve (AUC) for glucose in these types of individuals, relative to the much smaller differences in fasting glucose levels.

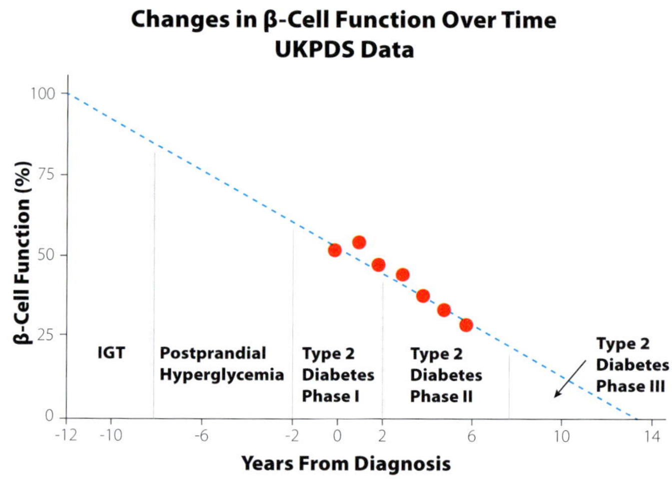

Figure 2 : Pancreatic β cell function through the progression of Type II diabetes
As metabolic reserve slowly diminishes due to the strain of insulin resistance and oxidative stress, beta cell dysfunction steadily progresses. Dashed line shows extrapolation forward and backward from years 0 to 6 based on HOMA data from UKPDS. From Lebovitz H. *Diabetes Rev.* 1999;7:139-53.

If **physiological resilience** defines the immediate capacity of cells, tissues and organ systems to respond to changes in physiological need, **metabolic reserve** defines the long-term capacity of tissues and organ systems to withstand repeated (chronic) changes to physiological needs. It is, in essence, the stored-up "reserve" available for each metabolic and organ system to maintain and rebuild its physiological resilience. As with any reserve, its capacity is vulnerable to depletion, but also capable of being resupplied and strengthened.

Related to the day-to-day physiological resilience that permits glucose disposal is the long-term depletion of the metabolic reserve in pancreatic beta cell function. In fact, by the time a person is diagnosed with type 2 diabetes, up to half of their pancreatic beta cell function is already depleted (see Figure 2). Insulin sensitivity and beta cell function are critical long-term reserve functions that can influence meal-to-meal physiological function.

Another well-known model showing the principles of metabolic reserve is that of bone mineral density. The constant back and forth of bone remodeling (osteoclasts/osteoblasts) responds to the immediate circumstances of the individual (physiological resilience). During menopause, internal and external signals favor changes that lead to a loss in bone mineral density. The eventual outcome for the individual is partly determined by the immediate changes in bone mineral density, but is greatly influenced by the level of bone mass built during the previous 50 years (peak bone mass-see Figure 3). The level of bone mineral (metabolic) reserve available when menopause starts will greatly impact the likelihood of osteoporosis. While building metabolic reserve can be done after menopause, the ability to build the reserve in the years between puberty and 30 is much greater.

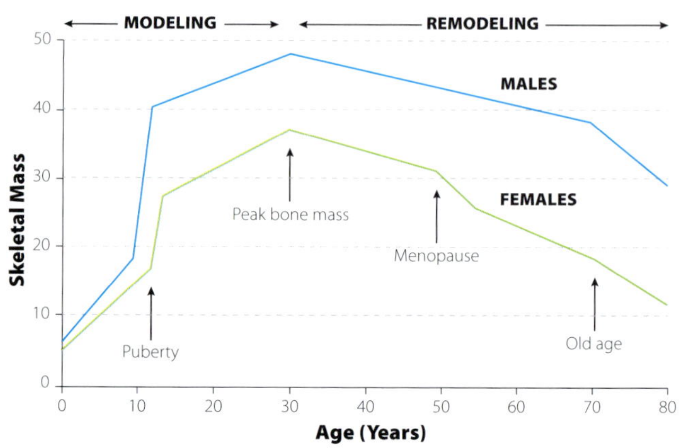

Figure 3 : Bone Mass in Women and Men over time
The general shape of this curve is similar in all women, but the height of peak bone mass and the slope of the bone loss later in life is determined by thousands of lifestyle decisions over her life.

Overall, lifestyle-based therapies should be designed to assess an individual's physiological resilience and metabolic reserve (using a variety of dynamic/functional tests and knowledge of the patient's history), emphasizing therapies known to specifically support the tissues and organ-systems for which the individual shows weaknesses. Since most basic lifestyle interventions support a variety of organ systems, building systemic metabolic reserve, clinicians can easily create programs that can be modified to suit nearly every patient needing chronic disease prevention and intervention.

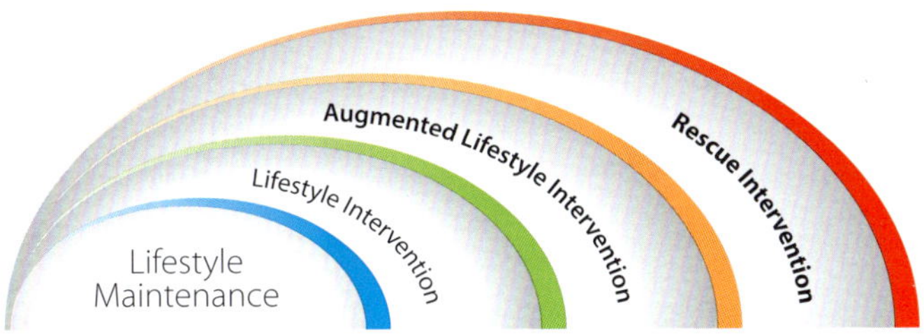

Lifestyle as Intervention

The approach in this guide recognizes many patients are well down the road of manifesting outcomes of dysfunction, where chronic disease prevention seems too late. Our premise is the same processes (building metabolic reserve and supporting physiological resilience) that protect tissues from the onset of chronic damage are even more vital when these tissues are metabolically stressed to the point of manifesting dysfunction, resulting in the diagnosis of a clinically defined "disease." While clinicians and patients may need to augment their lifestyle interventions with targeted therapies or even rescue medication, the promotion of the healthy signals designed to elicit healthy outcomes (lifestyle signals) should always remain the foundation of programs intended to support long-term health outcomes.

Therefore, implementation of lifestyle medicine within a wide range of clinical starting points requires a hierarchy of therapies that span early prevention to late intervention. Our Prevention to Intervention Hierarchy defines four points along this continuum: Lifestyle Maintenance, Lifestyle Intervention, Augmented Lifestyle Intervention and Rescue Intervention. Let us give a brief description of each.

Lifestyle Maintenance: Simply put, this is healthy life signals maintaining our metabolic reserve: eating right, keeping fit, sleeping well and avoiding the signals that sap our vitality. The longer we can rely on a prudent life maintaining our health, the more reserve we build against chronic disease.

Lifestyle Intervention: This is what most clinicians and patients think about when they describe lifestyle therapy. Using the same signals that maintain our health, we now increase both the intention and the dose of the lifestyle signals. We are specific about dietary choices (or changes), becoming fit, modulating stress and kicking bad habits known to be harmful to our health. There is still reliance on our body's capacity to build (or rebuild) metabolic reserve, but the greater focus is on risk prevention based on a specific vulnerability.

Augmented Lifestyle Intervention: Having discovered many of the specific mechanism(s) that link our lifestyle decisions to our health, we are capable of designing therapies to target those mechanisms. These therapies are the heart of functional medicine: such as nutritional and nutraceutical therapy, osteopathic or chiropractic manipulation, detoxification protocols and many more. For instance, recognizing omega-3 fatty acid consumption is a key signal in a healthy diet has led to our ability to augment, through supplementation, the consumption of omega-3 fatty acids. See Table 1 for more such examples. Clinicians reading this guide may find the majority of their patients will need augmented therapies for quite some time (perhaps indefinitely), depending on the severity and history of the chronic diseases experienced by the patient.

Rescue Intervention: These are interventions that have become common-place in our modern medical system. Essentially, these are drugs and surgery that are reasonable tools to prevent death, organ damage or major debility in order to rescue the patient. However, when the same paradigm of rescue interventions is used to ameliorate chronic conditions, a person's metabolic reserve and physiological resilience are rarely enhanced (in fact, they often depleted). Since the pharmaceutical burden weighs heavy upon most patients diagnosed with chronic diseases, wise clinicians who intend to use lifestyle therapies as the core of their intervention strategy must understand how to manage patients who have been treated with (or are currently on) these rescue interventions.

The Prevention to Intervention Heirarchy

	Lifestyle Maintenance	Lifestyle Intervention	Augmented Lifestyle Intervention	Rescue Intervention
Vitamin D & Bones	Sunlight: Work and Play	Sun Therapy/ Diet	Vitamin D Supplement	Osteoporosis Drugs
Antioxidant Defense	Wholesome Diverse Diet	↑Fruits & Veggies	Supplement Vitamins C and E/ Quercetin etc.	N/A
Back Health	Normal Physical Activity	Exercise and Flex Training	Chiropractic/ Physical Therapy	Surgery/Pain Medications
Joint Health	Physical Activity/Hydration	Weight Loss/ Flexibility	Glucosamine/ Chondroitin Sulfate	Drugs, Knee Replacement
Cancer Prevention	Wholesome Diverse Diet	↑Fruits & Veggies (Cruciferous)	Supplement Sulforophane or I3C	Antineoplastic Drugs
Detoxification	Wholesome Living	Avoidance/ Organic Focus	Supplement Agents that ↑Detoxification	Drugs to Combat Toxin Symptoms

Table 1: This table shows examples of the relationship between each point along the Prevention to Intervention Hierarchy. Notice that as we move from left to right along the continuum, the intention is to add signals, not replace them. For instance, the key to cancer prevention from a dietary standpoint is to eat a wholesome and diverse diet with many signals that support immune function and build the metabolic reserve that protects DNA from damage. Some individuals with higher risk or family history may choose to be more specific about increasing their "dose" of certain fruits and vegetables to maximize the dietary signals that help prevent cancer. An example of augmented lifestyle therapy is the use of concentrated phytonutrient supplements derived from these plants (e.g., sulforophane from broccoli) that have been tested for their ability to reduce cancer. In every case, a wholesome and diverse diet sets the foundation for each point along the continuum. Note that rescue interventions rarely trigger the same sorts of mechanisms as those designed to be triggered by lifestyle signals.

Seven Spheres of Lifestyle Signals

If nearly every aspect of our physiology can be modulated by lifestyle and environmental signals around us, we could easily define thousands of different signals. In a clinical setting, this vast number of potential variables can overwhelm the therapeutic decision-making process. It is helpful, therefore, to consider signals that can be defined in a limited number of categories. For this purpose, we define seven categories (or spheres) of signals based loosely on their origin. Since some lifestyle decisions are complex, they may include signals from multiple categories.

This Road map will focus almost exclusively on the signals coming from the "Diet and Nutrition" sphere of signals. A complete discussion of the signals and mechanisms of the other six spheres, written in language accessible to most patients, can be found in *The Original Prescription.*

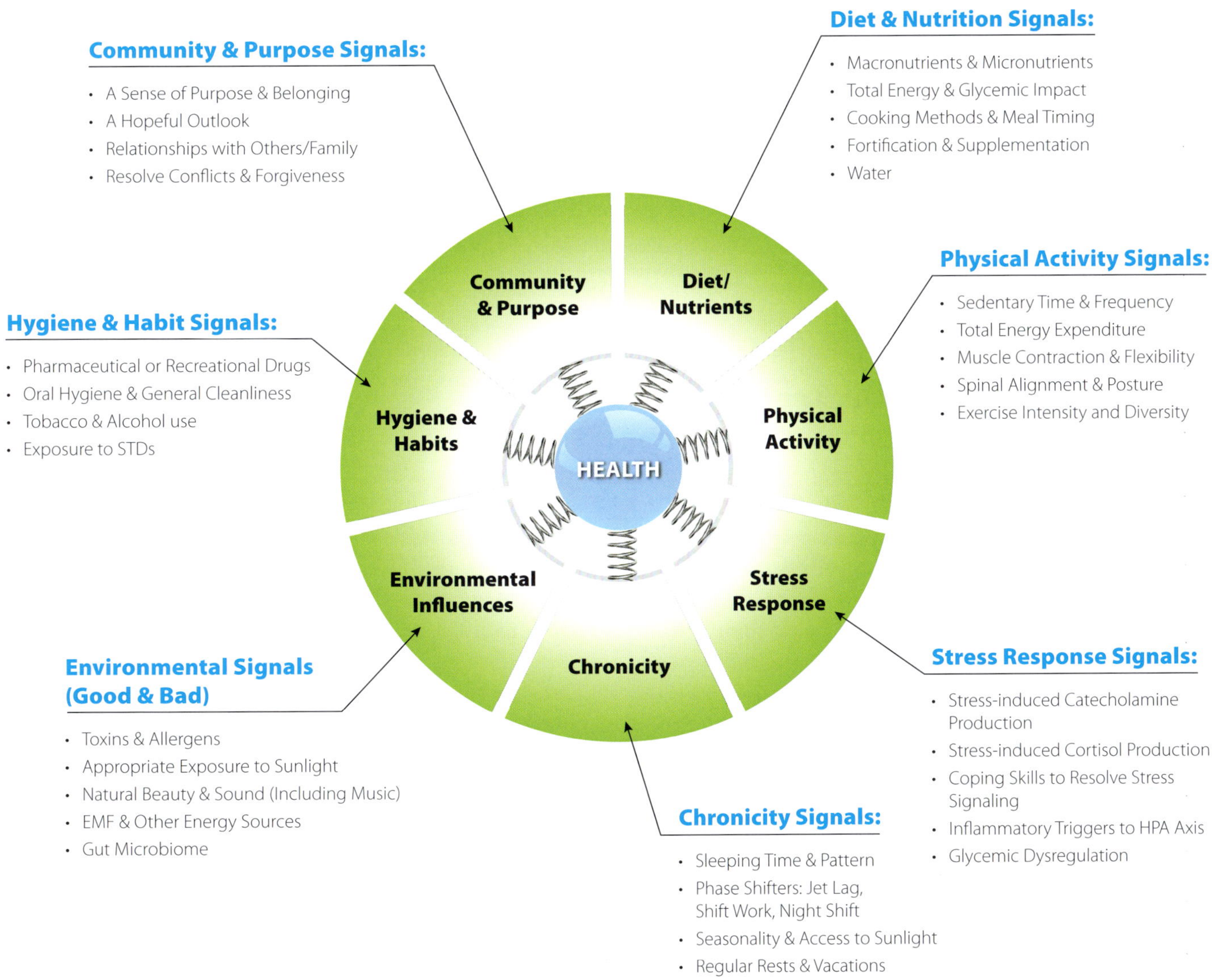

Optimal Nutrition

Building Physiological Reserve and Metabolic Reserve Through Diet and Nutrient Supplementation

There are few things more fundamental to building our metabolic reserve than the nutrients we consume on a daily basis. Over our lifetime, about 50 tons of food is consumed by the average American. The day-to-day dietary choices made throughout our lives prove to be either one of the primary ways in which we sustain our cellular function, or the means by which to burden those systems into dysfunction. Likewise, choosing to augment our dietary decisions with special components, such as functional foods, vitamin/mineral supplements, herbals/botanicals, probiotics, fatty acid supplements and nutraceuticals (i.e., CoQ_{10}, lipoic acid), has also become a fundamental health strategy.

Our aim in this Road map is to link fundamental dietary principles (as one of the spheres of the lifestyle synergy model described previously) to the structures and functions that build metabolic reserve, our major physiological protection against chronic disease. We will also break down signals "within" the diet (macronutrients, micronutrients, etc.) to explore different ways of using supplementation to target key cellular signaling mechanisms. Our goal is to anticipate the most frequent issues clinicians face when helping patients make decisions about their basic nutrient needs and the role of dietary supplementation.

Optimal Nutrition: How Is It Defined and Can It Be Achieved?

As with many other health-related phenomena, nutritional needs have been historically explored and defined within the context of deficiency-related diseases. Because of this history, *adequate nutrition was considered to exist where known symptoms of nutritional deficiencies* ***appeared*** *to be absent.* Consequently, the ability to use specific foods to treat or prevent specific "disease" conditions (scurvy, rickets, etc.) helped us discover and isolate most of the compounds we define as "vitamins" today. But does this history help us clinically, and exactly how should "adequate" nutrient intake be defined?

Undoubtedly, our understanding of nutrition has advanced well beyond the notion of *minimal* quantities to prevent deficiency diseases (even if it often appears the USRDA recommendations do not reflect these advances). We now recognize a wide range of nutritional insufficiencies that prevent optimal physiological function are influenced by many acute and chronic conditions. From a nutrient-deficiency-disease standpoint, these insufficiencies may be deemed "subclinical," but individually and collectively they create a major physiological burden and are a significant contributor to diminishing an individual's metabolic reserve and their resilience against both acute and chronic diseases.

While traditional guidelines do not recognize all of the following distinctions, for the purpose of this Road map, the following distinctions should be kept in mind when evaluating nutrition in the context of patient's situation:

Deficiency: The intake of the nutrient is below the threshold required to maintain minimal physiological functions required by that nutrient. Individuals with long-term deficiencies will exhibit traditional signs and symptoms associated with the nutrient deficiency. These levels are generally (although not always) similar across genders, ethnicities and ages. In financial terms, this would be bankruptcy.

Insufficiency: Nutrient intake is above the level where frank deficiency-related disease is present (or diagnosable) but the level is still inadequate to maintain all necessary functions performed by the nutrient. In financial terms, this is being behind on payments and having a low credit score.

Functional Insufficiency: Nutrient intake is below the individual's *current* physiological need (even if the intake amount is deemed sufficient by dose), a situation caused by one of the conditions below. When one or more of these conditions is combined with intermittent low intake, clinical symptoms of deficiency are not uncommon. Financially speaking, your income looks good on paper but you are spending more than you take in (or someone is embezzling from your account).

- Poor absorption caused by:
  - Food matrix
  - Poor eating habits (inadequate chewing, etc.)
  - Low stomach acid, enzyme production or other factors needed for absorption
  - Bowel transit time (usually too fast)
- Improper metabolism of nutrient to active or transport forms
- Increased elimination/detoxification of nutrient
- Drug- or toxin-induced depletion
- Increased physiological need (e.g., athletic need)
- Genetic defect or polymorphism alters need (nutrigenetics- see page 21)
- Deficiency in a different but physiologically related nutrient
- Overconsumption of some food or nutrient, reducing function or absorption
- Obesity
- Stress- or sickness-induced depletion

Adequate Intake: Nutrient intake level that prevents clinical or subclinical symptoms of nutrient insufficiency and compensates (for the moment) for any functional nutrient needs listed above. These levels are physiologically adequate but may not create the optimal function that allows for increased metabolic reserve for future physiological challenges. In financial terms, you are living paycheck to paycheck and have no official debt—just don't plan a big vacation, and hope that the furnace doesn't give out.

Optimal Intake: Nutrient intake is adequate to satisfy the individual's current physiological needs and to overcome chronic or transient causes of functional insufficiency; and promotes metabolic, cellular and organ reserve. In financial terms, all the bills are paid and there is enough savings to plan a vacation without detrimentally impacting your retirement plans.

Therapeutic Intake: There are times when high doses of certain nutrients will be used as targeted therapies in some patients. These nutrients are essentially being used for pharmacological, rather than physiological, potential (e.g., high-dose niacin for lipid management). Sometimes referred to as orthomolecular medicine, this sort of therapeutic use of nutrients is not done to manage nutrient deficiencies per se, but to act as a strong signal intended for a physiological response.

Excessive Intake: This occurs when intake of any nutrient interferes with optimal physiology or results in toxicity. While many nutrients have a Tolerable Upper Intake Level (UL), defined by the Institute of Medicine, these levels are often conservative (below safe therapeutic levels used in many clinical trials) and do not consider the use of these nutrients as therapeutic agents. Although rare, clinicians should be aware that patients who self-diagnose and self-medicate with dietary supplements may be getting an excessive intake of some nutrients. Although high-doses of several nutrients are safe and clinically justified, clinicians should be aware of the UL for vitamins and minerals (see appendix page 158) and be familiar with common signs and symptoms of excessive nutrient intake if they recommend nutrients and dietary supplements at doses above the UL.

What About Guideline Recommended Intakes?

As most are aware, there are guideline recommendations for appropriate intake of most essential nutrients. These have been variously described over the years by RDA (recommended daily allowance) or DRI (dietary reference intake) values or other such acronyms. How are these determined?

According to the Food and Nutrition Board of the Institute of Medicine (IOM, now the National Academy of Medicine), daily reference intake (DRI) is the general term for a set of reference values used to plan and assess nutrient intakes for healthy people. These values, which vary by age, gender and pregnancy/lactation status include:

- ***Recommended Dietary Allowance (RDA):*** *the average daily level of intake sufficient to meet the nutrient requirements of nearly all (97% – 98%) healthy people.*
- ***Adequate Intake (AI):*** *established when evidence is insufficient to develop an RDA and is set at a level assumed to ensure nutritional adequacy.*
- ***Tolerable Upper Intake Level (UL):*** *maximum daily intake unlikely to cause adverse health effects.*

As shown in the figure below, RDA levels are related to each nutrient's estimated adequate requirement (EAR), a level expected to satisfy the needs of 50% of the people in that age group based on a review of the scientific literature. The RDA, then, is the EAR + (2X the standard deviation of the EAR), which, if correct, should capture 98% of the population.

Several potential problems exist with this approach to nutrient guidelines and recommendations: 1) Individuals with acute or chronic diseases are known to have depletions of specific nutrients; these intake recommendations are for "healthy" individuals. 2) Body mass is growing with each generation; some (although not all) nutrient intake is greatly affected by total body mass (or fat mass). 3) Agreement as to which scientific literature should be used to set estimated adequate requirements is far from certain. In fact, most estimates are based on expert opinion, instead of recently published data. 4) Some individuals are genetically predisposed to require additional nutrient intake (nutrigenetics, see page 21). 5) Intake recommendations are linked with dietary estimates, not tied to measured blood or tissue levels.

Throughout this Road map we will discuss various guideline recommendations for nutrient intake as a reference, but will often point to literature that may suggest applications of various nutrients sometimes well below or above these recommendations. Ultimately the clinician and patient need to decide the best target of nutrient intake from diet and supplementation to achieve the necessary therapeutic goal.

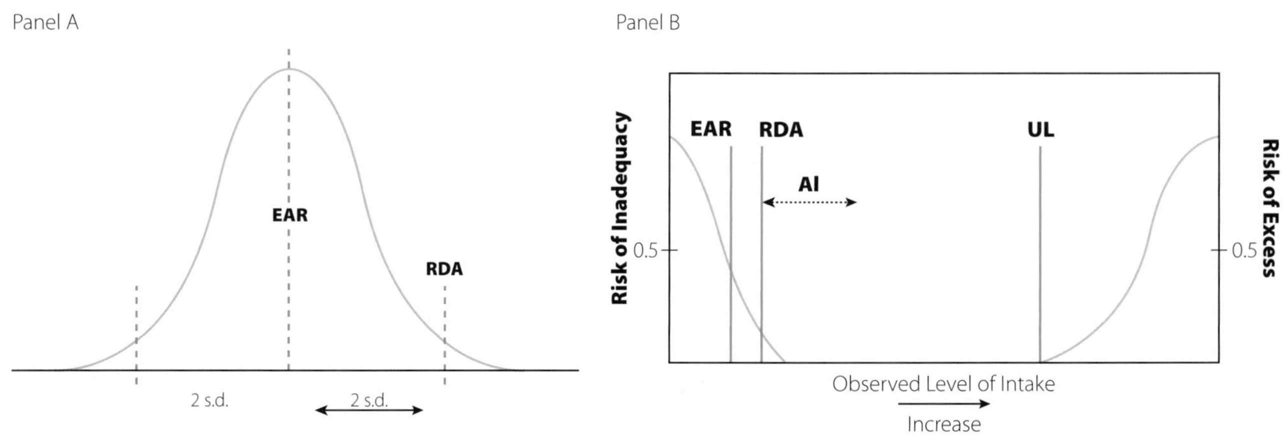

Relationship between DRI components. Panel A shows the basic relationship between the Estimated Average Requirement (EAR) expected to satisfy the needs of 50% of healthy people and the Recommended Daily Allowance (RDA); the intake at which the risk of inadequacy is predicted to be very small (2% – 3%) in healthy subjects. Panel B: The Adequate Intake (AI) does not bear a consistent relationship to either the EAR nor the RDA because it is set by expert panels when there is no data to estimate the average requirement (nutrients with no EAR). It is assumed that the AI is at or above the RDA, if one could be calculated. At intakes between the RDA and Tolerable Upper Intake Level (UL), risks of inadequacy and of excess are both close to zero. At intakes above the UL, the risk of adverse effects may increase in healthy subjects, though it may also include the therapeutic range of several nutrients in unhealthy or nutrient deficient subjects.

Translating DRIs to Label DVs

Clinicians should be aware that the DRIs (either an RDA or AI) set by the IOM differ slightly from the daily value (DV) numbers that FDA mandates for calculating the "%DV" found in the supplement facts box (SFB) or nutrition facts box (NFB) of dietary supplement and food labels. In addition, many of the DVs used by FDA are being updated in 2018, along with other significant formatting changes to the SFB/NFB.

The table shows each of the four categories used to determine the % DV for product labels and the level deemed to be "100%" for each based on the changes after July 2018.† The DV is set using the highest value in each respective category according to the IOM's list of DRIs (see tables in appendix pages 156-157). For example, the IOM's RDAs for vitamin C range from 25 mg/day for children 4-8 y and as high as 90 mg/day for males >19 y; thus the DV for this category (adults and children >4) is set at 90 mg. The table below also includes the levels used to calculate % DV prior to July 2018 for adults and children above 4 years of age (the most commonly used measure for foods and dietary supplements) for comparison. Two important changes should be noted. The first are actual changes (increase or decrease) in the daily value amount (e.g., vitamin C changes from 60 mg to 90 mg in the adult DV) (see arrows in table). Secondly, to normalize the unit of measure with the IOM and other groups worldwide, there are changes to the unit of measure used for several nutrients. Each of these changes (i.e., changing from international units-IUs- to mg or mcg units for vitamins A, D, E) are noted in the table and in each monograph for the respective nutrient. DVs for added sugars and choline have also been added.

† Note: The compliance date for implementing these labeling changes may be delayed well-beyond the 2018 deadline by FDA, due to regulatory discretion.

Component (unit of measure, in bold if units changed)	Adults and Children >4		2018 DV Pregnancy/ Lactating Women	2018 Children DV	
	Pre-2018	2018 DVs		0-12 mo	1-3 yrs
Total Fat (g)	65	▲ 78	78	30	39
Saturated Fat (g)	20	20	20	N/A	10
Cholesterol (mg)	300	300	300	N/A	300
Sodium (mg)	2,400	▼ 2300	2300	N/A	1500
Total Carbohydrate (g)	300	▼ 275	275	95	150
Dietary Fiber (g)	25	▲ 28	28	N/A	14
Added Sugars (g)***	N/A	50	50	N/A	25
Protein (g)	50	50	N/A	N/A	13
Vitamin A (mcg RAE)*	**5,000 IU**	**900**	**1300**	**500**	**300**
Vitamin C (mg)	60	▲ 90	120	50	15
Calcium (mg)	1,000	▲ 1300	1300	260	700
Iron (mg)	18	18	27	11	7
Vitamin D (mcg)*	**400 IU**	**20**	**15**	**10**	**15**
Vitamin E (mg α-tocopherol)*	**30 IU**	**15**	**19**	**5**	**6**
Vitamin K (mcg)	80	▲ 120	90	2.5	30
Thiamin (mg)	1.5	▼ 1.2	1.4	0.3	0.5
Riboflavin (mg)	1.7	▼ 1.3	1.6	0.4	0.5
Niacin (mg NE)*	**20 mg**	**▼ 16**	**18**	**4**	**6**
Vitamin B6 (mg)	2	▼ 1.7	2	0.3	0.5
Folate (mcg DFE)*	**400 mcg**	**400**	**600**	**80**	**150**
Vitamin B12 (mcg)	6	▼ 2.4	2.8	0.5	0.9
Biotin (mcg)	300	▼ 30	35	6	8
Pantothenic Acid (mg)	10	▼ 5	7	1.8	2
Phosphorus (mg)	1,000	▲ 1250	1250	275	460
Iodine (mcg)	150	150	290	130	90
Magnesium (mg)	400	▲ 420	400	75	80
Zinc (mg)	15	▼ 11	13	3	3
Selenium (mcg)	70	▼ 55	70	20	20
Copper (mg)	2	▼ 0.9	1.3	0.2	0.3
Manganese (mg)	2	2.3	2.6	0.6	1.2
Chromium (mcg)	120	▼ 35	45	5.5	11
Molybdenum (mcg)	75	▼ 45	50	3	17
Chloride (mg)	3,400 mg	▼ 2300	2300	570	1500
Potassium (mg)	3,500 mg	▲ 4700	5100	700	3000
Choline (mg)***	N/A	550	550	150	200

Note: Manufacturers must be in compliance with the new daily values by July 26, 2018 or a year later, depending on the company's annual food sales.†

*Note: Units changing for vitamin A, D, E, niacin and folate. See "Old DV" column for previously used units, the new units are listed in the "Component (new DV units)" column. See individual monographs for further information on unit changes.

▲/▼ denote an increase or decrease in the DV comparing the new to the previously used values.

*** Denotes new category added to the DV by FDA.

Dietary Nutrients as Signals: Genetics, Genomics and Epigenetics

Cell function could be described simply as a complex rearranging of nutrients: proteins (as enzymes, structural components and hormones), carbohydrates (to modify protein function and, of course, as a source of cellular energy), fats (as long-term energy stores, cell membranes and mini-hormones-prostaglandins), vitamins (as enzyme cofactors), and minerals (as structural components, enzyme cofactors and to manage electrical potential within the cell). The moment-by-moment functions of each cell is tightly regulated by predetermined processes within the cell and signals the cell receives from other cells, organs and the outside environment.

For most cells, a change in function is dependent on turning specific genes on or off within the nucleus. In some cases, increasing or decreasing gene expression by just 25% in a single gene may influence metabolic function of the cell. There are many nutrients known to change the expression of not just one gene, but hundreds of genes, sometimes altering their expression two-to-three fold (or more), resulting in tremendous impact on cellular function and clinical outcomes.

The effect of nutrients on gene expression is known generally as **nutrigenomics**. Within this overall term are several other terms that define how a nutrient signal is converted into a change in cellular function. The change in messenger RNA transcripts is called *transciptomics*; the change in proteins expressed is called *proteomics*; and the resultant change in the metabolites produced, *metabolomics*. Much of the current understanding of nutrient function within specific cells comes from the molecular biology techniques that define nutrigenomics.

Our cells are designed to function when the appropriate signals (triggered either by circadian signals, dietary nutrients, cell receptor binding, etc.) turn on the appropriate genes at the appropriate time. However, the abundance, or the depletion, of certain nutrients determines whether the cell is capable of fully responding to those signals. For instance, when liver cells are signaled to increase detoxification processes to remove a load of harmful toxins, they attempt to produce more glutathione to deal with the higher production of cellular reactive oxygen species (ROS or oxygen "free-radicals"). The necessary amino acid precursors, water- and fat-soluble antioxidants and related sulfur compounds necessary for the production of reduced glutathione, are just some of the necessary building blocks the cell will need. If any of these are in short supply, availability of reduced glutathione will be diminished, leaving the cell vulnerable to oxidative damage and the body's detoxification capacity weakened.

Going one step further in our glutathione example, some nutrients can act in a manner that increases the very enzymes responsible for glutathione production (through the Nrf2 pathway system). This multilevel function of nutrients explains why we find different levels of biological activity for a wide range of substances based on different "doses." Sometimes a nutrient is acting as a nutrigenomic signal, sometimes as an enzyme cofactor, and sometimes as a substrate for metabolic function.

The Language of the Basic Levels of Genomics

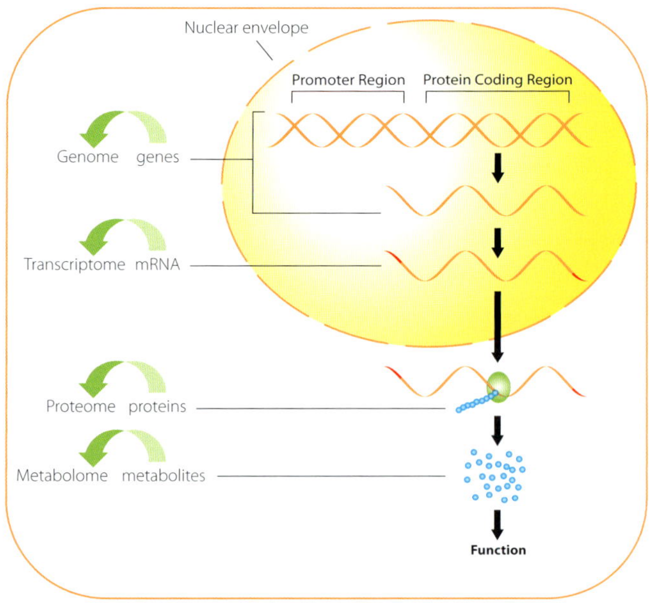

Figure 4 : The Language of the Basic Levels of Genomics
Gene expression determines cell outcomes. Almost any substance thought to influence health (positively or negatively) can be tested for the influence it has upon the total mRNA expression (called the transcriptome), the pattern of proteins expressed (proteome), and the resulting metabolites (metabolome) of the cell.

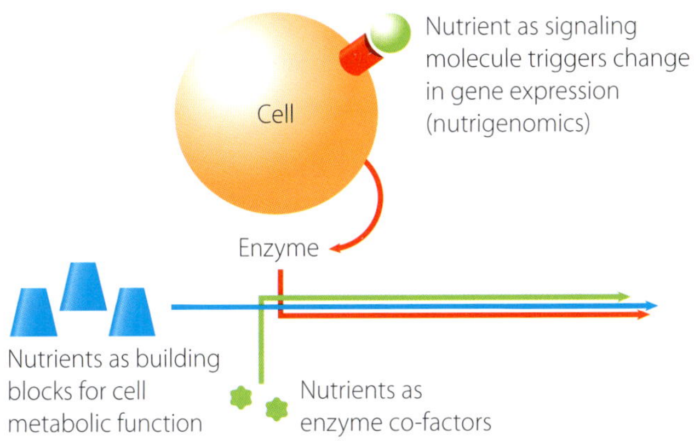

Figure 5 : How Nutrients Signal Cell Function
Nutrients function at numerous levels in the body. They can act as cell-signaling molecules, as genomic triggers of gene expression, as cofactors for important enzymatic reactions or as building blocks of important cellular structures.

Nutrigenomics vs. Nutrigenetics

If **nutrigenomics** defines how gene expression is altered by specific nutrients (just as toxicogenomics describes the changes in gene expression from toxin exposure), then **nutrigenetics** describes how a person's specific genetic sequences can affect their nutritional needs and responses to nutrient intake. Here, advances in genetic testing for a wide variety of genes are beginning to allow us to understand why specific individuals may need, for example, higher intake of vitamin D, folate or CoQ_{10}.

One of the best-characterized, clinically relevant examples of the influence of nutrigenetics is the single nucleotide polymorphism (SNP) located in the gene that expresses methylenetetrahydrofolate reductase (MTHFR is a protein that converts folic acid into its active biological molecule, methyltetrahydrofolate). Most common is the MTHFR C677T polymorphism, which results in an alanine to valine amino acid change at the 222 position of the protein. This small change in the protein actually alters its characteristics, resulting in a less efficient synthesis of active folate compounds. Most individuals in the U.S. are homozygous for the normal variant (677CC), but up to 10% of the population may be homozygous for the other variant (677TT). These individuals often have noticeably less efficient methylation, accounting for higher risk for certain diseases and a higher need for dietary folate consumption or folic acid supplementation (see page 75 for a detailed discussion).

As each year passes, more and more studies reveal an increasing number of genetic polymorphisms that may influence a carrier's need for a particular nutrient. Clinicians and patients now have numerous options for genetic testing that can help identify the need for additional nutrient supplementation, although it should be noted clinical studies showing specific changes in health outcomes related to supplementing these individuals are limited and often exaggerated by supplement manufacturers selling certain forms or doses of nutrients.

The Epigenetic Influence of Nutrients

One of the most important discoveries in genetics over the past few decades are the mechanisms described collectively as epigenetics. These are heritable changes in our genetic material that do not affect the actual sequence of DNA itself; they do, however, influence the genetic expression and function of the cell. The three mechanisms currently described as epigenetic changes are: DNA methylation, histone modification and microRNA interference. Without getting into the details here (see Figure 6), DNA methylation usually targets the promoter region of a gene, usually reducing gene expression;

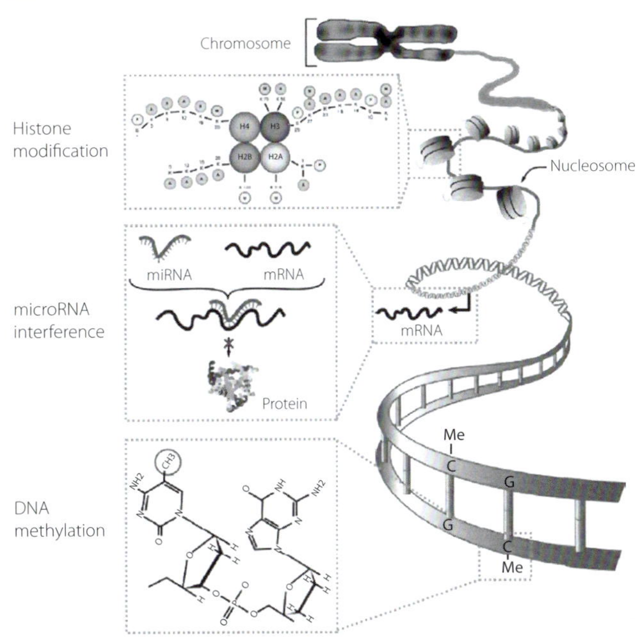

Figure 6 : The Three Main Mechanisms of Epigenetics.
See text for further explanation. Adapted from: Sawan C, Vaissiere T, Murr R, Herceg Z. Epigenetic drivers and genetic passengers on the road to cancer. *Mutat Res.* July 2008; 642(1-2): 1-13.

histone modification (e.g., acetylation) affects how easily the DNA unwinds to permit access to a single gene or cluster of genes; and the formation of small microRNA molecules can act to interfere with messenger RNAs before they can be translated into proteins, effectively reducing protein expression and changing cell function.

When nutrients act in such a way as to change gene expression (nutrigenomics), they often up-regulate or facilitate changes in the epigenome. This might occur simply by providing methyl-donors for DNA methylating enzymes or by changing the regulation of enzymes that acetylate (or deacetylate) histones. We know a bit less about how nutrients impact microRNA expression, although many nutrient-influenced miRNAs have been identified and more are being discovered every day.

As clinicians approach their recommendations for dietary changes and nutrient supplementation, each of these factors must be considered. Dietary intake must include minimum basic building blocks and key nutrients to prevent deficiency diseases. Equally as important is an understanding that contained within a healthy dietary pattern are a myriad of signals designed to work with our cells to manage short-term gene expression and long-term epigenetic patterns, some of which we might pass on to the next generation. The more we learn about specific signaling molecules within nature (nutrigenomic) and an individual's genetic ability to respond to those signals (nutrigenetics), the more targeted and personalized augmented lifestyle therapies can be.

Vitamin D Signaling Affects Nearly Every Cell

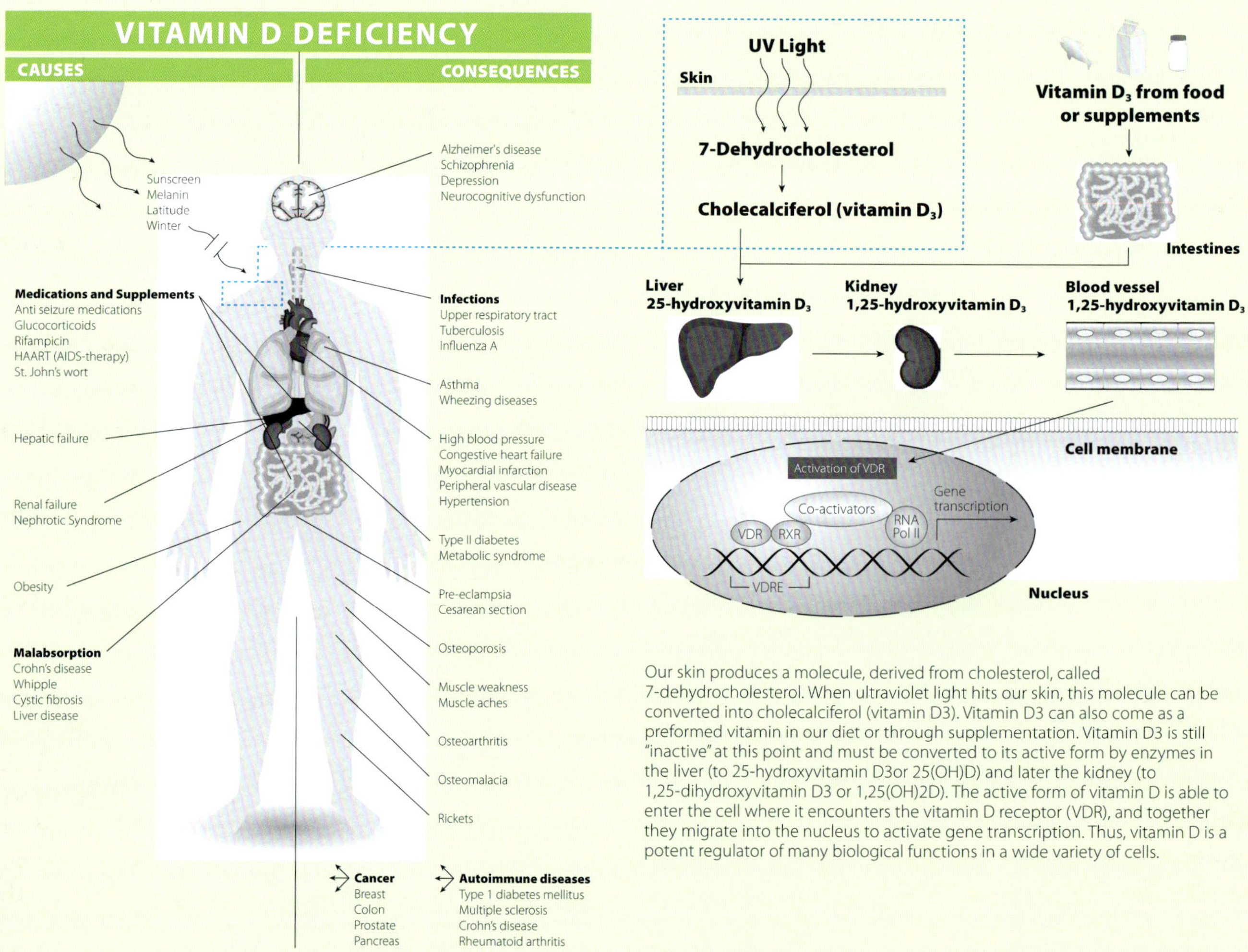

Our skin produces a molecule, derived from cholesterol, called 7-dehydrocholesterol. When ultraviolet light hits our skin, this molecule can be converted into cholecalciferol (vitamin D3). Vitamin D3 can also come as a preformed vitamin in our diet or through supplementation. Vitamin D3 is still "inactive" at this point and must be converted to its active form by enzymes in the liver (to 25-hydroxyvitamin D3or 25(OH)D) and later the kidney (to 1,25-dihydroxyvitamin D3 or 1,25(OH)2D). The active form of vitamin D is able to enter the cell where it encounters the vitamin D receptor (VDR), and together they migrate into the nucleus to activate gene transcription. Thus, vitamin D is a potent regulator of many biological functions in a wide variety of cells.

Dietary Patterns that Promote Health

In this section, we will discuss the clinical relationship of recommending broad dietary advice based on fundamental principles and information. This will help clinicians make appropriate clinical recommendations concerning supplemental nutrients for patients at various points along the prevention to intervention hierarchy. As a reminder, this is not a textbook on nutrition. It is a summary of those issues we consider most helpful in the day-to-day practice of recommending appropriate supplemental nutrition within a functional medicine practice.

Dietary Patterns and Principles

Before we attempt to examine food choices as discrete dietary components (macronutrients, micronutrients, etc.), it is important to understand the best overall way to promote nutritional advice is with broad dietary principles. Helping patients to honestly assess their own dietary habits and patterns, and then design and implement a more healthy pattern of eating, may be one of the most challenging and valuable roles a healthcare provider can play.

Assessing a patient's diet

One of the more difficult tasks in giving dietary advice to patients is getting an honest assessment of their current dietary habits. Dietary recall diaries and food frequency questionnaires, even in the hands of clinical trial experts, are not as reliable as we would like them to be. Yet, having a formal way (or even a consistent informal way) to assess a patient's dietary habits is critical in order to give competent clinical support. Two important factors are key to this assessment: getting accurate information that is as complete as possible to assess how a patient's dietary habits may affect their risk potential; and getting the patient to consciously acknowledge those habits. Therefore, the best clinical tools are those that have been validated across a number of different clinical trial settings, and those that provoke easy follow-up questions between a healthcare provider and the patient.

The Seven Principles for Diet and Nutrition, from *The Original Prescription*

Principle #1: Choose a healthy dietary pattern that governs 80% of your decisions.

Principle #2: Let your body tell you when to stop eating. Listen to your body.

Principle #3: Don't skip meals. Start each day with a balanced breakfast.

Principle #4: Eat real food! Limit prepared and packaged food.

Principle #5: Invest appropriately in your food selections; your life may depend on it.

Principle #6: Drink enough water and limit your liquid calories.

Principle #7: Prepare for cravings that can jeopardize your plans for success.

A single tool is rarely perfect for all patients and all situations. Therefore, we have provided several different tools in the appendix of this book to facilitate an assessment of a patient's dietary pattern and eating habits.

- 24-hour Diet and GI symptom Diary (page 188)
- Food Frequency Questionnaire (page 189)
- Validated MedDiet Score Sheet (page 192)

Depending on the situation and the patient, one or more of these may be used to "score" a patient's diet or connect certain symptoms with specific foods (e.g., GI complaints, food allergy suspicion or migraine-triggering foods). Beyond this, however, these tools can help initiate a meaningful dialogue about how diet and lifestyle habits may contribute to a patient's current health status.

Here are some quick, "on-the-fly" lifestyle questions to consider asking your patients, perhaps while checking their BP:

» How much soda (including diet sodas) do you drink in an average day/week?
» Have you been measuring your exercise in minutes or miles? How's it been going?
» How many servings of vegetables have you had since Sunday (or yesterday)?
» How many meals do you eat at home per week?
» How do you keep track of how much water you drink each day?
» Describe your typical breakfast. How often do you skip breakfast?
» What foods do you eat that you know are "bad" for you?

Questions should be specific. Vague questions like "So, how has your diet been lately?" will almost always be of little value: "It's been fine" or "Not too bad" provide little in the way of follow-up. Be prepared with a short piece of advice once they give an answer; try to add some humor. "Would you hurt me if I told you to try to go a month without…(soda, ice cream, etc.)?" "Mr. Smith, find a spot a half of a mile from your house and see how long it takes to walk back and forth. Once you get used to this, try to find a spot a mile away." "Mrs. Jones, here is a list of 10 healthy breakfast menus that provide at least 500 calories. Did you know that moving more of your calories to breakfast will help improve your daily metabolism, help you stay trim and lower your risk of chronic disease?"

For more information and referenced reviews of dietary changes as an intervention strategy for a wide range of chronic diseases, go to www.pointinstitute.org.

The Fundamental Dietary Principle: Improving the "Signal to Noise" Ratio

In our view, the most important overall principle for dietary advice is to increase and diversify the number of good signals coming from our diet, but not in a way that increases the amount of energy (calories) or noise (bad signals). In essence this means increasing the good signal-to-calorie ratio. This ensures the genomic and epigenetic signals that maintain our health and build our metabolic reserve will never be more than a meal or two away. The key is to recommend a dietary pattern that includes diversity, seasonality, color (natural, not artificial) and freshness.

Without a doubt, the diet that best meets these principles and has been tested as an intervention strategy amongst Western subjects consuming a primarily Western dietary pattern is the Mediterranean diet (MedDiet). It is our view this diet, or a modified version of the MedDiet as shown below, can be implemented by most patients in most communities regardless of their socioeconomic status.

Mediterranean Diet: The General Pattern

- Fresh and cooked vegetables
- Generous use of herbs and spices
- Legumes/plant proteins, such as beans and lentils
- Whole grains, such as bulgur, rice, quinoa and wheat berries
- Fresh fruit at each meal
- Lean meats, such as fish, chicken and lamb
- Monounsaturated fats in the form of nuts and olive oil
- Moderate dairy products, mostly as yogurt and cheese
- Moderate intake of red wine or phytonutrient-rich juices, such as pomegranate, berries, etc.
- Reduced consumption of red meat, refined grains and sweet foods
- Avoidance of prepackaged foods

The goal is to increase the number and diversity of healthy signals. This dietary pattern will improve the omega-3:6 ratio, increase the amount of the monounsaturated fat oleic acid (olive oil), provide a solid foundation of vitamins and minerals and, perhaps most importantly, provide a wide range of phytonutrients that are potent nutrigenomic-signaling molecules. Of course, the benefit of the diet cannot simply be broken down into its ingredients; although the synergistic benefits repeatedly seen in clinical trials can be understood by what we know of mechanisms attributed to foods contained within the diet.

The MedDiet cannot be accomplished merely by picking one or two recipes and eating these every day; this defeats the notion of diversity. Encouraging patients to experiment with new ingredients, recipes and cookbooks; and suggesting a more seasonal dietary pattern, which forces changes, will go a long way to accomplishing the goal of diversity.

MedDiet Signals that Build Metabolic Reserve

MedDiet Benefit	Dietary Components
Increases peripheral insulin sensitivity	Phytonutrients, spices
Reduces glycemic impact	Fiber, whole grains, spices
Alters gene expression	Phytonutrients from fruits/vegetables, olive oil, sunlight (vitamin D)
Improves fatty acid metabolism	Olive Oil, fish, low SFA
Reduces inflammation	Phytonutrients, fiber, MUFAs, PUFAs
Increases plasma antioxidant levels	Fruits and vegetables, wine, olive oil

Reducing Glycemic Impact

For most patients considering a diet change, weight loss or weight maintenance is a personal (or clinical) goal. When comparing weight-loss success in a variety of clinical trials, subjects who restrict carbohydrates or maintain a low-glycemic-index selection of foods have a high likelihood of reducing fat mass and body weight, at least for the first 6 – 12 months. While the MedDiet is not necessarily a low-calorie diet, for most Americans, emphasizing foods with a low-glycemic impact will generally result in a reduced calorie diet.

Dietary Recommendations for Reducing Glycemic Impact:

- Increase both soluble and fermentable fiber content. Supplement the diet, if necessary, with soluble and fermentable fibers such as inulin, flaxseeds, beta-glucans, psyllium, etc.
- Reduce the frequency of refined carbohydrate consumption—white bread, white pasta, muffins, cakes and cookies—and focus on whole grains.
- If helpful, limit total carbohydrates to less than 40% of total calorie intake.
- Increase phytonutrients by using brightly colored vegetables, spices and herbs to improve insulin sensitivity.
- Do not skip breakfast; this meal sets the tone of blood sugar stability for the day.
- Consider small, high protein snacks between meals to keep blood sugar stable.
- Remember, even small decreases in weight or increases in physical activity can have tremendous benefits, and emphasis should be placed upon improving insulin sensitivity and decreasing inflammation.

What about the DASH Diet?

The Dietary Approaches to Stop Hypertension (DASH) diet is often considered, along with the Mediterranean diet, to be the healthiest diet by vote of diet experts. This dietary pattern is similar to the MedDiet; many menus would fulfill both dietary patterns equally. Here are the differences between the two diets, according to the dashdiet.org website:

The Mediterranean diet is rich in fruits, vegetables, nuts/beans/seeds, and heart healthy fats. It contains whole grains, fish, limited amounts of poultry, red meat, and dairy (primarily cultured or cheese products). It may also include moderate amounts of red wine. And since it is the Mediterranean, the people get lots of vitamin D, courtesy of the sun....The main difference between the Mediterranean diet and the original DASH diet research is the higher amount of heart healthy fat. And, if you want to make room for red wine, take care to avoid adding extra calories. [Our new DASH diet] is based on newer DASH research, and is more similar to the Med diet. In fact, when we incorporate more of the heart healthy fats, and less of the refined starchy or added-sugar foods, we can improve blood pressure even better than with the original DASH plan. It is especially good for heart health, and targets people who carry their excess weight around their middle, people with metabolic syndrome, high triglycerides, diabetes, prediabetes, and/or hypertension, who are postmenopausal, or who have PCOS.

Objectively speaking, the newer DASH diet is essentially the MedDiet!

The "Paleo" Med

While space does not permit us to evaluate the merits of the "Paleo" diet approach, the popularity of this approach continues to grow here in the U.S. Essentially this diet is intended to approximate a pre-agricultural, hunter-gatherer diet using currently available foods. While foods permitted in this diet are also considered quintessential to the MedDiet (fruits, vegetables, fish, nuts, seeds and healthy oils), the major difference comes with the list of things not considered part of the pre-agricultural diet. Namely cereal grains of any kind, dairy of any kind, legumes (including peanuts), potatoes and salt. Red meat is encouraged on this diet, although grass-fed or wild animal meat is emphasized.

Since virtually no clinical trial data is currently available to test the principles of this dietary approach as an intervention for a wide range of individuals and clinical outcomes, we cannot recommend this approach as a long-term dietary pattern. However, since the vast majority of patients consume diets that are laden with "industrial" foods (prepackaged and full of refined flours, sugars and oils) and/or have become sensitive to grain or dairy products, this approach can be a good strategy to bring a more immediate elimination of unhealthy food selections. On the other hand, we do not believe there is evidence to suggest the vast majority of humans are inherently intolerant to prudent cereal grain and dairy consumption. Recommendations for lifetime restriction of these foods should be reserved for those who are confirmed to require such restrictions.

The Paleo-Med approach described here is simply a diet that is firmly based on the patterns and principles of the MedDiet, while at the same time avoiding food products that were not generally available to our ancestors prior to organized agricultural practices.

Other Dietary Habits to Recommend

Dietary advice almost always boils down to merely menu selection: What are you supposed to eat? But often, it is the "Where, why, how and with whom" of eating that can impact someone's health just as much.

The following should also be considered when advising patients about diet and nutrition:

- Do their refrigerator, freezer and pantry contain the foods needed to keep them on track with healthy choices? Adherence to a healthy eating pattern is poor when making the right food choice is complicated by not having healthy foods readily available, or when unhealthy convenient foods are readily at hand. Clinicians should have copies of patient handouts, books or a list of recommended websites for patients to take with them when they leave the office.
- Patients should be reminded to explore new foods and spend more time in food preparation and eating. Part of making good food choices is spending enough time to interact with our food.
- Eating slowly and mindfully will help patients realize when they are full; helping to improve the signal to calorie ratio. Whether eating out or at-home, most Americans need help estimating portion sizes and limiting calorie intake.
- While prepackaged food appears to be convenient and cheap, helping a patient understand that investing their time and resources toward their health—perhaps by planting a garden— is priceless.
- Patients should be encouraged to shift their caloric load toward the beginning of the day. Eating larger breakfasts (at least one-third of their daily calories or more), and modest-sized lunches and dinners will improve overall metabolism, promote proper circadian gene expression, and reduce cravings throughout the day.
- Snack options should be preplanned so patients do not sabotage a well-planned, three-meal day (see appendix for low-glycemic impact snack handout).
- Food preparation techniques can influence the health of any food choice. Frying, over-heating and charring foods can often limit nutrients or add inflammatory signals to otherwise healthy foods.
- Encourage patients to sit down and eat meals with people they enjoy being around. Eating alone, or with those who create tension, will counteract many of the healthful benefits of the food.

Organic Foods: What are the Advantages?

When discussing the "signal-to-noise" ratio of foods, a critical question is raised about potential negative health consequences of consuming foods grown with chemical additives, namely herbicides, pesticides, fungicides and antibiotics. How do these negative "signals" offset the benefits of consuming these otherwise healthy foods? These questions often get clouded by other related questions, which attempt to ascertain the measurable differences in nutrient content between organic and non-organic foods. We will try to address these questions one by one, allowing for a reasoned approach.

What makes a food "organic"?
The simple answer in the U.S. is based on the USDA regulatory definition that allows foods to be labeled as either "100% Organic," "Organic," or "Made with Organic ingredients."[1] Here is a brief description of the differences in these labeling designations.

"100% Organic": This highest organic labeling status requires that all ingredient and processing aids be certified organic. The product label may use the "USDA Organic" logo and must state the certifying agency.

"Organic": The USDA allows products to be labeled as "Organic" if greater than 95% of a product's ingredients are certified organic, as long as the other (less than 5%) nonorganic ingredients are within a specified list of approved ingredients. Genetically modified ingredients are not allowed in a product labeled "Organic."

"Made with" Organic Ingredients: Products that contain greater than 70% certified organic ingredients can declare the product is "Made with organic ingredient X," as long as the other nonorganic ingredients meet certain criteria (including no GMO ingredients). While the statement above is permitted on the label, these products cannot use the "USDA Organic" logo.

Individual Ingredients within Supplement Facts Box: Certified organic ingredients included in a product that contains less than 70% organic composition can be labeled as "organic" within the supplement facts panel or the ingredient list of the product. These products do not need to meet any other requirements (meaning they might contain other GMO ingredients) and cannot use the "USDA Organic" logo or represent themselves as organic products.

These labeling rules have been mostly beneficial to consumers, although they come with some unintended consequences. Obviously, having a single set of labeling rules and auditing regulations for certifying products has reduced the confusing array of "organic" definitions that existed prior to these guidelines. On the other hand, since these specific labeling guidelines have come into place, it is now possible to produce "industrialized" foods that still meet the official regulatory definition of "organic," a situation some would claim harms the original intent of defining products truly sustainable and "natural."

This nuance may seem trivial to some, but it is possible to purchase USDA organic produce grown in nutrient-depleted soil and picked weeks before optimal ripening to ship across the country. These not-so-trivial details must be kept in mind as we look at the published data comparing "conventionally grown" and "organic" foods in the rest of this section. Here are the most common questions concerning organic foods or supplements.

Are their fewer toxins in organic foods?
A number of studies have looked into the harmful levels of toxins in organic vs. conventional foods, or in individuals who routinely eat these foods. Studies have consistently shown produce labeled as "organic" have significantly fewer residues of pesticides, herbicides, fungicides and synthetic fertilizers (organic meats contain less residual antibiotics and, paradoxically, less antibiotic-resistant micro-organisms).[2] This should come as little surprise; the prohibition of these substances is at the core of organic food production.

Perhaps the most often cited study to show the impact of consuming organic foods and pesticide exposure is a paper published in 2006 from Emory University in Atlanta, Georgia.[3] In this study urinary biomonitoring was used to measure dietary organophosphorus pesticide exposure in a group of

1. For a complete description of all the requirements, see USDA's National Organic Program Website, www.ams.usda.gov/nop.

2. Smith-Spangler C et al. Are organic foods safer or healthier than conventional alternatives?: a systematic review. *Ann Intern Med.* 2012 Sep 4;157(5):348-66.

3. Lu C, Toepel K, Irish R, Fenske RA, Barr DB, Bravo R. Organic diets significantly lower children's dietary exposure to organophosphorus pesticides. *Environ Health Perspect.* 2006 Feb;114(2):260-3.

23 elementary school-age children. The researchers substituted most of the children's conventional diets with organic food items for five consecutive days and collected two spot daily urine samples, first-morning and before-bedtime voids, throughout the 15-day study period. The researchers found median urinary concentrations of the specific metabolites for malathion and chlorpyrifos decreased to non-detectable levels immediately after the introduction of organic diets and remained undetectable until the conventional diets were reintroduced. As one would expect, organic foods simply contain fewer chemical residues than conventionally-grown foods.

Which conventionally grown fruits and vegetables have the most toxic residues?

Since organic foods are more expensive, it may be of some value to inform patients about conventionally grown foods traditionally associated with the most (and least) use of chemicals. The Environmental Working Group (www.ewg.org) publishes a list of fruits and vegetables known to contain the highest and lowest amounts of pesticides called The Dirty Dozen and Clean 15 to help consumers prioritize their organic food budget. A free app for mobile devices is also available so this list can be handy when patients are standing in the produce aisle trying to remember these items.

Are there more nutrients in organic foods?

This question is more difficult to answer, as studies from various countries using a variety of fruits and vegetables have resulted in a range of differences in some measured nutrients. Reviews and meta-analysis of studies comparing organic vs. conventionally grown fruits and vegetables have generally concluded there is little difference in the measurements of most nutrients.[4]

However, subtleties of agricultural practices, seasonality and harvest-to-market timing may diminish the ability to detect these benefits.[5] In contrast, organic dairy products have consistently shown improved nutritional content, likely due to the necessary changes to animal feed required for organic dairy production.[6]

It is possible that the consumers' desire for cheap and ubiquitous agricultural crops has forced many large organic producers to adapt quick-to-mature organisms (plants and animals) to the organic model. While these products often meet the requirements of organic labeling, they are not always conducive to maximizing nutrient value. Purchasing produce and meats from local growers, especially those using heirloom seeds and animal stock (harvested at their nutritional peak) may prove to be more nutritious and affordable to most.

Dirty Dozen *Buy These Organic* (WORST)		**Clean 15** *Lowest in Pesticides* (BEST)	
1	Strawberries	1	Sweet Corn**
2	Spinach	2	Avocados
3	Nectarines	3	Pineapples
4	Apples	4	Cabbage
5	Peaches	5	Onions
6	Pears	6	Sweet peas frozen
7	Cherries	7	Papayas**
8	Grapes	8	Asparagus
9	Celery	9	Mangos
10	Tomatoes	10	Eggplant
11	Sweet bell peppers	11	Honeydew Melon
12	Potatoes	12	Kiwi
13	Hot Peppers*	13	Cantaloupe
		14	Cauliflower
		15	Grapefruit

(www.ewg.org)

*Dirty Dozen PLUS

**The EWG notes: "A small amount of sweet corn, papaya and summer squash sold in the United States is produced from genetically modified seeds. Buy organic varieties of these crops if you want to avoid genetically modified produce."

Is wildcrafting better than cultivating?

Wildcrafting, or foraging for foods and herbal products, is popular in many regions of the country. Whether it is seasonally harvesting game animals and fowl or collecting mushrooms, asparagus, wild berries and nuts or a host of medicinal plants and roots; wildcrafting is both a business and hobby for millions of Americans. Some wildcrafted products may even meet the USDA's requirements for "Organic" labeling.

Since wildcrafted products are seasonal and local, no systematic studies have been performed to compare their nutrient content with cultivated products, whether organic or conventional. Even so, it should be noted many of the secondary metabolites in plants, especially those deemed to be medicinally beneficial, are often produced by plants to help them deal with a harsh, naturally competitive environment. Cultivation by any measure provides the plants with consistent water and nutrient supplies, pest control, weed control and ample space to grow. These plant "luxuries" trigger fewer of the secondary metabolites usually needed to survive in the wild and may end up producing foods with a lower concentration of the bioactive phytonutrients traditionally associated with these plants.

In addition to select organically grown foods, wildcrafted foods, when harvested ethically and sustainably, can certainly be a fun, educational and healthy part of a well-rounded diet.

4. Dangour AD, Dodhia SK, Hayter A, Allen E, Lock K, Uauy R. Nutritional quality of organic foods: a systematic review. *Am J Clin Nutr*. 2009 Sep;90(3):680-5.

5. Crinnion WJ. Organic foods contain higher levels of certain nutrients, lower levels of pesticides, and may provide health benefits for the consumer. *Altern Med Rev*. 2010 Apr;15(1):4-12.

6. Benbrook CM, Butler G, Latif MA, Leifert C, Davis DR. Organic production enhances milk nutritional quality by shifting Fatty Acid composition: a United States-wide, 18-month study. *PLoS One*. 2013 Dec 9;8(12):e82429.

The Signals Within the Food

This section will focus on what we have learned about the various signals within foods. Again, we will limit our focus to practical issues for clinical decision-making, not a comprehensive review of each subject.

Total Energy Content and Glycemic Impact

Since dietary advice is often given for weight loss and management, it is important to note total energy intake, measured by calories, is a critical "signal" sent by our daily dietary choices. It is often said "a calorie is a calorie is a calorie," meaning the source of the energy (fat, protein, carbohydrate) is irrelevant for purposes of weight control. According to this theory, consuming the same number of caloric energy in our food as we burn through our daily activities will result in no weight gain or loss. This may be true if each system in the body is maintained with 100% efficiency and no loss in metabolic reserve or physiological resiliency has occurred; however, this is rarely the case. In the U.S. alone, 25 million people have been diagnosed with diabetes and another 75 million are considered pre-diabetic—that is one-third of the country's population.

So what does this mean?

Even though weight gain and loss is related to energy consumption and energy expenditure, in overweight and insulin-resistant subjects, metabolic responses to certain nutrients (especially carbohydrates) is shunted toward storing rather than burning energy. However, when these subjects are forced to consume much lower intakes of energy than their metabolism requires, the relative difference in their functional metabolic use of various macronutrients is much less relevant. Macronutrient ratio is simply less important when energy intake is substantially lower, or higher, than energy output (see Figure 7). Therefore, when a patient is undergoing a severe calorie-restricted diet (reduced by 500 calories or more), the ratio of carbohydrate, protein and fat intake is much less relevant. However, when attempting to maintain that weight, macronutrient selection and glycemic impact will influence the overall metabolic effect.

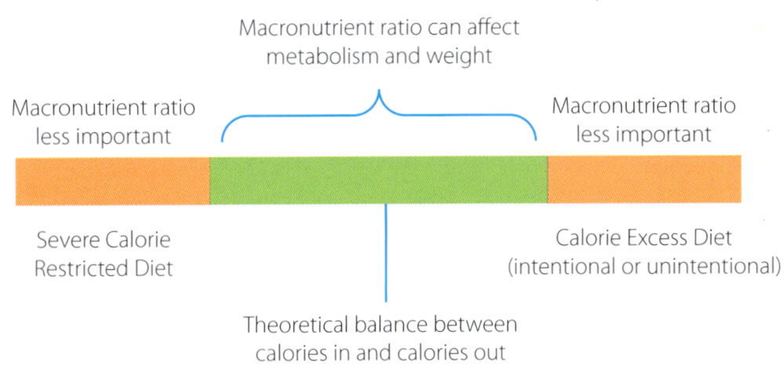

Figure 7 : When Macronutrient Ratio Matters
Macronutrient ratio becomes less relevant to weight loss/weight maintenance the farther the caloric intake is from that needed to offset calories burned (higher or lower).

One of the best studies to show this phenomenon was done in more than 750 overweight subjects living throughout eight different countries in Europe.[1] This was a two-phase weight loss, weight maintainence trial. Initially 938 subjects enrolled in a very-reduced-calorie diet (800 to 1000 kcal per day) for eight weeks. Subjects who were able to achieve an 8% weight loss were randomly assigned to one of five diets to maintain their weight and followed for an additional 26 weeks.

1. Larsen TM et al. Diets with high or low protein content and glycemic index for weight-loss maintenance. *N Engl J Med.* 2010 Nov 25; 363(22):2102-13.

The five diets were:

1. Low in protein (13% of total energy consumed) with a low glycemic index
2. Low in protein with a high glycemic index
3. High in protein (25% of total energy consumed) with a low glycemic index
4. High-protein and high-glycemic-index diet
5. A control diet that followed dietary guidelines in each participating country; a moderate protein content with no instructions to participants with respect to the glycemic index

None of the dietary recommendations included calorie restriction, since part of the intent of the trial was to detect whether macronutrient and glycemic index advice had an effect on calorie consumption and satiety.

As Figure 8 shows, subjects consuming either the control diet or the low-protein/high-glycemic-index diet (LP-HGI) began gaining weight within the first several weeks of the trial and added the most weight over the full 26 weeks. Adding either a high-protein (HP) or a low-glycemic-index (LGI) emphasis did delay the added weight gain. However, when combining both a high-protein diet with a low-glycemic emphasis, subjects were able to keep their weight at or below their original 8% weight loss for the full 26 weeks.

In contrast, trials that attempt to compare macronutrient-related effects on weight loss within the context of very-reduced-calorie diets rarely show consistently different outcomes related to macronutrient ratios or glycemic index changes. This has led many people to miss the beneficial differences of appropriate macronutrient balance for weight maintenance in calorie neutral or unmonitored-calorie situations, leading to the false notion that "all calories are equal." Therefore, for long-term weight maintenance and long-term weight loss where only modest reductions in energy intake over expenditure are required, we believe patients should be instructed to reduce their intake of high-glycemic-index foods and attempt to get 25 – 30% of their calories from protein. While this pattern is also likely to be helpful for more aggressive weight-loss goals (using restricted calorie intake and high energy output); in short-term weight-loss studies, the subject's adherence to dietary limits and exercise goals is often the best measure of success, regardless of dietary pattern.

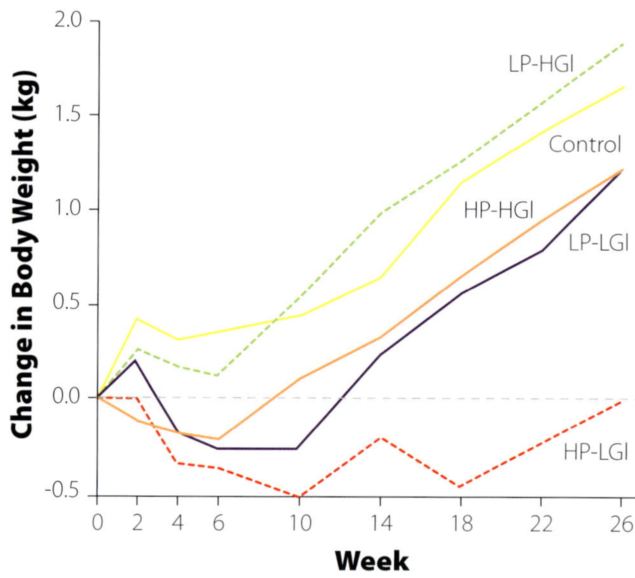

Figure 8 : Protein and GI-effect on Weight Maintenance
Change in Body Weight after 8% weight loss based on macronutrient and glycemic index instructions. See text for details. From Larsen et al. 2010.

Type 2 diabetic subjects and even more sensitivity to changes in glycemic index

Many researchers and clinicians have dismissed the notion that glycemic index education will greatly impact health. They do so because most glycemic index research has been done using relatively healthy (and cash-strapped) college students with adequate glucose tolerance. On the other hand, when you compare the glucose and insulin impact of foods that differ in their glycemic impact in type 2 diabetic subjects, a much greater impact is realized. Figure 9 shows that when subjects with normal glucose tolerance consume white (milled) rice, they have a slightly higher blood glucose excursion than when they consume brown (unmilled) rice.[2] However, a much greater influence in glucose excursion is seen in type 2 diabetic subjects given the same challenge of milled or brown rice. By removing the fiber and some of the vitamins and trace phytonutrients in the milling process, the same caloric load provides a different "signal" and a different physiological response. In this case, as the physiological resilience related to glucose disposal is weaker in the type 2 diabetic subjects, these subtle changes are magnified.

2. Panlasigui LN, Thompson LU. Blood glucose lowering effects of brown rice in normal and diabetic subjects. *Int J Food Sci Nutr*. 2006 May-Jun; 57(3-4):151-8.

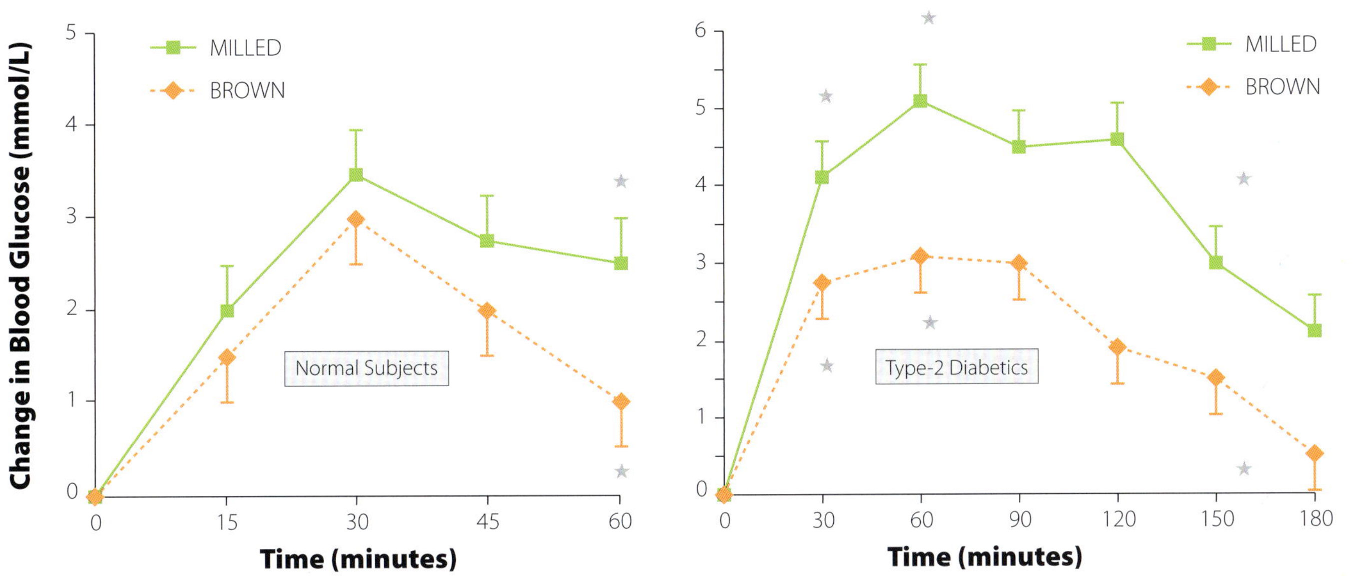

Figure 9 : Glycemic Impact is Exaggerated as Insulin Resistance Increases.
Change in blood glucose over 60 minutes after consuming unmilled (brown) rice and milled (white) rice in normal, healthy subjects (left) and type 2 diabetic subjects (right). Note that the AUC for blood glucose is elevated for over three hours in the diabetic subjects consuming milled rice (normal subjects only followed for 1 hour). Adapted from Panlasigui LN, Thompson LU. Blood glucose lowering effects of brown rice in normal and diabetic subjects. *Int J Food Sci Nutr.* 2006 May-Jun;57(3-4):151-8.

Clinicians should advise all patients who are overweight, insulin resistant or diabetic (type 1 and 2) about the role of glycemic impact on their health and provide them with tools to help them select foods that have a lower glycemic impact.

Meal Timing and Frequency

Space does not permit us to review the literature that attempts to answer questions about optimal meal timing and frequency in humans. A growing body of literature continually confirms the benefit of eating breakfast for both men and women and, as mentioned earlier, moving a larger proportion of the caloric intake to breakfast while reducing caloric intake later in the evening. This is not only to provide energy that will likely be used during the day, depending on the sedentary nature of the subject, but also acts as a circadian regulator of metabolism.[3,4,5]

Ideal meal frequency, a subset of meal timing, is also a hotly debated subject among researchers, clinicians and patients. Various camps advocate for frequencies ranging from intermittent fasting or one meal per day all the way to a dozen or more small snacks throughout the day, each with their own physiological theory as to why the frequency they suggest is best. A survey of the literature will suggest that when daily caloric intake, glycemic index and macronutrient ratios are the same, it is virtually impossible to see a consistent pattern of benefit using a meal frequency that is different than the traditional three meals per day.[6]

One could conclude from this that meal frequency doesn't matter, which is perhaps true from a clinical trial perspective. However, from a clinical

3. Garaulet M, Gómez-Abellán P, Alburquerque-Béjar JJ, Lee YC, Ordovás JM, Scheer FA. Timing of food intake predicts weight loss effectiveness. *Int J Obes* (Lond). 2013 Apr; 37(4):604-11.

4. Sherman H, Genzer Y, Cohen R, Chapnik N, Madar Z, Froy O. Timed high-fat diet resets circadian metabolism and prevents obesity. *FASEB J.* 2012 Aug; 26(8):3493-502.

5. Froy O, Miskin R. Effect of feeding regimens on circadian rhythms: implications for aging and longevity. *Aging* (Albany NY). 2010 Dec 11; 2(1):7-27.

6. Leidy HJ, Campbell WW. The effect of eating frequency on appetite control and food intake: brief synopsis of controlled feeding studies. *J Nutr.* 2011 Jan; 141(1):154-7.

application perspective, this means flexibility in choosing a meal frequency that works best for the patient is unlikely to diminish their success when choosing a healthy dietary pattern. The only exception to this would be if their frequency consisted of regularly skipping breakfast or pushing most of their calories toward evening.

What about small, frequent meals helping to maintain stable blood sugar? This is the most common argument given for recommending small frequent meals, one we have given in the past. It appears, in well-controlled settings, this is not necessarily the case. However, in an uncontrolled setting (i.e., real life), advising someone to eat frequent, smaller meals may prevent them from gorging themselves on the typical three-meals-per-day pattern. Technically then, this is using more frequent meals to reduce daily calories and would only work if the patient actually achieved the goal of consuming fewer calories, resulting in a lower overall daily glycemic impact.

While it is possible frequent meals may benefit certain subjects such as highly trained athletes or highly insulin-resistant individuals, there is not enough evidence—and in some cases, even contradictory evidence—to depend on a meal-frequency strategy solely based on avoiding the traditional three-meals-per-day pattern.

What about snacking?

By definition, snacks are foods consumed between meals, using the traditional three-meal-per-day pattern. The implication is these are small amounts of food, intended to "tide me over" until the next meal. The reality can be quite different. Patient success doesn't mean abandoning snacks altogether; in fact for many, appropriate snacking can help reduce later meal over-consumption. In one study that measured weight-loss success in postmenopausal women, they found those who frequently consumed snacks in the morning were less likely to succeed in their weight loss and were more likely to have multiple snacks per day, while those who only snacked in the afternoon were more likely to eat fruits and vegetables and, therefore, succeed in their weight-loss goals.[7] While this study didn't make a direct analysis of breakfast meals in comparison to mid-morning snacks, we know mid-morning hunger is related to low satiety after breakfast (skipping breakfast or consuming a high-glycemic breakfast will do this) and food availability. We recommend you help your patients understand their own vulnerability to cravings (what, where, when, with whom) and help them plan to have healthy snack options, with appropriate serving size, at hand for the occasion.

Healthy Snack Ideas:

- Small handful of mixed almonds and walnuts (preferably unroasted)
- 1 handful assorted dried fruits such as dates, figs or apricots
- 12-15 low-fat blue corn chips with ¼ cup salsa or guacamole
- ¼ cup hummus and ½ cup vegetable sticks
- 1 medium sliced apple with 1T almond butter
- 1 low-fat cheese stick with whole grain crackers
- 2 brown rice cakes with tahini and jam spread
- Healthy protein bar (read label carefully)
- ½ cup celery sticks with 1 T peanut butter
- 1 hard-boiled egg and ¼ cup carrot sticks
- ½ cup mixed berries and cherries
- 1 handful of spiced dried green and chick peas
- 4-6 rye crackers and roasted vegetable dip
- 1 berry smoothie made with 6 oz of nut milk and ½ cup fruit and flax seeds

7. Kong A, Beresford SA, Alfano CM, et al. Associations between snacking and weight loss and nutrient intake among postmenopausal overweight to obese women in a dietary weight-loss intervention. *J Am Diet Assoc.* Dec 2011; 111(12):1898-1903.

Macronutrients: Proteins

Unlike many developing countries, protein sources are abundant in the Western diet, especially among the meat-eating majority. Protein provides us with the building blocks (amino acids) to reassemble into our own proteins for use as enzymes, hormones, extracellular matrix materials, cell receptors and much, much more. While humans are capable of synthesizing several of the necessary amino acids used for protein synthesis, there are a number considered to be essential dietary components in humans: valine, phenylalanine, threonine, leucine, lysine, tryptophan, isoleucine, methionine and histidine. For purposes of intake guidelines and food nutrient labeling, protein is generally calculated to contain four calories per gram.

USRDA	Men (Adults)	Women (Adults)
Protein	56 grams (225 calories)	46 grams (184 calories)

In our opinion these guideline numbers are below the level that forms a healthy glycemic impact for most Western adults. Independent of total calories consumed, protein consumption should make up 20 – 30% of that intake. For a male consuming 2,000 calories, this means total protein intake would be 400 – 600 calories, or 100 – 150 grams of protein per day.[1] For a female consuming 1,600 calories, this would be 80 – 120 grams of protein per day. CDC data collected between 2007 and 2010 record that the average American male consumes 16% of his 2,500 daily calories as protein, which equals 100 grams per day; the average American female consumes 15.6% of her 1778 calories as protein, equaling 70 grams per day. These data suggest the average American consumes well more than the USRDA recommendation of protein (and calories) already and would meet our suggestion for protein intake and percent of dietary calories merely by reducing their caloric intake of carbohydrates and fat.

High Protein Foods:
Grams of Protein Per 100 Calories

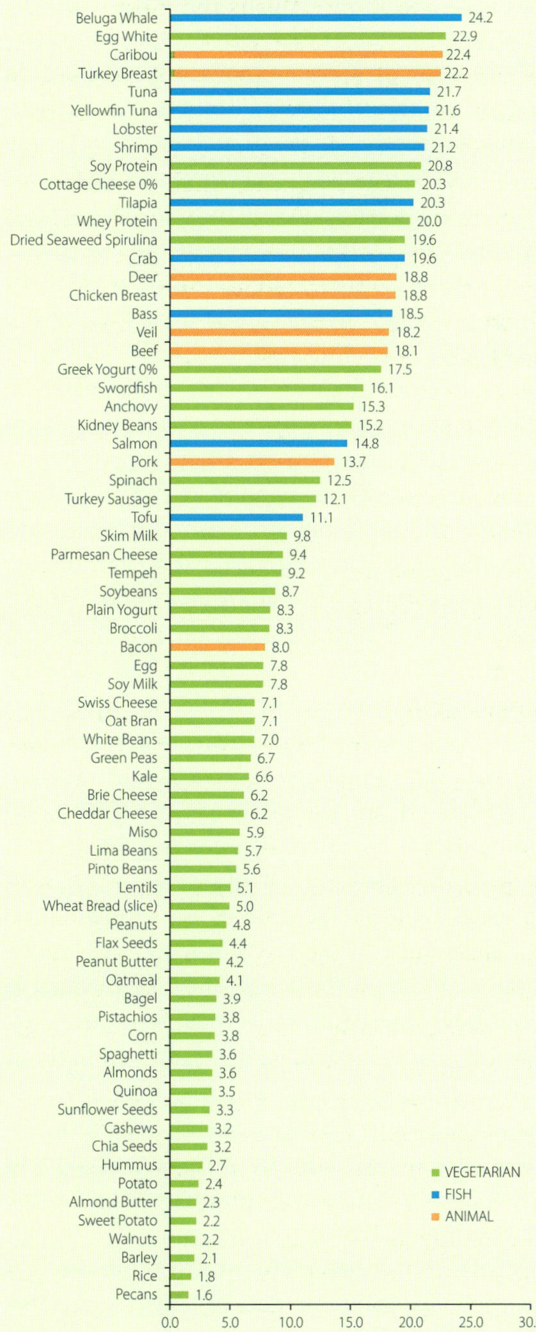

Data taken from USDA Food Database as compiled by nutritiondata.self.com

1. These recommendations are for healthy adults with average physical activity. Athletes and very large individuals may require even higher levels, while those with poor kidney function should consume less.

Supplemental Protein Sources

A wide variety of protein supplements are available labeled either as functional foods or dietary supplements, some even claiming to be medical foods. These proteins are often combined with a variety of ingredients and sold as meal replacements; multivitamin drinks; fiber-containing, glycemic-control shakes; or simply as protein supplements. These products can range dramatically in protein content per scoop, depending on the purpose of the product. Products intended to deliver as much protein as possible (typical of some products for building muscle mass) contain large scoops and can provide 20 – 60 grams of protein per serving. Products intended to deliver proteins in the context of other nutrients often deliver 8 –20 grams of protein per serving. These protein powders can be mixed with milk or milk substitutes (rice milk, almond milk, soy milk, etc.) to provide even more protein when consumed.

Clinicians and patients have many supplemental protein choices today, since powder-based supplements/meal replacements are growing in popularity. While these powder products will not replace the use of capsules and tablets in the majority of patients, the ability to deliver supplemental micronutrients—vitamins, minerals, etc.—in the context of the added healthy protein can be an advantage for many patients, especially when the dose of certain micronutrients would make an equivalent capsule count burdensome. Not surprisingly, physician-only brands of dietary supplements have a wide selection of products blended in ready-to-mix, protein-based powders using different protein sources and flavors.

Table 2 shows the amino acid profile of the most commonly used commercial sources of supplemental protein available (raw material) compared to food-source proteins. Most of these commercially available sources have been concentrated to contain over 60 – 80% protein, some protein isolates are as high as 90%. Clearly, these products do not contain the whole nutrient profile of their parent source and, depending on the purpose of the supplement, must be complemented with other macronutrient and micronutrients to achieve an appropriate signal balance.

Clinicians choose supplemental protein sources based on various parameters: total protein delivered, amino acid profile, allergy concerns, vegan-friendly, organic status; or on the absence of phytates, estrogen-like compounds or heavy metals. The limited amount of research available comparing supplemental protein sources (e.g., whey vs. soy) for a wide range of surrogate markers of health make it difficult to recommend one source for all clinical applications. For instance, while whey protein supplements have been shown to help promote positive metabolic changes and weight-loss in a variety of clinical trials, these studies often don't compare the effects (head-to-head) with other protein sources (soy, rice, pea, etc.). In any case, many clinicians prefer to avoid dairy-source protein for allergy-related or philosophical reasons (e.g., the paleo approach).[2]

Although the *therapeutic* role of isolated amino acids, of which there are many, is beyond the scope of this Road map; we do not believe there is compelling evidence to use combinations of isolated amino acids in place of dietary or supplemental proteins in healthy individuals. The addition of certain amino acid isolates to enhance a supplemental protein concentrate is, however, sometimes warranted. As with dietary signals, products that contain a blend of protein sources are likely to create an amino acid/protein balance typical of what the body receives in a normal diet.

2. Pal S, Radavelli-Bagatini S. The effects of whey protein on cardiometabolic risk factors. *Obes Rev.* 2013 Apr; 14(4):324-43.

	Rice Protein[1]	Pea Protein S85 F[2]	Soy Protein SF-P[3]	Whey Protein[4]	Egg White Protein[5]	Whole eggs, scrambled[6]	Fish, Salmon, dry heat[7]	Chicken cooked[8]	Beef/ Steak[9]	Breast Milk
Typical protein % of ingredient	**80%**	**80%**	**90%**	**80%**	**80%**	**10%**	**25.82%**	**29%**	**34%**	**1.03%**
Typical Amino acid Profile Essential Amino acids (as % of protien)										
Tryptophan	0.8	1	5.3	1.92	NA	1.39	1.15	1.12	0.69	1.66
Threonine	3.8	3.8	3.8	8.86	4.34	4.42	4.52	4.02	4.20	4.50
Isoleucine	5.03	4.7	4.6	6.21	4.53	5.32	4.47	5.04	4.79	5.48
Leucine	9.4	8.2	8.1	12.42	7.53	8.61	8.39	7.18	8.38	9.31
Lysine	3.6	7.1	5.7	9.62	5.87	7.05	9.48	8.05	8.90	6.66
Methionine	2.8	1.1	1.5	2.61	4.90	2.97	3.05	2.63	2.74	2.05
Phenylalanine	6.8	5.5	6.2	3.4	5.31	5.35	4.03	3.81	4.16	4.50
Valine	5.4	5	4.7	5.81	6.45	6.76	5.32	4.74	5.22	6.17
Histidine	2.3	2.5	2.4	1.85	2.18	2.45	3.04	2.96	3.36	2.25
Non Essential Amino acids										
Alanine	5.01	4.3	4.1	4.57	7.5	5.66	6.24	5.19	6.40	3.52
Arginine	8.7	8.7	7.4	2.42	5.25	6.23	6.18	5.74	6.81	4.21
Aspartic acid	9.06	11.5	11.6	12.76	10.46	10.34	10.57	8.47	9.60	8.03
Cysteine	1.5	1	1.1	0.76	NA	2.05	1.10	1.23	1.36	1.86
Glutamic acid	17.2	16.7	19.6	19.48	13.12	13.78	15.41	14.60	15.82	16.46
Glycine	4.3	4	3.6	2.06	3.28	3.35	4.95	4.68	6.42	2.54
Proline	3.8	4.3	4.7	7.76	3.53	4.53	3.65	4.03	5.02	8.03
Serine	5.4	5.1	5.3	5.91	6.40	7.42	4.21	3.31	4.15	4.21
Tyrosine	5.1	3.8	5.3	3.32	NA	4.02	3.48	3.22	3.36	5.19
Hydroxyproline	NA	NA	NA	0.1	NA	NA	NA	NA	1.10	NA

Table 2: Typical Amino Acid Profile of Commercially Available Protein Supplements and Foods.

Protein sourced from:

1. Rice protein isolate (Oryzapro; Pevesa)
2. Pea protein concentrate (Nutralys)
3. Soy protein isolate (Pevesa)
4. Whey protein concentrate (Wisconsin Specialty Protein)
5. Egg white protein (Healthco)

6–10. USDA /ARS / National Nutrient Database for Standard Reference
http://ndb.nal.usda.gov/ndb/foods/show/837?fg=&man=&lface t=&count=&max=&sort=&qlookup=&offset=&format=Full&new=&measureby=

Meal Replacements: Advantages and Disadvantages

In the clinical application of macronutrient supplementation, products specifically labeled or used as "meal replacements" are common. While the regulatory definition of meal replacement products are murky (some claim medical food status, etc.), the question we would like to investigate here pertains to whether these products are appropriate for use in clinical practice and what, if any, disadvantages there are in recommending these products to patients.

Much of the early work on meal replacement application came from the space program, where a compact liquid "meal" that provided all the necessary daily nutrients was critical. From there, meal replacements were expanded to deliver special nutrient combinations for the hospitalized, institutionalized or person's with inborn errors of metabolism requiring them to supplement (or avoid) particular nutrients. Today, a wide variety of products are available that are called (or used as) meal replacements. These products are typically in the form of ready-to-eat liquid drinks, ready-to-mix powder drinks, or as bars.

The basic advantage of any meal replacement product is simple: control. By knowing exactly what a patient is consuming, both the clinician and patient eliminate the ambiguity of implementing a portion of the dietary regimen. For instance, if a patient routinely skips breakfast or often chooses foods with high glycemic impact for breakfast, recommending a high-protein, high-fiber breakfast shake with a known caloric and glycemic impact will allow the patient to control these factors without difficulty. The most common use of meal replacements is their ability to aid individuals in calorie reduction for weight-loss/weight-maintenance. Clinical studies over the past several decades have shown that in obese subjects (including type 2 diabetic subjects), those able to use meal replacement products were more likely to reach their daily calorie reduction and weight loss goal than those given only dietary means to restrict calories. In the Look AHEAD trial, obese type-2 diabetic subjects consuming the highest number of meal replacement products had nearly twice the weight reduction compared to those consuming the least, over a one-year follow-up.

There are, however, potential disadvantages that must be considered when using meal replacements. The first is the overall poor quality of many products currently available. Macronutrient ratios are often heavily skewed toward carbohydrates (mostly through added sugars), while protein, fiber and (good) fat levels are rarely adequate. Clinicians should look for products that contain a well-designed balance of macronutrients, perhaps even using proteins from multiple sources. While it is difficult to get true "diversity" using the same product on a daily basis, some products are designed with more inherent signal diversity than others. Depending on the desire to use these products for calorie-restriction, clinicians and patients should be aware that milk and milk substitutes (rice, soy, almond or coconut milk are the most common liquids used to reconstitute powdered products) contain approximately 100 calories per serving.

One final concern is that the use of meal replacements on an ongoing basis may prevent the transition of the subject toward appropriate food (meal) selection and generate an overreliance on meal replacements for dietary restraint. This, of course, is common of any augmented lifestyle therapy. By way of analogy, 45 minutes on a treadmill is an artificial means to approximate an equivalent amount of running/walking in one's daily life. However, like meal replacements and dietary signals, treadmills can be a convenient and consistent way to facilitate most of the walking "signals." Meal replacement products (and all supplement products in general), like treadmills, are intended to augment lifestyle signals, not replace them.

- Heymsfield SB. Meal replacements and energy balance. *Physiol Behav.* 2010 Apr 26;100(1):90-4.
- Hamdy O, Zwiefelhofer D. Weight management using a meal replacement strategy in type 2 diabetes. *Curr Diab Rep.* 2010 Apr;10(2):159-64.
- Wadden TA, West DS et al. One-year weight losses in the Look AHEAD study: factors associated with success. *Obesity Silver Spring.* 2009 Apr;17(4):713-22.

Macronutrients: Carbohydrates

Carbohydrates are major nutrient compounds such as monosaccharides, disaccharides, polysaccharides and starch. In foods and supplements, all other organic compounds other than fats and proteins (e.g., polyol sugars, fiber, plant cellulose, etc.) are measured as carbohydrates, all calculated as four calories per gram.

USRDA	Men (Adults)	Women (Adults)
Carbohydrates	130 grams (520 calories)	130 grams (520 calories)
"Added sugars"	(Up to 25% of total calorie intake)	

As you can see from the USRDA numbers, intake levels of both carbohydrates and "added sugars" creates quite a large "fudge-factor" for total carbohydrate intake based on calorie consumption. Ultimately, this combination is similar to the other common advice given by nutritional guidelines; to consume 45 – 65% of your calories as carbohydrates. If a woman consuming 1,700 calories were to consume 130 grams (520 calories) of carbohydrates and another 25% of her calories as "added sugar," she would consume a total of 945 calories as carbohydrates, accounting for 55% of her daily calories. CDC data gathered from 2007 – 2010 estimates the average American consumes 48 – 51% of their calories as carbohydrates.

While carbohydrate counting is not necessarily a recommended target of this guide, some patients still prefer this method. Overall, we believe helping patients understand how to consume the correct types of carbohydrates, those with a low glycemic impact and a high amount of fiber, is much more important for long-term health than merely counting carbohydrate calories. Nonetheless, for those desiring carbohydrate counting advice, we believe maintaining carbohydrate totals between 40 – 50% of total caloric intake is a good starting point for most individuals. We advise those attempting weight-loss or maintenance, when counting carbohydrate calories, not to exceed 40%. Some low-carb diet plans may even suggest dropping down carbohydrates to less than 20% of total calories.

Carbs in Context

One important thing to grasp about carbohydrates is there are virtually no unhealthy carbohydrate molecules, but there are many unhealthy ways to consume them—that is, carbohydrates of all kinds, when consumed with a balance of other nutrients (protein, fiber, vitamins, phytonutrients) are rarely "bad" for our health. Problems arise when individuals consume high amounts of refined carbohydrates (refined flours, refined sugars, HFCS, etc.) with virtually no other nutrients to temper the body's glycemic response. Having previously discussed the glycemic response based on the glycemic index of certain foods (pages 29-31), here we will briefly discuss how glycemic index and glycemic load are calculated, since they directly relate to the carbohydrate content of the food being measured.

Glycemic Index (GI): This number corresponds to the tested glycemic response, using healthy subjects, of a particular food portion containing a measured amount, typically 50 grams, of available carbohydrates (carbohydrates minus fiber), compared to the glycemic response of glucose *in the same subjects*. This number is "indexed" to glucose, arbitrarily set at a GI of 100. Foods with a GI above 70 are usually considered high-GI foods, while those below 55 are considered low GI.

Glycemic Load (GL): This is essentially the measurement of the glycemic burden of a food based on the total amount of available carbohydrates per serving, multiplied by its GI. This takes into account not all foods with a high GI will contain high amounts of carbohydrates, like watermelon, while other foods, like a bagel, contain high amounts of high-GI carbohydrates creating a large GL.

Glycemic Impact -What to Tell Patients: While glycemic load is likely more relevant to a person's glycemic response, few individuals are walking around with a scale and calculator to decipher the glycemic load of their meal. In the end, the goal is to reduce the glycemic impact of the meal by increasing the signal-to-calorie ratio, or here, the signal to available carbohydrate ratio. The best way to do this is to give patients simple advice such as:

- Reduce or avoid added sugars and anything made with white flour
- Reduce or stop drinking sweetened (or artificially sweetened) soft drinks and juices
- Consume more fiber
- Eat food as close to its natural state as possible
- Have a handy list of high-glycemic index foods, read it, and avoid them
- Take a leisurely walk after a large meal

What About Natural Non-Nutritive Sweeteners?

While controversy still remains about the risk of consuming *artificial* sweeteners, we recommend they be avoided by all individuals. We do know obesity and type 2 diabetes are more prevalent in subjects who consume more artificially sweetened beverages than their healthier counterparts, even though these compounds elicit no apparent insulin response. Whether these compounds are acting physiologically or psychologically, leading users to indulge in more extravagant eating habits, has yet to be determined. Although less controversial, the role of "natural" non-nutritive sweeteners is also unsettled in the minds of many health-minded consumers and physicians. Frankly, while the general use of these compounds have been shown to be safe, extensive research on subtle changes in long-term glycemic control or insulin sensitivity are lacking in most cases.

More challenging is the idea that questions how the use of any sweetening agent reinforces the "need for sweet" craving to which individuals have grown all too familiar. It is a delicate balancing act between consuming products designed to deliver healthy ingredients, while offsetting the bitter or off-putting flavors with something that is sweet on the tongue. The reality is many patients will simply not consume products they do not like (taste, smell, mouth-feel, aftertaste, etc.). For that reason, we will give a brief overview of some of the sweeteners commonly used in therapeutic products—functional foods, powders, bars and chewable tablets—available through healthcare professionals.

Agave nectar (syrup): We list this here only because some of the marketing material for products containing agave-derived sweeteners implies it is low in calories. In fact, agave syrup is one of many natural sweeteners mostly made of fructose, which is lower in GI than glucose. We consider agave products to be similar in nature to honey and maple syrup, and do not consider it to be worse than HFCS. As with other natural sweeteners, the total amount used and the context of the food containing the ingredient will determine its overall glycemic impact. Agave syrup is often from organic-sourced plants.

Fructose: We are not talking here about natural fructose in general, from consuming fruits, but the commercially available fructose ingredients used as added sugar for bars, powders and tablets. Fructose is one of the most popular added sugars for these products because it is sweet, has a natural mouth-feel, dissolves well, has a relatively low GI and is cheap to use. Fructose is also commonly recommended, over glucose and sucrose, as a "diabetes-friendly" sugar because it results in less post-prandial glucose and insulin. However, regular and long-term consumption of fructose has been linked with insulin resistance, obesity, metabolic syndrome and diabetes.

Because data on added fructose alone and that of high-fructose corn syrup are often combined, it is difficult to distinguish the health-related outcomes of one from the other. Therefore, we advise fructose be used in moderation; and since other sweeteners are available, fructose should be limited when consuming products designed to promote health. Nearly all available commercial fructose is derived via a multistep process from cornstarch, although it may also be converted from cane or beet sugar sucrose or, sometimes, directly from fruit juice sources. While GMO-free fructose is becoming more available, most fructose available in the U.S. is likely to be derived from a genetically modified source.

Polyol sugars: Sugar alcohol molecules, or polyol sugars as they are called (e.g., xylitol, sorbitol), are technically counted as part of total carbohydrates (for label carbohydrate and calorie measurements), but are often subtracted, along with fiber, to produce what some call "net carbs" on food labels since these "sugars" contain fewer calories than the standard four calories per gram.[1] These polyol compounds are used to sweeten gum, chewable tablets, bars and powders; the sweetness and GI of each varies (see Table 3). Some people do not tolerate certain polyol sugars; GI complaints, such as bloating, gas, and diarrhea, are not uncommon when these sugars are used in large amounts. Erythritol appears to be the best tolerated, but individual tolerance of each varies.

Ingredient	Sweetness	GI	Cal/g
Sucrose (table sugar)	100%	60	4
Maltitol Syrup	75%	52	3
Hydrogenated Starch Hydrolysate	33%	39	2.8
Maltitol	75%	36	2.7
Xylitol	100%	13	2.5
Isomalt	55%	9	2.1
Sorbitol	60%	9	2.5
Lactitol	35%	6	2
Mannitol	60%	0	1.5
Erythritol	70%	0	0.2

Table 3 : Comparing Polyol Sugars
Sweetness, Glycemic Index (GI) and calories per gram (U.S. calculation) for polyol sugars used in foods and supplements. Data from: Livesey G. Health potential of polyols as sugar replacers, with emphasis on low glycaemic properties. *Nutr Res Rev.* 2003 Dec;16(2):163-91.

With the exception of lactitol (derived from cow's milk), polyol sugars can be made from a number of different vegetable materials; although corn is the most frequently used starting material. Other materials sometimes used include cassava root, sucrose or hardwood pulp. If you are using products containing polyol sugars, you should be able to ask the supplier about the raw material source and the GMO-status of the raw material, as some of these products, even some corn-derived versions, are made from GMO-free sources. Since many products with added flavorings are often bitter, requiring some form of additional sweeteners for palatability, modest levels of polyol sugars appear to be without documented issues in most people, though they are not calorie-free as some advertise.

Stevia: The leaves of *Stevia rebaudiana* are extracted to concentrate the naturally occurring steviol glycosides for use as a non-nutritive sweetener. Foremost amongst the sweet glycosides is rebaudioside A, often the only glycoside in highly purified products. After limiting how stevia could be used and labeled for years, the FDA approved the use of stevia extracts as an additive in food and supplements in 2008. Stevia concentrates can be up to 300 times as sweet as sugar, yet appear to elicit no blood-glucose or insulin response. Concentrated stevia products can taste bitter to some consumers; most often it is used to accent the sweetness of other natural sweeteners.

Numerous studies have looked at various physiological effects of stevia extracts in humans and animal models. While long-term studies of stevia's effects on glucose, insulin and other metabolic outcomes are limited, nearly all short-term studies, along with an abundance of animal studies exploring stevia's metabolic effects, have suggested either no effect, or even an improvement in markers of insulin and metabolic function.[2]

Licorice root extracts (glycyrrhizin): Licorice root *(Glycerrhiza glabra L.)* has been used as both a sweetening agent in foods or candy and a medicinal plant for millennia.[3] Glycyrrhizin can be concentrated and used in foods and supplements, as it is between 30 – 50 times sweeter than sugar. Unlike other sweeteners, the sweetness of glycyrrhizin lingers on the tongue for much longer. Excessive use of glycyrrhizin, as with overconsumption of black licorice candy, can result in water retention and hypertension. These symptoms may be an issue when consuming greater than 100 mg of glycyrrhizin per day, equivalent to 50 grams of licorice candy. Rarely would glycyrrhizin be used in quantities this high as an added sweetener in supplements.

1. "Net carbs," or similar terms, have no official definition for labeling and these terms are not recognized by the FDA. The use of this calculation (total carbs minus fiber and polyol sugars) became popular during the resurgence of diets emphasizing very-low-carbohydrate intake. This term can be misleading since the glycemic impact of a food product may be affected by other factors: fiber content, type of fiber, protein content and insulin-sensitizing nutrients.

2. Goyal SK, Samsher, Goyal RK. Stevia (Stevia rebaudiana) a bio-sweetener: a review. *Int J Food Sci Nutr.* 2010 Feb; 61(1):1-10.

3. Asl MN, Hosseinzadeh H. Review of pharmacological effects of Glycyrrhiza sp. and its bioactive compounds. *Phytother Res.* 2008 Jun; 22(6):709-24.

A Balanced Approach to Sweeteners in Supplements

The use of both nutritive and non-nutritive sweeteners is often a concern for clinicians who believe these compounds are either unnecessary inactive excipients or downright harmful to consume. It is our view that these sweeteners allow for the delivery of many agents in powders, liquids and chewable tablets that would be virtually impossible for some patients to consume in "tasteless" capsules and tablets. Clinicians need to be realistic with their expectation of their patients' tolerances for consuming unsweetened products, realizing the amount of added sugars (or natural non-nutritive sweeteners) used in supplements is often miniscule compared to the USRDA allowance for added sugars. A balanced combination of nutritive sweeteners—sucrose, fructose, agave syrup, rice syrup, honey, etc. —low-calorie/GI polyol sugars, and natural non-nutritive sweeteners, such as stevia and licorice root, can be part of the necessary delivery of health-promoting nutrient supplements.

Macronutrients: Fiber

Dietary fiber is defined as all non-starch plant polysaccharides, with the addition of plant lignins. This includes celluloses, gums, pectins and mucilages found in fruits, vegetables, legumes and grains. Plant fiber is nearly indigestible in humans and is often referred to as "roughage," although this term is losing favor the more we learn about the immune-signaling power and microbial-feeding actions of many fiber compounds. Dietary fiber can be further divided into soluble and insoluble fiber. This characteristic does not mean true solubility (in the chemical sense), but describes fibers dispersible in water. The soluble fibers, such as pectin and gums, have a high water-holding capacity and often form a gel when mixed with water. Insoluble fibers hold little water and will usually fall to the bottom of a glass when mixed in water. Most non-isolated plant fibers within food will be a combination of both soluble and insoluble fibers.[1]

Adequate Intake	Men (Adults)	Women (Adults)
Fiber	38 grams/day	25 grams/day
In young children, recommendations are typically determined by adding five to the child's age to get the recommended grams per day (e.g., child age 7=12 grams/day).		

Many clinicians and nutritionists believe these recommended levels are much too low to maintain optimal health, recommending instead 45 or even 50 grams per day. However, even at current RDA levels, most Americans are not getting adequate levels of dietary fiber. A report from the Institute of Medicine (IOM), which deems 14 grams/1,000 calories as the adequate intake, says only 3% of Americans are consuming adequate amounts of fiber and average consumption is only half the recommended amount (i.e., only seven grams/1,000 calories).[2] According to the latest national survey data, fiber intake for men is around 18 grams/day, while for women it is around 14 grams/day. How important is fiber intake? In both men and women, the risk is significantly lower for metabolic syndrome (23%), inflammation (34%) and obesity (23%) in the highest quintile of fiber consumption (>22.5 grams) compared to the lowest quintile of fiber consumption (<8.1 grams).[3]

The benefits of fiber are many. Foods high in fiber are rich in other phytonutrients, some which are bound within the matrix of the fiber itself. Certain fibers are also important nutrients for healthy microbial organisms in the gut and have been termed "prebiotics" for their ability to stimulate bacterial growth, especially *Bifidobacteria*. Beyond their water holding capacity, soluble fibers influence functions such as stool viscosity, microbial fermentation to short-chain fatty acids, positive influence on digestive enzymes, bile acid binding capacity and anion exchange capacity.

Decreased fiber intake as a function of modern food practices is suggested to be the leading cause of idiopathic constipation. While this has been empirically shown in adults for more than a century, this has recently been researched specifically in children. In one study in Brazil, children with chronic constipation typically ingested 20 – 30% less fiber than age- and gender-matched controls with normal bowel habits.[4] In a larger sample group of children in Greece, dietary fiber alone was independently and inversely correlated with chronic constipation, despite the child's age or age of onset of constipation.[5] Furthermore, a study conducted in the U.S. showed constipated children were consuming less than one-fourth of the age-plus-five recommended

1. For a complete referenced article reviewing fiber and other agents as therapeutic agents for constipation, see The Standard: Maintaining Regularity: Constipation, Fiber and Natural Laxatives (Volume 5, No. 2) at www.pointinstitute.org.

2. Clemens R et al. Filling America's fiber intake gap: summary of a roundtable to probe realistic solutions with a focus on grain-based foods. *J Nutr.* 2012 Jul; 142(7):1390S-401S.

3. Grooms KN et al. Dietary Fiber Intake and Cardiometabolic Risks among US Adults, NHANES 1999-2010. *Am. J. of Med.* 16 October 2013- published online ahead of print.

4. Morais MB, Vítolo MR, Aguirre AN, Fagundes-Neto U. Measurement of low dietary fiber intake as a risk factor for chronic constipation in children. *J Pediatr Gastroenterol Nutr.* 1999 Aug; 29(2):132-5.

5. Roma E, Adamidis D et al. Diet and chronic constipation in children: the role of fiber. *J Pediatr Gastroenterol Nutr.* 1999 Feb; 28(2):169-74.

intake, even though they had been instructed "to eat a high-fiber diet." It seems in children, as well as adults, increasing dietary fiber is a difficult lifestyle change many simply decline to make. The use of supplemental dietary fiber in patients in elderly care facilities, where less individual control over diet is practiced, has been shown to decrease laxative use and increase bowel frequency.

The role of dietary fiber from food is vital for maintaining balanced blood sugar levels, especially in type 1 and type 2 diabetics. The mechanism is thought to be related to fiber's ability to slow glucose absorption from the small intestine and to reduce postprandial blood glucose levels. In a study published by the *New England Journal of Medicine* in 2000, type 2 diabetic patients were placed on two different diets; each for six weeks. Each diet was identical with the exception of dietary fiber; one provided 24 grams of fiber (8 gm soluble, 16 gm insoluble) and the other provided 50 grams of fiber (25 gm soluble, 25 gm insoluble) per day. The additional fiber statistically lowered mean daily blood glucose, daily urine glucose excretion, insulin concentration, triglycerides and VLDL particles. In a report comparing type 1 diabetic patients consuming less than 20 grams of fiber with those consuming more than 30 grams of fiber per day, a significant decrease in blood glucose, glycosylated hemoglobin, as well as number of hypoglycemic events was seen in patients taking more fiber. These data suggest it would be wise to advise all diabetic patients, as well as those with any cardiometabolic risk (metabolic syndrome), to seriously evaluate and increase their dietary fiber intake.

Fiber Used for Supplements/ Functional Foods

Since at least 80% of the U.S. population consumes less than 22.5 grams of fiber per day, most clinicians can easily recommend patients *add* at least 20 grams/day of fiber through targeted changes in their dietary choices, and for many, fiber supplements. A patient handout that shows a chart of foods based on their fiber content/ serving can be used to help the patient choose high-fiber (low-glycemic index) foods. Patients can be given a total daily goal of 35 – 50 grams/day from food and supplements, gradually moving from their current daily amount to the targeted amount over a few months, as adding high amounts of fiber quickly can cause GI gas, bloating and cramping.

The most common supplement forms of fiber are psyllium (seed and husks), flaxseeds, beta-glucans (oats or other grains), inulin and oligofructans, fruit pectin concentrates, chitosan (shellfish), gums (guar gum), and a variety of celluloses. Combining soluble, insoluble and fermentable fibers (all contribute to the dietary fiber total), is the best way to promote the wide-ranging benefits of increased fiber intake. Clinicians should have specific recommendations or formulary availability of several fiber-containing supplements. Products sold as "powders" to be mixed in water or juice will be easier to consume in higher doses, although some patients prefer encapsulated or tableted products. Clinicians should be aware that it often takes 12 or more capsules or tablets to reach the same dose as a single scoop of many commercially available fiber powders.

Clinicians should also consider the need for a children's product, which might include some of the fibers above or may even include extracts of fruits known to contain gentle fiber laxatives, such as plums, figs or various seeds. These products are helpful to alleviate constipation due to low fiber (and water) intake, but they should not be considered as a substitute for dietary sources of fiber that should be increased through changes in dietary habits.

Macronutrients: Fatty Acids

USRDA	Men (Adults)	Women (Adults)
Total Fat	20-35% of total calories	20-35% of total calories
Linoleic Acid (w-6)	17 grams	12 grams
α-Linolenic Acid (w-3)	1.6 grams	1.1 grams
Trans Fat	As little as possible	As little as possible
Cholesterol	As low as possible	As low as possible

Nutritional advice on fatty acid intake has gone through a vast upheaval over the past few decades. Not so long ago, the standard (and seemingly only) recommendation was to limit nearly all fat intake; a "low-fat" diet was presumed to be preferable to reduce the risk of most diseases, especially cardiovascular disease. This advice is no longer standard and, thankfully, the discussion around fat intake has been transformed by the understanding of the essential nature of consuming healthy fats, as well as the dangers of replacing healthy fats with refined carbohydrates (as the original food pyramid often was implemented). We will discuss the details of the various fatty acid structures and function and then discuss the varieties of fatty acid supplements, but purely from a nutrient and labeling standpoint, fat provides nine calories/gram: more than twice that of carbohydrates and protein.

The Basics of Fatty Acids

Fatty acids are simply a string of carbon molecules of varying length with a carboxylic acid group on one end, sometimes called the delta end. A saturated fatty acid is one in which all the other carbons along the chain have two hydrogen molecules bonded to them, with the exception of the very last carbon, which has three hydrogen molecules attached—this is called the omega carbon. In other words, they are "saturated" with hydrogens. Because of this, saturated fatty acids have no double bonds, making them fairly rigid and giving them a higher melting point than unsaturated fats. Saturated fats are ubiquitous in animals and plants, but high dietary amounts come mostly from butter, coconut oil, palm kernel oil and animal fats.

Each fatty acid has a scientific name, although many also have common names, usually related to their most common or first discovered source. In many cases, fatty acids are often simply described by a numerical shorthand designation based on the total number of carbons and by the number and location of each double bond. In the case of the saturated fatty acid in Figure 10, containing 18 carbons and zero double bonds, this would be designated 18:0. The name for this fatty acid is octadecanoic acid, or also commonly known as stearic acid. Figure 10 lists the most common fatty acids and their number designations.

Triglycerides

Most dietary fatty acids are consumed as triglyceride molecules (TG), where three fatty acids (saturated, monounsaturated or polyunsaturated) are bound together along a three-carbon glycerol molecule. Upon digestion, fatty acids are removed from the glycerol backbone to form free fatty acids and monoglycerides, where they can then pass into the enterocytes. This process requires several lipase enzymes and the actions of bile to help the water-soluble enzymes interface with the lipid-soluble fatty acids.

Once in the enterocyte, fatty acids are reassembled into TG molecules and packaged into chylomicrons, lipoprotein complexes that include TG, cholesterol esters, free cholesterol, phospholipids and proteins. These chylomicrons are then released into circulation and are modified by the liver to form VLDL particles.

Unsaturated fatty acids

If saturated fatty acids are defined by having each carbon "saturated" with hydrogen, then unsaturated fatty acids describe those that are missing some hydrogens, allowing for carbon-carbon double bonds instead. Monounsaturated fatty acids are those with only one double bond, while polyunsaturated fatty acids contain more than one. The nomenclature for unsaturated fatty acids is based on the number of carbons and double bonds with one additional feature: a notation to describe where along the fatty acid the first double bond is located—measured from the last or omega carbon (e.g., omega-3 or sometimes n3 or w3). Figure 11 shows a special diagram of four different 18-carbon fatty acids: Stearic acid (18:0), Oleic acid (18:1:w9), Linoleic acid (18:2:w6) and Alpha-Linolenic acid (18:3:w3). Each double bond creates a bend in the molecule, which greatly decreases its melting point and increases its fluidity.

Cis and trans fatty acids

Cis (or trans) refers to the location of hydrogen molecules on either side of a double bond within, in

FATTY ACID PRIMER

STRUCTURES

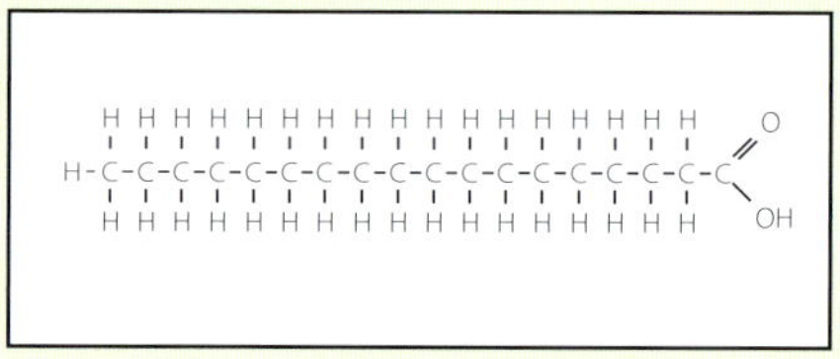

Fatty Acid (18:0)

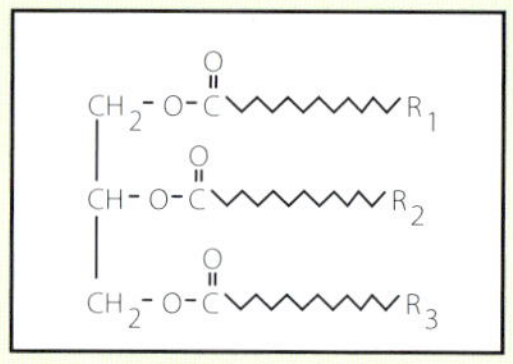

Triglyceride

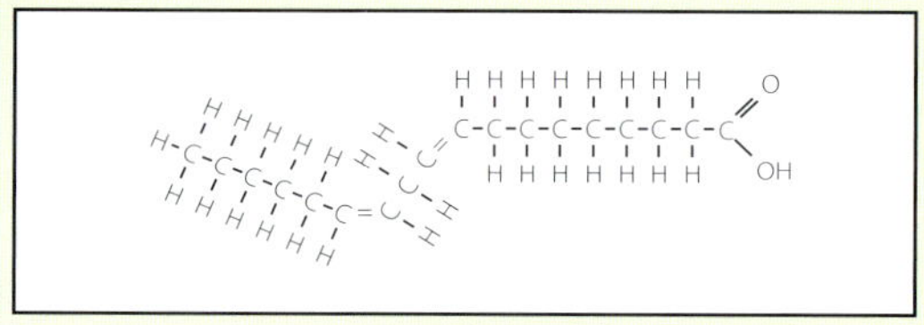

Linoleic Acid

NAMING FATTY ACIDS

Common Name	Shorthand
Oleic	18 : 1 w9
Linoleic	18 : 2 w6

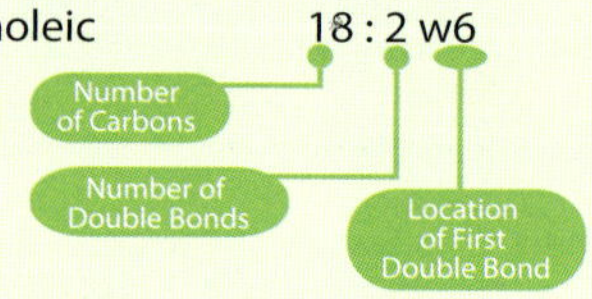

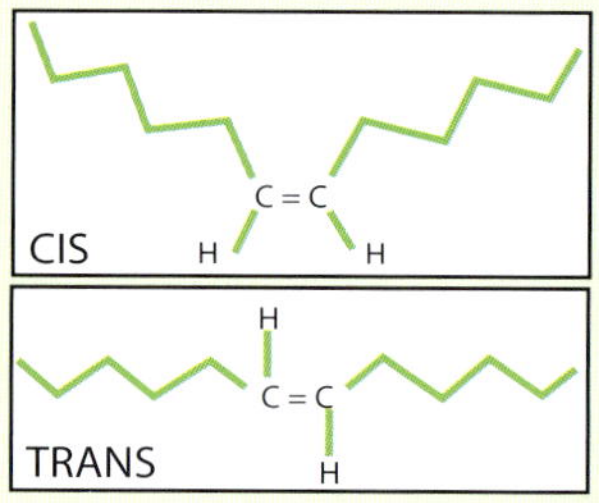

An unsaturated fatty acid double bond is normally in the cis conformation (both hydrogens on the same side). This gives the molecule a bend or kink at each double bond. These bends increase the fluidity or mobility of the fatty acid. When these molecules are heated, exposed to damaging light or oxygen; or partially hydrogenated, trans bonds form. These cause fluid oils to become more rigid (margarine). These new molecules are difficult for the body's enzymes to metabolize. There are significant levels of research looking into the connection between the increased dietary intake of trans-fatty acids and the increased incidence of chronic illnesses.

Saturated Fatty Acids:

Butyric Acid	[4:0]
Caproic Acid	[6:0]
Caprylic Acid	[8:0]
Capric Acid	[10:0]
Lauric Acid	[12:0]
Myristic Acid	[14:0]
Palmitic Acid	[16:0]
Stearic Acid	[18:0]

Monounsaturated Fatty Acids:

Oleic Acid	[18:1w9]

Polyunsaturated Fatty Acids:

Linoleic Acid (LA)	[18:2w6]
Alpha-linolenic acid (LNA)	[18:3w3]
Gamma-linolenic acid (GLA)	[18:3w6]
Arachidonic acid (AA)	[20:4w6]
Eicosapentaenoic acid (EPA)	[20:5w3]
Docosahexaenoic acid (DHA)	[22:6w3]

Typical Fatty Acid Profile of Various Fats & Oils
(% of total fat)

	Saturated			Mono-unsaturated		Polyunsaturated			
	4:0-14:0	16:0	18:0	18:1w9 Oleic	Other MUF A	18:2w6 LA	18:3w3 LNA	20:5w3 EP A	22:6w3 DHA
Butter	22	26	12	25		2.2	1.4		
Milk Fat	23.5	30.6	12.5	26.9		3.1	1		
Chicken Fat	0.9	21.6	6	37.3		19.5	1		
Beef Fat	3.7	24.9	18.9	36		3.1	0.6		
Olive Oil	-	11	2.2	72.5		7.9	0.6		
Corn Oil	-	10.9	1.8	24.2		58	0.7		
Safflower Oil	-	4.3	1.9	74.6		14.4	0		
Canola Oil	-	4	1.8	56.1		20.3	9.3		
Soybean Oil	0.1	10.3	3.8	22.8		51	6.8		
Sesame Oil	-	8.9	4.8	39.3		41.3	0.3		
Sunflower Oil	-	5.4	3.5	45.3		39.8	0.2		
Cottonseed Oil	0.8	22.7	2.3	17		51.5	0.2		
Coconut Oil	58.7	8.2	2.8	5.8		1.8	0		
Palm Oil	1	43.5	4.3	36.6		9.1	0.2		
Fish-Herring	7.3	11.7	1	12	34	1.1	0.7	6.2	4.2
Fish-Salmon	3.3	9.8	4.24	17	12.3	1.5	1	13	18
Walnut Oil	0	7	2	22.2		53	10.4		
Flax Seed Oil	-	5.5	4.5	18		15	55		
E. Primrose Oil	-	-	2	6.4		73.2	9.4*		

* - as gamma linolenic acid (18:3w6) not ALA (18:3w3)

w3 and w6 FATTY ACIDS COMPETE FOR ENZYMES DURING METABOLISM

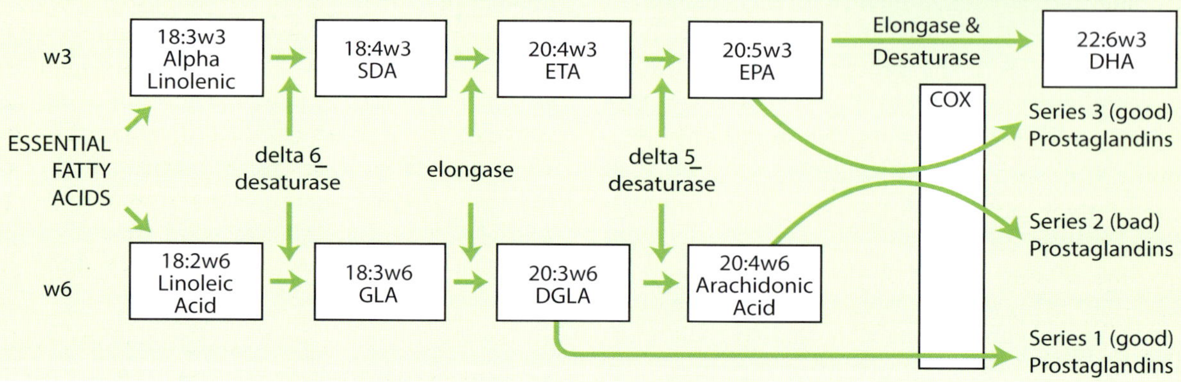

SDA - Stearidonic Acid, ETA - Eicosatetraenoic acid, DGLA - Dihomogammalinolenic Acid, COX - Cyclooxygenase

Figure 10 : Fatty acid structures, nomenclature, common sources and pathways of elongation, desaturation and conversion to prostaglandins. See text for more detail.

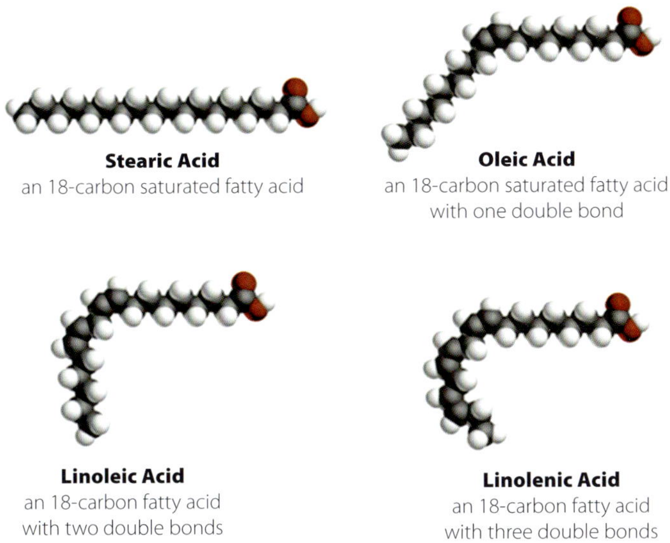

Figure 11 :
Three-dimensional space filling models showing four 18-carbon fatty acids. Notice how the shape of the molecule changes as more cis double bonds are added to the fatty acid.

this case, an unsaturated fatty acid. In nature, when a double bond is created, the hydrogen molecules end up on the same side, forming what is called a cis bond. Like the repelling force of mini-magnets, these hydrogen molecules push away from each other and create the bend in the fatty acid. However, when hydrogen molecules of a polyunsaturated fatty acid are rearranged in a process known as partial hydrogenation (e.g., partially hydrogenated soybean oil), these hydrogen molecules attach opposite of one another, forming a *trans* bond (see Figure 10). These trans-bonded fats no longer bend, creating a fatty acid that acts like a saturated fatty acid while technically remaining a polyunsaturated fatty acid. Decades ago these fats were thought to be a healthy alternative to saturated fats like butter and lard or coconut oil. As it turns out, we now know these unnatural fats are associated with increased risk for numerous disease processes and are being eliminated (in some cases by legal means) from most of the human food supply. One well-known exception to this rule is conjugated linoleic acid (CLA), found mostly in grass-fed meat and dairy, which has both naturally occurring cis and trans double bonds. Supplements containing CLA use fatty acids derived originally from safflower oil converted into "bio-identical" CLA molecules.

<u>Essential fatty acids: omega-3 and omega-6</u>

There are two fatty acids considered essential: linoleic acid (LA, 18:2w6) and alpha-linolenic acid (LNA, 18:3w3). They are essential in that they are absolutely required for human health but cannot be synthesized by humans. In this respect, these two fatty acids can be considered "vitamins." Like all mammals, we are incapable of forming double bonds at either the omega-3 or omega-6 position, although we can synthesize longer and more unsaturated fatty acids once we have consumed these essential fatty acids through our diet.

Over the past 100 years a dramatic change has occurred in our diet, especially in our fatty acid intake. Industrially prepared foods shipped to consumers via supermarkets increased the need to extend "shelf life." Essential fatty acids (EFAs) on the other hand, greatly diminish shelf life because they have a tendency to go rancid, or oxidize, when exposed to heat, light and oxygen. At the same time, large commercial oil manufacturers began producing the refined vegetable oils we are now so familiar with. Currently, four oils—soybean, cottonseed, corn and canola—account for more than 90% of the vegetable oil use in the U.S. The w6:w3 ratio of these combined oils is between 12:1 and 25:1.

An estimate of the w6:w3 ratio in our diet 100 years ago is considered to be between 3:1 and 5:1. The dramatic shift toward w6 oil consumption since that time, coupled with the alteration of these fats via hydrogenation and oxidation, is thought to be one of the leading factors in the rise of chronic illnesses, especially cardiovascular diseases over the past century. Modern agricultural practices also have a dramatic effect on the EFA ratios of animal products. For example, a free-range chicken egg has a w6:w3 ratio of nearly 1:1, while a corn-fed USDA chicken egg has a w6:w3 of 19:1.[1]

The current USRDA recommendations suggest a w6:w3 intake of 11:1. We think this is much too high. Instead, we recommended a minimum of 25 grams/day in men and 20 grams/day women of w6 and w3 fatty acids be consumed in a ratio of less than 5:1. However, most individuals don't count their intake of fats, nor do they have a convenient way to determine the ratio of w6:w3 fat consumption. Therefore, reducing the w6:w3 ratio in the diet is best accomplished by supplementing omega-3-containing oils, while at the same time reducing excess omega-6 intake from the

1. Simopoulos AP, Salem N Jr. n-3 fatty acids in eggs from range-fed Greek chickens. *N Engl J Med* 1989; 321(20):1412.

diet by intentionally avoiding packaged food with corn, sunflower, cottonseed and soybean oils.

Fatty Acid Supplements

Flaxseed oil (or linseed oil): This oil has the highest amount of the essential omega-3 fatty acid alpha-linolenic acid (18:3w3), containing 55% on average. No other edible oil comes close (hemp oil is probably the closest at ~22%). Consumption of flaxseed oil (or ground flaxseeds) would benefit nearly every person, lowering the unhealthy w6:w3 ratio they are likely consuming. Fresh, expeller-pressed flaxseed oil can be added to salad dressings, protein shakes, fruit smoothies, or with just about any non-cooking use of vegetable oil. The taste should be pleasant and slightly nutty, and many people just take a spoonful directly. Flaxseeds and flaxseed oil can be used in some baked goods; the heat is usually not enough to destroy the oil (except in crust). Do not fry using flaxseed oil; this highly unsaturated oil will oxidize quickly. For many people softgel capsules are a convenient and easy way to take flaxseed oil. Most products contain about one gram of oil, delivering about 550 mg of LNA. Regardless of the package instructions, flaxseed oil should be refrigerated after opening to help preserve freshness.

The conversion of LNA (18:3w3) into the long-chain omega-3 fatty acids (e.g., EPA 20:5w3 and especially DHA 22:6w3) is inefficient in many individuals, especially those consuming high amounts of omega-6 fatty acids. Therefore, individuals desiring elevated levels of EPA and DHA should be directed to consume EPA and DHA directly from fish or fish oil supplements. It is equally true, however, that consumption of EPA and DHA will not compensate for low dietary levels of LNA and should not be considered a replacement for dietary or supplemental sources.

Other sources of supplemental LNA include hemp oil (w6:w3 ratio of 2:1) and walnut oil (w6:w3 ratio of 5:1), along with diets generally high in green vegetables, nuts and seeds.

Fish oil (marine-derived omega-3): The research on marine-derived omega-3 fatty acids, mostly EPA and DHA, from fish and fish oil supplements is extensive and will not be reviewed here. Needless to say, the use of fish oil or related supplements has become commonplace in most healthcare settings worldwide. Here in the U.S., a wide range of EPA and DHA products are available from a variety of fish and non-fish (krill, squid, algae, mussels) sources; there are even several products currently available as prescription drugs.

For the clinician, choosing or recommending the appropriate EPA and DHA supplement for a patient's therapeutic need is important. Clinicians are often concerned about bioavailability; toxins; dosing; the use of EPA, DHA or a combination; sustainability issues; and the potential for allergic reactions. The appendix contains a complete monograph addressing most of these issues:

- Choosing the Best Marine-derived Omega-3 Products for Therapeutic Use: An Evaluation of the Evidence [Page 175]

Our current recommendation for therapeutic EPA and DHA is to use concentrated reesterified triglyceride (rTG) versions of fish oil, and to have a range of products available that differ in their EPA and DHA content. A summary of our current recommendations for using EPA, DHA or a combination are shown in the Table 4.

Olive oil (omega-9): In the debate over appropriate dietary w6:w3 ratios and the overall advice on fatty acids, one fatty acid often gets left out: oleic acid. This 18:1w9 fatty acid makes up over 70% of the content of olive oil and is a likely to be one of the critical "signals" contributing to the healthy success of the MedDiet. The best way to encourage olive oil consumption is simply through dietary advice: "consume more olive oil." Olive oil-based salad dressing should be used in place of other vegetable oils; olive oil should be the oil of choice for lightly sautéing, rather than canola or other vegetable oils, and can replace butter when consuming bread. One of the easiest ways to help patients consume more oleic acid is to get them to adopt a Mediterranean dietary pattern, as most cookbooks focused on the MedDiet emphasize the use of olive oil.

When it comes to olive oil quality, and cost, there can be significant differences. Extra-virgin olive oil, which is slightly green and has a smooth, pleasant aroma and taste, contains more healthful qualities than olive oils that are clear and slightly bitter. Patients should be advised to invest a little more to purchase higher quality olive oil, one that is protected from light with a dark bottle or can.

We are often asked, "Do you recommend the use of omega-9 supplements?" There are products available to consumers that claim to provide omega-3, omega-6 (usually GLA, see below) and omega-9 in an "ideal" ratio. Unfortunately these products provide low doses of fatty acids that need to be consumed in gram levels and do so at a high cost. Since oleic acid is the only omega-9 used in any supplement—from olive, borage or other oils—the best way to consume this is by simply increasing the daily consumption of olive oil.

Supplementing Omega-6s

Since individuals consuming a mostly Western diet are rarely deficient in omega-6 fatty acid consumption, supplementing these fats seems contradictory. However, one particular w6 fatty acid has garnered most of the attention: gamma-linolenic acid, or GLA. Like alpha-linolenic acid, GLA is an 18:3 fatty acid, but its first double bond is after the sixth carbon, hence it is 18:3w6. This structure gives it slightly different biological functions than the closely related essential fatty acids LNA and LA. In particular, GLA is a substrate for elongation to produce the fatty acid dihomogammalinolenic acid (DGLA, 20:3w6), which can act as a precursor to anti-inflammatory prostaglandins [see Figure 10].[2] Since conversion of LA (18:2w6) to GLA is considered to be limited in many individuals, direct consumption of GLA is considered helpful in many subjects.[3] The two oils usually associated with GLA supplementation are evening primrose oil (EPO) and borage oil, although black current seed oil also contains a high amount of GLA.

Evening primrose oil is extracted from the seeds of the evening primrose plant *(Oenothera biennis L.)*, a yellow flowering plant found throughout North America. The oil is one of the highest in omega-6 fatty acids, with over 70% LA and between 9 – 11% gamma-linolenic acid. Most of the initial research looking into the biological effects of GLA was done using evening primrose oil. While the published therapeutic outcomes of evening primrose are limited, the popular view is that its GLA content drives much of the therapeutic effect. On the other hand, borage oil (*Borago officinalis L.*, 24% GLA) and black current seed oil (*Ribes nigrum L.*, 18% GLA) have not gained the popularity of evening primrose oil, although they contain more GLA content. Overall, the review of published data using GLA-containing oils for atopic and rheumatic conditions has been disappointing. The use of evening primrose oil for female-specific concerns—mastalgia, menopausal or premenstrual symptoms—shows a bit more promise, but it is rarely used as a monotherapy for these concerns.

GLA-containing oils should not be considered as daily supplements for most individuals. Limited data suggests they may be helpful in some individuals with rheumatic or atopic conditions, but since other agents are likely to perform better for such conditions, we generally advise against this use. Evening primrose oil for use in women has a long tradition and slightly more favorable outcomes in clinical trials. Clinicians should consider the use of evening primrose when their clinical judgment suggests it may be favorable.

Condition	EPA-Rich	EPA/DHA	DHA-Rich
General Health		★★	
Improving w3:w6 ratio		★★	
Low-Risk CVD prevention		★★	★
High CVD Risk/Atherosclerosis		★	★★
Inflammatory Diseases		★★	
Depression	★★	★	
Macular Degeneration			★★
Alzheimer—Dementia		★	★★
Maternal—Childhood Development		★	★★

Table 4 : Condition-specific recommendations for EPA and DHA use. General recommendations for the differential uses of EPA and DHA. An "★★" recommendation is used when clinical trial and/or mechanistic data suggest better outcomes using a product rich (although not exclusively) in EPA or DHA. The data used to make these suggestions can be found in a whitepaper on our website http://www.pointinstitute.org/white-papers/.

2. Kapoor R, Huang YS. Gamma-linolenic acid: an anti-inflammatory omega-6 fatty acid. *Curr Pharm Biotechnol.* 2006 Dec; 7(6):531-4.

3. Das UN A defect in the activity of Delta6 and Delta5 desaturases may be a factor in the initiation and progression of atherosclerosis. *Prostaglandins Leukot Essent Fatty Acids.* 2007 May; 76(5):251-68.

Macronutrients: Water

Water is one of the quintessential nutrients of life and yet is often one of the most commonly neglected. Despite its great importance for nearly every bodily function, many clinicians and patients are still at a loss when it comes to knowing how much to drink each day and, furthermore, which beverages count towards our daily needs. All this confusion about water needs comes as no surprise considering the first official recommendation for adequate intake (AI) of water was only established in 2004 by the Institute of Medicine, which coincided with an increase in popular awareness about water needs for preventing diseases, such as cancer and heart disease, and for promoting weight loss. Prior to that, the USRDA concluded it was impossible to set a recommendation for water needs and the National Research Council used a general rule of thumb of one ml/kcal (two liters of water per 2,000 calories consumed).

Today's recommendations for daily water requirements are based on average water consumption as defined by NHANES III data. The Institute of Medicine says adequate intake of total water per day is 3.7 liters for men and 2.7 liters for women. The "Eight by Eight rule" (eight glasses of eight oz. each) equates to about two liters. It is important to note these adequate intake recommendations are for *total water in temperate climates*. All sources (according to IOM) can contribute to total water needs: beverages including tea, coffee, juices, sodas and drinking water, and moisture found in foods, which likely accounts for about 20% of total water intake.

Throughout history humans have relied on water as their primary source of hydration, struggling to ensure an abundant and clean source was available for their survival. This struggle still exists in many locations around the world today. In the West, water abundance, at least for drinking, is rarely in jeopardy, and yet many choose other options. Countless individuals have replaced water with soft drinks to attempt to quench their thirst and, as a result, sweetened beverages have become one of the major sources of calories in the American diet. To make matters worse, the calories provided by soft drinks often fail to satisfy hunger the way solid food does, nor do they quench our thirst in the way water can, making sugary beverages a key player in the obesity epidemic. Patients should be encouraged to limit the number of calories they consume through beverages.

- Recommend patients drink mostly water to keep hydrated.
- Ensure they have a water source that is clean and free of contaminants.
- Tea and coffee are generally fine for most people in moderation. The diuretic properties of caffeine-containing drinks appear to be less substantiated than popularly thought.[1]
- Alcohol is dehydrating and should not be counted as a hydrating liquid.
- Water-based soups and stews, herbal teas and low-sugar fruit juices are excellent sources.
- Hydrate more frequently when physically active and when the weather turns hotter.

1. Maughan RJ, Griffin J. Caffeine ingestion and fluid balance: a review. *J Hum Nutr Diet.* 2003 Dec; 16(6):411-20.

Supplementing Micronutrients

The majority of products used for nutrient supplementation are primarily designed to deliver micronutrients. In fact, more than 40% of dietary supplement sales are products described as vitamin or mineral supplements, or a combination of both. The reasons individuals use such supplements, or clinicians recommend them, are wide ranging: from filling in nutrient gaps in individuals with mostly healthy diets, as insurance for those whose diets are far from healthy, or as therapeutic agents designed to trigger specific metabolic functions. Likewise, the products and doses available in this category are wide ranging: from single nutrient supplements dosed at 1,000% of the DV, to comprehensive multi-nutrient products with more than 50 ingredients.

While we will not review the detailed function of each nutrient, nor the clinical data available for each, this section will cover some of the most frequent issues clinicians face in selecting and recommending micronutrient supplements for their patients. Once we cover these pertinent issues, we will list each of the major vitamin, mineral and nutrient ingredients, covering relevant details unique to each.

Micronutrient Supplementation in "Healthy" Subjects: An Overview

Before we discuss the nuances of supplement ingredients, forms and doses, we want to address one of the basic questions, and criticisms, of nutrient supplementation in "healthy" populations: Do so-called "healthy" subjects really need micronutrient supplementation? After all, every few months or so news reports recount a "failed" nutrient study followed by a medical journal editorial repeating the mantra that vitamin and mineral supplements are a "waste of money." Are these criticisms fair?

In evaluating this issue, recall the discussion in the first section of this Road map, where a distinction was made between determining the amount of a nutrient a person consumes, usually through dietary estimations; compared to ascertaining an individual's "adequate" or "optimal" requirement for that nutrient based on the person's particular health need: weight, health status, genetic predisposition, or a host of other factors that may create an increased need for one or more nutrients. Most research is simply based on epidemiological estimates of population intakes, which then gives rise to estimated adequate requirements (EAR) and daily reference intakes (DRI). However, even using these limited estimates, the number of Americans not meeting the intake guidelines of important nutrients is alarming.

Further complicating matters is that while many nutrients are found in low levels in foods, many methods of food preparation diminish those naturally occurring nutrients. Recognizing this, many processed foods have nutrients added back (enriched)—in some cases, higher than natural amounts added (fortified) before distribution. The NHANES (National Health and Nutrition Examination Survey) data attempts to calculate nutrient intake from food, whether naturally occurring, fortified or enriched, as well as from dietary supplementation, when estimating the level of nutrient intake in the U.S. population. According to these data, the number of Americans over the age of two not consuming guideline levels of vitamin D, calcium, vitamin A, vitamin C, vitamin E, thiamin, folate and magnesium from natural sources is more than 40%—that's well over 100 million Americans.[1] Even after including fortification and supplementation, this is still the case for vitamin D, vitamin E and magnesium (see nutrient monographs for details on each nutrient). Considering that these data assume that the guideline EAR levels are "adequate" for only 50% of individuals, these numbers are even more problematic.

1. Fulgoni VL 3rd, Keast DR, Bailey RL, Dwyer J. Foods, fortificants, and supplements: Where do Americans get their nutrients? *J Nutr.* 2011 Oct;141(10):1847-54.

In view of the overwhelming safety of micronutrient supplementation (exceptions discussed for some below) and the inadequate intake of basic guideline levels of certain nutrients among a large population of Americans, routine supplementation of most patients is clinically justified. Since most micronutrients are critical to the basic activities that allow cells to function and build the metabolic reserve needed to delay or prevent chronic diseases in the first place, micronutrient supplementation can be a vital foundation for a variety of therapeutic interventions in today's clinical practice, if for no other reason than to increase the likelihood a patient is consuming the minimum guideline amounts of most nutrients. It should be noted, however, that broad, non-specific nutrient supplementation alone in individuals without known deficiencies in a particular nutrient is unlikely to result in measurable disease-related clinical outcomes.

This does not mean there are not studies that show clinical benefits for specific vitamins or minerals, but there are varying opinions as to which studies should be used to determine micronutrient efficacy. In some cases, like the Physician's Health Study-2, the same one-a-day multivitamin that showed a small, but statistical reduction in the risk for cancer and cataracts[2,3] showed no benefit for other outcomes like cognitive performance.[4] In either case, there were many other variables that might account for these outcomes, not the least of which is the fact that the multivitamin supplement used in this study was not specifically designed for any of these outcomes and none of the subjects were known to have vitamin or mineral deficiencies.

Generally speaking, the types of studies and end-points used to evaluate the efficacy of pharmaceutical agents, for FDA approval, with regard to disease management are inappropriate and unsuitable to test the relative benefit of "optimal" nutrient supplementation. Drug trials can be managed to ensure subjects in the control group have never consumed the pharmaceutical agent being tested, something untrue and even unethical in nutrient studies. The clinical goal of multivitamin-mineral supplementation, therefore, is not to reduce the risk of a particular outcome but to diminish the likelihood the patient will have limited metabolic capacity due to inadequate availability of a necessary nutrient.

Overall, nearly half of the U.S. population consumes vitamin and mineral supplements on a regular or semi-regular basis. Even the Physicians Health Study showed long-term use of supplements amongst this cohort (male physicians) was 36%, and healthcare professionals interested in, or knowledgeable about, dietary supplements were much more likely to use and recommend dietary supplements.[5]

Multivitamins: A wide range in available doses

Comparing one multivitamin-mineral product with another is often a daunting and confusing task, even for those well-versed in nutrient supplementation. For the most part, the greatest difference in these products is the number of total ingredients, the dose of each ingredient and, in many cases, the form of those ingredients. Most one-a-day multivitamins are designed to provide 100% of the DV of as many ingredients that will fit in one tablet or capsule. This turns out to be feasible for nearly all vitamins, but is impossible when attempting to supplement key minerals like calcium and magnesium. When these products do add minerals, they are almost always in cheap forms that are inferior for absorption (oxides, carbonates, etc.).

On the other hand, a number of products designed for physician use are available; these products typically include higher doses of most vitamins, higher doses and quality of minerals, as well as additional nutrients with no official DVs. Compared to the one-a-day approach, these additional ingredients are delivered in higher numbers of capsules—three, six, eight or sometimes more. Clinicians should realize that while some patients may benefit from adhering to the full dose, six-plus capsules per day, of certain multivitamin-mineral supplements, many patients would be adequately served by using half the dose, which, in many cases, still provides most nutrients above the DV/DRI.

2. Gaziano JM, et al. Multivitamins in the prevention of cancer in men: the Physicians' Health Study II randomized controlled trial. *JAMA.* 2012 Nov 14;308(18):1871-80.

3. Christen WG, et al. A Multivitamin Supplement and Cataract and Age-Related Macular Degeneration in a Randomized Trial of Male Physicians. *Ophthalmology.* 2013 Nov 20.[Epub ahead of print].

4. Grodstein F, et al. Long-Term Multivitamin Supplementation and Cognitive Function in Men: A Randomized Trial *Ann Intern Med.* 2013;159(12):806-814-814.

5. Gardiner P, Woods C, Kemper KJ. Dietary supplement use among health care professionals enrolled in an online curriculum on herbs and dietary supplements. *BMC Complement Altern Med.* 2006 Jun 12;6:21.

Generally, nutrient supplements should be taken with meals

Usually we recommend taking micronutrient supplements with meals whenever possible. We do so for three basic reasons. First, when eating a meal, the body naturally begins producing the necessary agents—acid, intrinsic factor, enzymes, bile, etc.—to digest and absorb macro and micronutrients. These agents are designed to deal with both fat-soluble and water-soluble nutrients within the matrix of a complex food environment. Second, many people report GI complaints when consuming high-dosed multivitamins apart from a meal, something usually solved by taking them with a meal. Third, since adherence to a multivitamin regimen is often related to forgetfulness and fear of GI side effects, adherence is often better when patients are initially told to use their nutrient supplements with meals.

Since the main purpose of micronutrient supplementation is long-term nutrient sufficiency, the answer here may not be applicable for very specific nutrient use in every patient, but should be helpful for the vast number of patients using multivitamin-mineral products. While it is true that certain foods or nutrient combinations can actually reduce the full benefit of some supplemental nutrients, usually by inhibiting absorption, long-term benefits of improved adherence with a simple recommendation may still have better long-term benefits than creating a schedule that attempts to optimize the absorption of each nutrient. [This advice may not apply to specific non-nutrient dietary supplements such as herbal extracts, concentrated phytonutrients or enzymes].

Supplemental nutrient needs for men and women

The guideline recommendations for daily intake of certain nutrients are slightly different for men and women (see DRI tables in the appendix). These recommendations are not generally based on scientific analysis of gender-based nutrient needs; they are based on estimated intakes and, in some cases, historical body weight differences between men and women (see specifics for prenatal needs below). Since there is no other evidence that men and non-pregnant women have substantially different *basic* nutrient needs, there is no scientific justification for products designed specifically for men or women. Some professional companies provide their multivitamin-mineral formulas with or without iron, allowing clinicians to use iron-free supplements for most men and post-menopausal women, while providing multivitamin-mineral supplements with iron for menstruating, pregnant and nursing women, vegetarians or those known to have low iron levels.

Still, there are many commercially available nutrient supplements marketed specifically for men or women. Many companies choose to add additional ingredients to their nutrient supplement formulas intended for gender-targeted marketing. Ingredients for prostate health are popular in products marketed to men, while ingredients designed to boost bone health or promote hormone balance are popular in products marketed to women. These ingredients, however, are rarely provided in doses needed to match therapeutic potential and, in some cases, include botanical agents that may increase the likelihood of allergic responses. While generally harmless, problems arise when patients believe these low-dosed additional ingredients neutralize their risk for gender-specific diseases, something not supported by clinical research.

Nutrient needs for pregnant and lactating women

While the guideline recommendations for nutrient intake is only slightly different in pregnant and lactating women, clinical urgency and patient awareness of micronutrient supplementation in these subjects is much greater. NHANES data from 1999 – 2006 suggest about 75% of pregnant women in the U.S. report taking nutrient supplements, mostly multivitamins with extra folic acid and iron.[6] One note of concern among these data is that supplement use increases with each trimester, from a low of about 55% in the first trimester to a high of nearly 90% in the third trimester. This pattern of supplement use resulted in the lowest folate status (RBC levels) in the first trimester of pregnancy, when the need for folate is most critical for the prevention of neural tube defects. As you might imagine, clinical research on pregnant subjects is limited in developed countries and most of the information available is based on observational data.[7]

6. Branum AM, Bailey R, Singer BJ. Dietary supplement use and folate status during pregnancy in the United States. *J Nutr*. 2013 Apr;143(4):486-92.

7. Sfakianaki AK. Prenatal vitamins- A review of the literature on benefits and risks of various nutrient supplements. *Formulary*. January 1, 2013.

In light of specific nutrient needs for pregnant women, many clinicians and institutions recommend nutrient supplementation for pregnant woman, usually in the form of a prenatal multivitamin.[8] Some products are designed to provide only limited prenatal needs, such as increased iron, folic acid, and B-vitamins; others attempt to provide a full multivitamin-mineral approach. In some cases, products will provide additional ingredients, such as DHA and choline for healthy brain development, or even herbs like ginger to help with nausea.

Clinicians should have a readily available recommendation for a prenatal vitamin/mineral supplement because the desire to find a product is usually an urgent concern for the patient. An iron-containing multivitamin-mineral product from a professional brand is likely to be adequate, though products designed specifically as prenatal supplements may have additional benefits for patients.

The nutrient needs of lactating women are similar to those of pregnant women, though the guidelines make a few distinctions. Vitamin A recommendations are nearly double for lactating women, as vitamin A stores are low in newborns, and the recommendation for vitamin C is nearly 50% higher at 120 mg.[9] Other small differences in nutrient needs reflect the higher calorie intake generally required for lactating/breastfeeding women.

Nutrient needs for children and adolescents

Once again, the guideline nutrient recommendations for children and adolescents (in the U.S.) are determined by estimates of intake and age. In some cases, rapid growth in adolescents accounts for a higher recommendation than in adulthood. For instance, the RDA for calcium is highest (1,300 mg) for adolescent boys and girls (nine –18 years old), lowest (1,000 mg) at maturity, and then increases (to 1,200 mg) after age 50 in women and 70 in men.

The specific nutrient recommendations for infants are much less certain, and are listed as adequate intakes (AIs), rather than RDAs. Infant nutrient needs and supplementation are also tied to other factors, such as whether the child is consuming formula or breast milk, and if breast milk, the nutritional status of the mother. In general, nutrient supplementation is not recommended for healthy infants, with the exception of vitamin D. According to the American Academy of Pediatrics, exclusively breastfed infants or babies drinking less than one liter of baby formula should receive 400 IU of vitamin D each day. Liquid products (typically in dropper bottles) are designed specifically for delivering this dose to children. Other micronutrients, probiotics or fatty acid supplements (e.g., DHA) are often recommended for infants and children, and can be found packaged and dosed specifically for these subjects.

Even though foods marketed to children are often fortified, NHANES data show American children between the ages of 2 –18 are consuming less than the EAR for vitamin D (73%), vitamin E (66%), magnesium (48%), vitamin A (25%) and vitamin C (28%).[1]

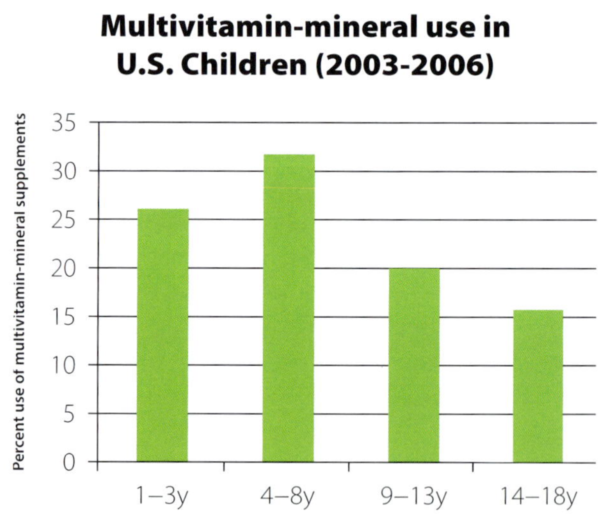

Figure 12 : Multivitamin use in children and adolescents (2003-2006).

Use of multivitamin-mineral supplements in U.S. children and adolescents ranges from 16 – 32%.[10] As Figure 12 shows, nutrient supplementation is highest in those four to eight years old, and lowest in the late teenage years. Since nutrient intake from foods is also lower in adolescents (nine – 18 years old), these individuals are known to have a higher prevalence of inadequate nutrient intake. While supplementation

8. Some, like the American College of Obstetrics and Gynecology, recommend supplementation for only iron and folic acid-believing the diet will suffice for the rest. See their FAQ: www.acog.org/~/media/For%20Patients/faq001.pdf .

9. Haskell MJ, Brown KH. Maternal vitamin A nutriture and the vitamin A content of human milk. *J Mammary Gland Biol Neoplasia*. 1999 Jul;4(3):243-57.

10. Bailey RL, Gahche JJ et al. Dietary supplement use in the United States, 2003-2006. *J Nutr*. 2011 Feb;141(2):261-6.

does not alleviate all inadequate nutrient intakes in children older than eight years, especially for calcium and vitamin D, dietary supplements added micronutrients to diets that would have otherwise been inadequate for magnesium, phosphorus, and vitamins A, C and E.[11] We believe these data are sufficient to recommend routine multivitamin-mineral supplementation in children over two years old, and especially in children ages nine to 18.

Popular children's multivitamins usually lack adequate levels of quality minerals and often have excessive zinc and copper; the most common nutrients consumed above the tolerable upper limit in children using supplements. Look for products that use natural sweeteners such as polyol sugars, sucrose, etc., and avoid artificial sweeteners, colors and flavorings.

Special needs for vegetarians and vegans

While there is much to commend in an appropriate vegetarian or vegan diet, there are also a few nutrient deficiencies more common in individuals who choose this lifestyle, recognizing that not all diets that exclude animal products are of equal nutrient content. The most commonly cited nutrient deficiencies are vitamin B_{12}, vitamin D, long-chain omega-3 fatty acids, calcium, iron, zinc, carnitine and protein.[12,13]

Vitamin B_{12} deficiency is probably the most studied of these deficiencies, where researchers have shown vegetarians to have elevated levels of plasma homocysteine (tied to low B_{12}) and related arterial dysfunction which can be mitigated by supplementing vitamin B_{12}.[14,15] These common deficiencies, along with the wide range of diets deemed "vegetarian," should compel clinicians to ask specific dietary questions (see questionnaires in the appendix) to determine nutrient supplementation needs in these individuals. Most multivitamin-mineral products are appropriate for vegetarian subjects, though some vegans may object to fish-derived omega-3 fatty acids or vitamin D_3 (see Vitamin D monograph).

11. Bailey RL, Fulgoni VL 3rd, Keast DR, Lentino CV, Dwyer JT. Do dietary supplements improve micronutrient sufficiency in children and adolescents? *J Pediatr.* 2012 Nov;161(5):837-42.

12. Craig WJ, Mangels AR. Position of the American Dietetic Association: vegetarian diets. *J Am Diet Assoc.* 2009 Jul;109(7):1266-82.

13. Craig WJ. Nutrition concerns and health effects of vegetarian diets. *Nutr Clin Pract.* 2010 Dec;25(6):613-20.

14. Kwok T, Chook P et al. Vitamin B-12 supplementation improves arterial function in vegetarians with subnormal vitamin B-12 status. *J Nutr Health Aging.* 2012;16(6):569-73.

15. Obersby D, Chappell DC, Dunnett A, Tsiami AA. Plasma total homocysteine status of vegetarians compared with omnivores: a systematic review and meta-analysis. *Br J Nutr.* 2013 Mar 14;109(5):785-94.

Food and Supplement Forms of Nutrients: How do they Differ?

Here we'll discuss a few issues that can be contentious within the world of marketing vitamins and minerals: the relative differences and benefits between various forms of vitamins, minerals or other nutrients (for a complete discussion of marine-derived omega-3 fatty acids, see the complete discussion on page 175). As it turns out, almost every vitamin or mineral we will list below can be delivered in different chemical forms. In some cases this might mean different isomers of the same molecule (d vs. d-l tocopherol), a modified form of a molecule (pyridoxal-5-phosphate vs. pyridoxine HCl) or different mineral forms (calcium carbonate vs. calcium citrate). In some cases, attempts to define nutrients based upon their supposed origins: "whole-food," "natural concentrate," "active-form" or "synthetic" create an additional level of differentiation.

Unfortunately, the terms "natural," "whole-food," "synthetic" and "active-forms" have different meanings to different people, and for the most part, are often used to mislead consumers about nutritional supplements. Here, we will provide clear definitions of each of these concepts, revealing the real potential differences between some nutrient forms, while showing most marketing information about these differences is unsubstantiated and, in some cases, false.

Synthetic vs. natural vitamins

Few terms are more loaded with implied meaning in the supplement world as the terms "natural" and "synthetic." The former is nearly always viewed as being better than the latter. Many supplement users would be surprised to learn that nearly all vitamins and minerals used for making dietary supplement products—and for food fortification—are not strictly "natural." This means the nutrient ingredient, as it is used in the capsule or tablet, has been changed in some way from the form found in nature, or is a bioequivalent (or chemically identical) molecule derived by organic synthesis. An example of this is ascorbic acid, the most common source of vitamin C in dietary supplements.

Vitamin C compounds, natural ascorbates, are found in a variety of fruits and vegetables and are fairly stable when the food source maintains its integrity. Ascorbic acid, on the other hand, is made from corn-derived sugars via a multistep process. While natural ascorbate compounds found in foods are often believed to be associated with other compounds, most notably bioflavonoids, there is no evidence that ascorbates/vitamin C from food and ascorbic acid are different chemically or biologically (see vitamin C monograph for details and references). Like the bioidentical "human" hormones derived "synthetically" from wild yam or soy compounds, there are many organically synthesized vitamins that function in a bioidentical or "bioequivalent" manner compared to their "natural" counterpart (some call these nature-identical). This is not to say that 60 mg of ascorbic acid will have all the biological effects of 60 mg of vitamin C from an orange, but any difference there may be (studies looking for such differences have not found any) would likely be due to the other, non-vitamin C ingredients in the orange. In the case of these "bioequivalent" vitamins or previtamins (see below), there is no known clinical difference between these compounds and their natural counterparts, except that the organically synthesized versions allow for higher doses at reasonable prices.

On the other hand, not all "synthetic" vitamins are bioidentical equivalents of their "natural" counterpart and are, in many cases, inferior biological alternatives. The best example of this is "synthetic" vitamin E, a blend of eight closely related isomers, only one of which is identical to natural d-alpha-tocopherol. The chemical differences are subtle but result in measurable differences in nutrient benefits (see vitamin E monograph). Similar diminished benefits might also be true of folic acid, synthetic beta-carotene, the retinyl form of vitamin A, vitamin D_2 and vitamin K_1, each discussed in their respective monograph.

Describing a vitamin within a dietary supplement product either as "natural" or "synthetic" needs to be considered on a case-by-case basis. While marketers of so-called "whole-food" or "natural" multivitamins will routinely vilify all "synthetic" vitamins as harmful, the evidence to support these claims is lacking. We are aware that industrial chemicals are often used in the processing of these vitamins, though these substances are not present in the finished vitamin ingredient added to foods or supplements (there are monograph standards that set limits for these). Moreover, nearly every research study on almost every vitamin, whether chemistry, basic science, cell culture, animal or human clinical trials, has been performed using these "synthetic" vitamins. For better or worse, the evidence-based knowledge of the dose, bioavailability, pharmacokinetics, deficiencies, toxicities, metabolites and supplementation has all been documented in reference to these nutrients, in these forms. While many of us may not consider most of these substances to be strictly "natural," there is no evidence to suggest our body's biochemistry would see these compounds, those that are truly "bioequivalent," as anything but.

Food or Supplements: Which is better?

Some who read this section may be confused about whether we are advocating the use of supplements in place of food nutrients, and how this fits in with the Lifestyle Synergy model we discussed in earlier sections of this Road map. Let us be clear: our bodies are designed with the necessary processes (digestion, absorption, enzymes, etc.) to extract from foods the essential nutrients our bodies need to function properly. For many individuals, the amount of food-derived nutrients obtained is below their functional nutrient needs due to poor dietary habits, poor food quality, insufficient digestion, nutrigenetics or a higher need for particular nutrients than a healthy diet can provide. In these cases, we advocate what we call augmented lifestyle therapy, where we rely on known signals, in this case nutrient signals, that can be isolated and provided in higher doses within the context of the original signal—another reason to take supplements with food.

Scores of research studies over a half-century or more have shown augmentation through the supplementation of isolated nutrients, or combinations of isolated nutrients through fortification and dietary supplements, has been remarkably helpful to human health in developed countries, even if only to compensate for decreased nutrient density from our agricultural practices and industrialized food supply, and has been instrumental for helping to alleviate nutritional deficiencies and save the lives of millions throughout the underdeveloped world. Clinicians are responsible for choosing the best therapeutic options for their patients using all available evidence. This means helping them choose and implement the optimal dietary pattern for their current and future health needs, and to help them determine the most appropriate supplemental ingredients, if needed, to target specific nutrient deficiencies or as a basis of a therapeutic intervention.

Provitamins and activated forms

We now need to take this one step further to understand how our body converts vitamins into vital nutrients. For the most part, vitamins consumed in foods and supplements are compounds the body turns into their final bioactive vitamin compound. Therefore, most vitamins are really what we might call previtamins or, as they are often referred to, vitamin precursors, vitamers or provitamins. Most people know that beta-carotene, and a few other carotenoids, are converted into vitamin A and are often referred to as previtamin A. Most others are less well known, like the vitamin riboflavin (or B_2), a precursor to two critical metabolic coenzymes, flavin mononucleotide (FMN) and flavin adenine dinucleotide (FAD); or niacin being converted to the coenzyme nicotinamide adenine dinucleotide (NAD and NADH). These and many more will be discussed in the monograph for each vitamin.

Establishing that many vitamins are converted from a previtamin form before use at the cellular level, researchers and manufacturers of vitamins have experimented with modified forms of several vitamins in an attempt to deliver vitamins in a readily usable or "activated" form. The most popular of these are niacinamide, methylated folate, phosphorylated riboflavin and B_6, and, for minerals, amino acid chelates. These ingredients are an attempt to mimic natural forms (mineral chelates) or an activated intermediate of the vitamin. In most cases, while some would deem these compounds "natural," they are almost universally synthesized from other so-called "synthetic" vitamins. For instance, pyridoxal-5-phosphate is derived from pyridoxine HCl, a common previtamin.

Are these so-called activated forms better than other food or supplement forms of vitamins? It depends on which one. A case can be made that a small, but consistent, benefit can be derived from the use of methylated folate, instead of folic acid, in subjects with genetic polymorphisms that reduce folate methylation, though this benefit is often exaggerated well beyond the published literature. However, phosphorylated B_6 and riboflavin must necessarily be dephosphorylated in the gut before entering circulation, making these products equivalent, except for added cost, to their non-phosphorylated versions. In the case of mineral chelates, intended to mimic the plant-based delivery of minerals, they often improve bioavailability over more commonly used mineral salts.

With few exceptions, "activated" vitamins as supplement ingredients add much confusion with little clinical benefit. More importantly, all vitamins function in the body by a constant conversion between various active and inactive forms. In many cases, active vitamins are converted to their inactive forms by specific enzymes in order to be transported from one part of the body to another. Inactivating the vitamin prevents it from reacting prior to reaching the target tissue. Even in the case of methylated folate, the amount of stored body folate that needs to be continually remethylated could never be overcome by oral methylfolate supplementation alone. We will make the case for or against the various activated forms within each vitamin monograph based on available biochemical, pharmacokinetic, animal and human study data.

"Whole-food" supplements: What are they?

Let us take this one step further as we discuss what are often referred to as "whole-food" nutrient supplements. This unofficial term can mean a few different things, depending on how the product is designed. It can describe a product (capsule, tablet or powder) made of dried powders of various foods, mostly fruits and vegetables. For instance, many products generally referred to as "green drinks" are made from a variety of grasses, dried fruit and vegetable powders, and added-phytonutrient/herbal powders. These types of products are often organic or mostly organic and promote themselves as ways of helping consumers receive the types of phytonutrients they may be missing from an abundant and diverse diet. Unless they are fortified, however, these products rarely provide minimal RDA levels of vitamins and minerals. So while these products may be excellent sources of key phytonutrients, something that may prove to be a clinical benefit to individuals with little diversity or under-consumption of fruits and vegetables, they may not be a substitute for the increased vitamin and mineral supplementation some patients need.

The largest group of products sold under the rubric of "whole-food" supplements are quite different and, in many cases, highly problematic. These are products that claim to deliver adequate levels of supplemental vitamins and minerals in capsules or tablets, which they claim are derived from whole-food sources. There are two basic problems with these products. One: They are almost never derived from what most people would consider a "whole food." Two: Those with any substantial level of vitamin or mineral claims have been "spiked" with the "synthetic" and concentrated forms of the vitamins they market their products against.

While there is some debate about whether truly whole-food supplements offer *clinical* benefits, there are three types of widely available products inappropriately, and fraudulently in some cases, marketed as "whole-food" supplements. They are: products whose ingredients are plainly not natural or whole-food derived; products that contain vitamins and minerals from unmodified natural sources that are not strictly foods or "whole" parts of those "foods"; and products whose "food" ingredients are intentionally spiked with synthetic vitamins and minerals prior to preparing the ingredients. We will explain each below.

1. Products sold as "whole-food," which clearly are not:

As we have seen in the sections above, and will detail for each vitamin in the next sections, spotting a vitamin or provitamin source is fairly easy. However, some manufacturers and marketers simply do not know the difference or, believing the public won't know the difference, sell "synthetic" ingredients as if they were whole-food or naturally derived. In many cases, they use alternative names or slightly unique forms to disguise this fact. For instance, look at the Supplement Facts box for a product widely marketed as a "whole-foods" multivitamin in Figure 13. While this formula may very well be a good multivitamin product, it is in no way delivering these vitamins and minerals as whole foods. In fact, of all the vitamins and minerals listed, only a few (beta-carotene, vitamin E, and iodine) are likely to be unmodified and "natural-sourced"; all the others have been modified in some way or are organically synthesized bio-equivalent compounds. Notice that while additional food ingredients have been added to the multivitamin, none of these ingredients are listed in the parenthesis for the vitamin claims. In other words, these food ingredients are not intended to be the source for any of the vitamin or mineral claims.

Another confusing issue for consumers and unknowledgeable manufacturers and marketers is the idea that using so-called activated forms or combined forms, in order to avoid the most obvious synthetic compound names, makes the product appear more natural. In this product, the use of mineral or vitamin ascorbates is used to obscure the fact that these compounds are merely salts (or mixtures) derived from commercial ascorbic acid—with calcium, magnesium, palmitic acid, or niacin. Also, while we are generally in favor of using mineral chelates (see mineral section), these compounds are chemically reacted to mimic the mineral-amino acid complexes found in plants; but would not be considered strictly natural- and are far from whole food.

There are a host of products with similar designs (adding fruit and vegetable powders to a standard multivitamin blend) masquerading as natural or "whole-food." Because the term "whole-food" is not defined from a regulatory stand-point, the marketers of these products have done a great disservice to the nutrient supplement world and added much confusion to patients and clinicians, intentionally or not. Thankfully, these products should be easy to spot due to the mandatory disclosure of ingredient sources within the supplement facts box- something that was not true prior to 1997.

Supplement Facts V1

Serving Size: 8 Tablets — Servings Per Container: 30

Amount Per Serving		%DV
Vitamin A (from natural beta carotene)	5,000 IU	100%
Vitamin C (as Calcium, Magnesium, Niacinamide, Ascorbates and Ascorbyl Palmitate)	500 mg	833%
Vitamin D-3 (as cholecalciferol)	5,000 IU	1,250%
Vitamin E (natural, as d-alpha tocopherol plus mixed tocopherols)	400 IU	1,333%
Thiamine (as Thiamine Pyrophosphate)	3 mg	200%
Riboflavin (as Riboflavin-5-Phosphate)	3.4 mg	200%
Niacin/Niacinamide (as Niacinamide Ascorbate)	40 mg	200%
Vitamin B-6 (as Pyridoxal-5-Phosphate)	4 mg	200%
Folate (as L-methylfolate, Metafolin®)	400 mcg	100%
Vitamin B-12 (as methylcobalamin)	100 mcg	1,667%
Biotin	900 mcg	300%
Pantothenic Acid (as d-Calcium Pantethenate)	30 mg	300%
Calcium (as Calcium Ascorbate, Citrate/Malate Complex)	250 mg	25%
Iodine (from Kelp)	200 mcg	133%
Magnesium (as Magnesium Ascorbate/ Amino Acid Chelate Complex)	500 mg	125%
Zinc (as Zinc Amino Acid Chelate)	15 mg	100%
Selenium (as Amino Acid Chelate Complex)	200 mcg	286%
Copper (as Copper Amino Acid Chelate)	50 mcg	3%
Manganese (as Manganese Amino Acid Chelate)	2 mg	100%
Chromium (as Amino Acid Chelate)	200 mcg	167%
Molybdenum (as Amino Acid Chelate)	100 mcg	133%
Potassium (as Potassium Krebstr and Amino Acid Chelate Complex)	99 mg	2%
Lutein (natural)	6 mg	*
Lycopene (natural)	6 mg	*
Zeaxanthin	1 mg	*
Other Minerals, Nutrients and Trace Elements		
Inositol	100 mg	*
Trace Elements (from Sea Vegetation) approx	100 mcg	*
Strontium (from 0.5 mg strontium carbonate)	297 mcg	*
Silica	100 mg	*
Choline (from 150 mg Choline Citrate/Bitartrate)	60 mg	*

Amount Per Serving		%DV
PABA (para-aminobenzoic acid)	50 mg	*
Boron (as Amino Acid Chelate Complex)	1.5 mg	*
Vanadium	50 mcg	*
Amino Acids and Enzymes		
L-Cysteine/N-Acetyl Cysteine	150 mg	*
Betaine (from 150 mg Betaine HCl)	114 mg	*
Bromelain (2,000 GDU/g)	50 mg	*
Glutamic Acid (from 25 mg Glutamic Acid)	20 mg	*
L-Methionine	12.5 mg	*
Bioflavonoids and Prosnthocyanidins		
Rose Hips	100 mg	*
Lemon Bioflavonoids	100 mg	*
Red Wine Proanthocyanidins/Pine Bark Extract	50 mg	*
Hesperidin	35 mg	*
Rutin	25 mg	*
Vegetables Fruits and Herbs		
Proprietary Blend	700 mg	*
Kale (leaf), Spinach (leaf), Carrot (root), Radish (root), Celery (leaf and stalk), Apricot (fruit), Blackberry (fruit), Cranberry (fruit), Grape (fruit), and Pineapple (fruit)		
Blueberry (fruit)	100 mg	*
Garlic (bulb, Pure-Gar® odorless	100 mg	*
Broccoli (entire plant)	100 mg	*
Cauliflower (entire plant)	100 mg	*
Spirulina	100 mg	*
Chlorella (broken cell wall)	100 mg	*
Green Papaya Extract (fruit)	100 mg	*
Green Tea Extract (leaf	50 mg	*
Sprouted Barley Juice (entire plant)	50 mg	*
Wheat Grass Juice (entire plant)	50 mg	*
Beet Extract (root)	50 mg	*
Apple Pectin (fruit)	50 mg	*

* Daily Value not Established

Figure 13 : Sample of Product Label Incorrectly Marketed as "Whole Foods"

If each vitamin and mineral in the supplement facts box does not list its source (in parenthesis) adjacent to the claim, they are almost certainly misleading the consumer by using standard multivitamin sources of nutrients, falsely marketing them as natural or whole-food.

2. Products made with mostly non-food yeast extracts or wheat germ:

Concentrating and stabilizing vitamins and minerals from whole foods, predominantly fruits and vegetables, is expensive and difficult, which is why many products that attempt to use only unmodified vitamins use mostly yeast extracts, often labeled as *Saccharomyces cerevisiae* or just *S. cerevisiae*, or wheat germ, which is less popular with today's gluten-free focus. These products will sometimes have a few other ingredients to supply vitamins not high enough in the yeast extract. These products, if they haven't been spiked with undeclared vitamins, will be limited in the dose of each vitamin, but especially low in mineral content.

While these types of products are designed to avoid ingredients they claim are "unnatural," the notion that a concentration of fermented yeast grown in a factory represents a natural food source is a bit of a stretch, and since these products deliver a limited amount of nutrients, their clinical utility is also limited. If these products are labeled correctly, clinicians and patients can decide if they are helpful in their quest for sufficient nutrient intake.

3. Products made with ingredients spiked with undeclared synthetic vitamins:

Marketers of "whole-food" nutrients quickly realized vitamins and minerals are difficult to concentrate and deliver from truly whole-food sources. So, when using non-yeast foods such as fruits and vegetables, it is difficult to deliver even measurable amounts well below the USRDA of key vitamins and minerals. Consequently a number of deceptive methods have been used to sell products higher in vitamins and (some) minerals, while claiming the ingredients to be food-derived or natural. This is accomplished by various techniques, usually described in marketing literature and websites as a patented or unique process, referred to as some form of "culturing" or "fermentation." Essentially what these marketers, or their raw material suppliers, are doing is adding large amounts of synthetic vitamins to the process (fermentation vessel of yeast or foods) at some point prior to "extraction" and then claiming the measured vitamin content is from the natural source. These products typically avoid making source claims within the Supplement Facts box, but vaguely describe patented or proprietary processed sources in a notation below or outside the box.

While these products may deliver the vitamin content they claim, these deceptive and fraudulent practices lead to confusion about nutrient supplementation and falsely imply that high doses of natural-sourced vitamins and minerals can be delivered in capsules for a reasonable price. By doing so, they falsely exaggerate the differences between whole-food sourced vitamins and those they deem harmful (synthetic isolates), while at the same time using these same ingredients to "fortify" their product by deceptively hiding behind their proprietary process.

USP/NF Ingredients: What are they?

Oftentimes you will see the designation USP or NF next to an ingredient or excipient within a food or dietary supplement. This means that the ingredient conforms to the standards set forth in monographs published by the United States Pharmacopeia/National Formulary (US Pharmacopeial Convention). These raw material monographs describe all the specific physical and chemical properties (including maximum levels of contaminants) of the ingredient, along with the specific testing methods required to ensure the ingredient conforms to the monograph. There are USP/NF monographs for at least one form of almost every vitamin and mineral. In some cases, USP has created no monograph for specific quality micronutrient sources (like mineral amino acid chelates).

The USP also has a dietary supplement verification program that can be used to certify some finished products as well. However, only certain limited-ingredient formulas have monograph standards available for such a certification.

The clinical utility of single nutrients: Is it appropriate?

The question often arises as to whether the use of single-nutrient therapies is clinically appropriate. This question stems from two key observations. First, since vitamin and mineral nutrients are typically consumed in various combinations within their normal food matrix, supplementing isolated nutrients appears to be inherently unnatural. The second is the perception that many clinical trials with negative findings are performed with single nutrients (similar to drug trials), and criticism of the design of these trials often points to the use of nutrients in isolation. While these observations may be valid, it's equally true that many foods provide only limited vitamins and minerals in dose and diversity, and our bodies are designed to appropriately store key nutrients for days, weeks or even months as a resilient mechanism to handle fluctuations in food availability and seasonality. The notion that our bodies depend on an ideal ratio of macronutrients, micronutrients and other compounds at each meal conflicts with what we know about the design and adaptability of nutrient usage in humans. Moreover, the vast majority of *positive* clinical trials are also done with isolated nutrients (e.g., studies on vitamin D, folic acid, DHA, CoQ_{10}, vitamin K, etc.). This is due to the fact that most intervention trials choose to use a limited number of variables in order to limit the range of interpretations, even if this is bad dietary advice.

Clinicians should have a diverse formulary of nutrient supplements available to meet the clinical needs of their patients. On the one hand, clinicians should utilize products that combine a variety of nutrients, such as high-dose multivitamins or multi-nutrient products designed for specific purposes, and also a handful of key single-nutrient products. It is common to see products that combine all the B-vitamins with their B-complex nutrients, or calcium-containing supplements with additional vitamin D. In some cases, isolated nutrients at high or therapeutic doses can result in an imbalance of other nutrients, such as when high doses of zinc depletes copper, or high-dose folic acid masks a vitamin B_{12} deficiency. Most well-informed professional supplement companies are aware of these issues and formulate to compensate for these well-known interactions. Of course, not every interaction can be anticipated in each patient; it is important to always be aware that high-dose therapy with any single nutrient, even if clinically warranted, has a higher likelihood of side effects, most of which are documented.

Nutrient Assessment using Laboratory Tests

It is common to use laboratory analysis for patient nutrient assessment, though the utility of laboratory results for making clinical and dietary recommendations is not universally agreed upon. Most frank nutritional deficiencies are easy to spot by a trained nutritional expert, but many still prefer laboratory analysis to confirm findings or discover subtle deficiencies and imbalances difficult to detect during physical examination or diet diary analysis.

Nutrient analysis can be performed using whole blood, serum, RBCs, lymphocytes, blood spot, tissue biopsy, urine, hair, stool or saliva, depending on the nutrient or metabolite being tested. In some cases, analysis of more than one type of sample, or analyte, is needed in order to capture the true status of that nutrient. In addition, nutrients can be measured directly, without challenge, much like a fasting blood glucose is done; after challenge or functional test, much like an oral glucose tolerance test; or by assessing related metabolites to understand the functional activity of the metabolite over time, much like glycated hemoglobin helps us understand blood glucose levels over weeks and months.

Several laboratories that serve the functional and integrative healthcare community have developed nutritional assessment test panels, which combine different testing methods using a variety of collected samples in a single report of nutritional status. Some laboratories even combine stool analysis, which can provide status of the gut microbiome and estimations of fiber intake and digestive efficiencies. In addition, many labs now provide a number of genetic tests that can point to the potential for specific nutrigenetic-driven supplementation protocols.

Since each laboratory provides different tests and reports, often using completely different technologies and philosophies of nutrient testing, it is important for the clinician to understand the test methods, the laboratory test results and the ways these results affect dietary or supplement recommendations. Clinicians should be familiar with several labs and laboratory methods, and consult closely with them to interpret their findings as it applies to specific patients.

Vitamin Monographs

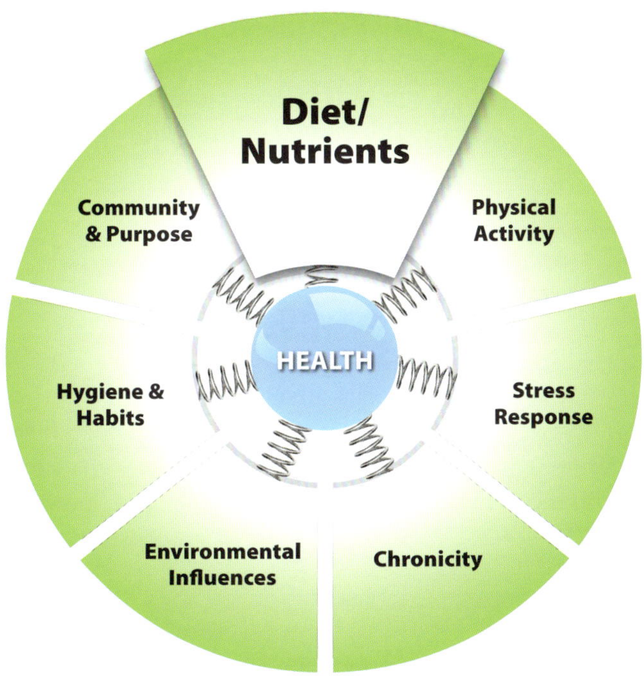

Vitamin A

Essential Nutrient Functions

Vitamin A refers to a wide range of fat-soluble nutrients, some referred to as preformed (retinol and derivatives), and those generally deemed vitamin A precursors (beta-carotene and other carotenoids). Ultimately, the isomers of the final bioactive form of vitamin A, called retinoic acid (RA), act as nutrigenomic "hormones" that alter gene expression and influence various physiological processes. Vitamin A is best known for its role in retinal function and vision, especially night vision, but is also well known for its effects on immune function.

Intake Guidelines

Recommended Dietary Allowances (RDAs) for Vitamin A

Age	Males mcg /day (IU/day)	Females mcg /day (IU/day)	Pregnancy mcg /day (IU/day)	Lactation mcg /day (IU/day)
0-6 months	400 (1,333 IU)	400 (1,333 IU)		
6-12 months	500 (1,667 IU)	500 (1,667 IU)		
1-3 years	300 (1,000 IU)	300 (1,000 IU)		
4-8 years	400 (1,333 IU)	400 (1,333 IU)		
9-13 years	600 (2,000 IU)	600 (2,000 IU)		
14-18 years	900 (3,000 IU)	700 (2,333 IU)	750 (2500 IU)	1,200 (4000 IU)
19+ years	900 (3,000 IU)	700 (2,333 IU)	770 (2,567 IU)	1,300 (4,333 IU)

Note: IU calculated as retinol

Unit(s) of Measure for Guidelines and Labeling

Unlike most vitamins, measuring vitamin A is complex; making it complicated for consumers by the conversion to international units (IU) on most Supplement Facts boxes. The basic unit of measurement, however, is micrograms (mcg) of retinol activity equivalents (RAE), with one mcg of retinol equal to one mcg RAE, and one RAE equal to 3.33 IU of vitamin A. Note the RDA levels are listed in mcg of RAE, the mandatory unit of measure on dietary supplement labels as of 2018, not in IU. This is important because dietary and supplemental sources of vitamin A differ in their retinal activity. This results in the following conversions:

- One IU retinol = 0.3 mcg RAE
- One IU beta-carotene from dietary supplements = 0.15 mcg RAE
- One IU beta-carotene from food = 0.05 mcg RAE
- One IU alpha-carotene or beta-cryptoxanthin = 0.025 mcg RAE

A RAE cannot be directly converted into an IU without knowing the source(s) of vitamin A. For example, the RDA of 900 mcg RAE for adolescent and adult men is equivalent to 3,000 IU if the food or supplement source is preformed vitamin A (retinol). However, this RDA is also equivalent to 6,000 IU of beta-carotene from supplements, 18,000 IU of beta-carotene from food, or 36,000 IU of alpha-carotene or beta-cryptoxanthin from food. So a mixed diet containing 900 mcg RAE provides between 3,000 and 36,000 IU of vitamin A, depending on the foods consumed.

General Levels of Deficiencies in the U.S.

NHANES data (2003 – 2006) show the percent of Americans over the age of two with dietary intake below the EAR is about 75%. This is reduced, but not eliminated, when considering intake from fortification (45%) and supplementation (34%). Patients taking Orlistat are known to have reduced ability to absorb dietary vitamin A.

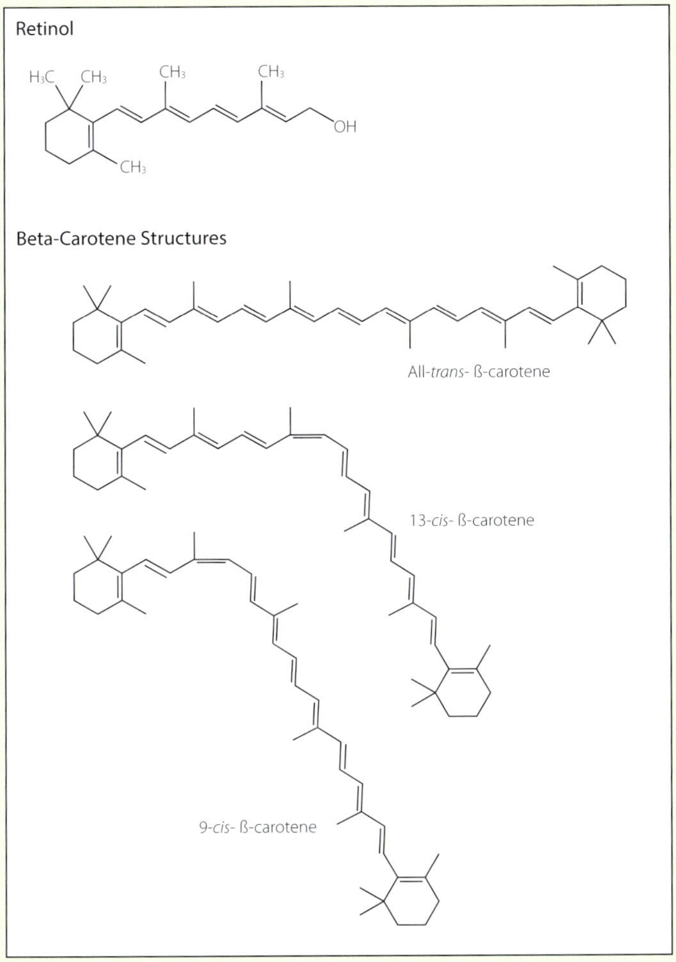

Natural and Supplemental Forms

The major forms of supplemental vitamin A are either retinol esters (retinyl palmitate or acetate) or beta-carotene. While retinol forms are found in some dietary sources—highest in animal or fish livers, lower amounts in eggs—the majority of dietary vitamin A comes from beta-carotene and other carotenoids. After ingestion, β-carotene is metabolized in the mucosa of small intestine by β-carotene dioxygenase into two retinyl molecules, which are then reduced to vitamin A (retinol).

There is also a synthetic form of beta-carotene used in food fortification, dietary supplements and, unfortunately, in a number of widely publicized clinical trials. The synthetic form differs from natural beta-carotene in that it contains only a single isomer (all-*trans* retinol), while natural beta-carotene contains several *cis*-isomers along with the all-*trans* isomer.

In the past few decades a natural beta-carotene source from the algae species *Dunaliella*, which is both adequately priced and highly concentrated with an approximately 50:50 blend of all-*trans* and 9-*cis*-isomers has become widely available. Limited animal and human studies show mixed results related to bioavailability between this natural form and the all-*trans* synthetic form of beta-carotene. While this form is more expensive than the synthetic beta-carotene alternative, the fact that it also contains several other carotenoid compounds, sometimes labeled as "mixed carotenoids," with health benefits unrelated to their conversion to vitamin A alone, we recommend using this form by itself, or in combination with preformed retinol (retinyl palmitate) for use in dietary supplements.

Potential for Toxicity

The potential for toxicity is different for preformed vitamin A and beta-carotene forms. Since both are fat-soluble and stored in the body, excess beta-carotene can be stored without full conversion to active retinol forms, though excess beta-carotene can turn skin a shade of yellow. Long-term intake of preformed vitamin A in doses above 15,000 IU should be avoided; however, short-term higher doses may be appropriate, under clinical supervision, for certain individuals with low immune function. Clinicians using high-dose retinol therapies should be familiar with signs of hypervitaminosis A. Acute vitamin A toxicity is relatively rare; symptoms include nausea, headache, fatigue, loss of appetite, dizziness, dry skin, desquamation and cerebral edema. Signs of chronic toxicity include dry and itchy skin, desquamation, loss of appetite, headache, cerebral edema, and bone and joint pain.

References:

- Vitamin A Page of Linus Pauling Institute Website: http://lpi.oregonstate.edu/infocenter/vitamins/vitaminA/.
- Office of Dietary Supplements- National Institutes of Health- Health Professional Information. http://ods.od.nih.gov/factsheets/VitaminA-HealthProfessional/.
- Patrick L. Beta-carotene: the controversy continues. *Altern Med Rev*. 2000 Dec;5(6):530-45.
- Ben-Amotz A, Mokady S, Edelstein S, Avron M. Bioavailability of a natural isomer mixture as compared with synthetic all-trans- beta-carotene in rats and chicks. *J Nutr.* 1989 Jul;119(7):1013-9.
- Ben-Amotz A, Levy Y. Bioavailability of a natural isomer mixture compared with synthetic all-trans beta-carotene in human serum. *Am J Clin Nutr*. 1996 May;63(5):729-34.
- Khoo HE, Prasad KN, Kong KW, Jiang Y, Ismail A. Carotenoids and their isomers: color pigments in fruits and vegetables. *Molecules*. 2011 Feb 18;16(2):1710-38.

Vitamin B_1/Thiamin

Essential Nutrient Functions

Thiamin, or thiamine, also known as vitamin B_1 or aneurine is a water-soluble nutrient. Isolated and characterized in the 1930s, thiamin was one of the first organic compounds to be recognized as a vitamin. Thiamin occurs in the human body as free thiamin and as various phosphorylated forms: thiamin monophosphate (TMP), thiamin triphosphate (TTP), and thiamin pyrophosphate (TPP). Thiamin is a precursor for thiamin pyrophosphate (TPP), the active form in the body, which is involved in several enzyme functions associated with metabolizing carbohydrates, branched-chain amino acids and fatty acids.

Intake Guidelines

Recommended Dietary Allowances (RDAs) for Thiamin

Age	Males mg/day	Females mg/day	Pregnancy mg/day	Lactation mg/day
0-6 months	0.2 (AI)	0.2 (AI)		
6-12 months	0.3 (AI)	0.3 (AI)		
1-3 years	0.5	0.5		
4-8 years	0.6	0.6		
9-13 years	0.9	0.9		
14-18 years	1.2	1.0		
19+ years	1.2	1.1		
All ages			1.4	1.4

Unit(s) of Measure for Guidelines and Labeling

Thiamin is simply measured by weight in mg of thiamin.

General Levels of Deficiencies in the U.S.

While clinical deficiency in thiamin (beriberi) is rarely diagnosed in Americans, NHANES data from 2003 to 2006 show the percent of Americans over the age of two with dietary intake below the EAR is about 50%, though fortification and supplementation bring this down to 4%. However, since the synthesis of TPP from free thiamin requires magnesium, functional deficiency of thiamin may be influenced by widespread low intake of magnesium. Consuming large amounts of tea and coffee, including decaffeinated varieties, as well as chewing tea leaves and betel nuts, have been associated with thiamin depletion in humans due to the presence of antithiamin factors.

Thiamin

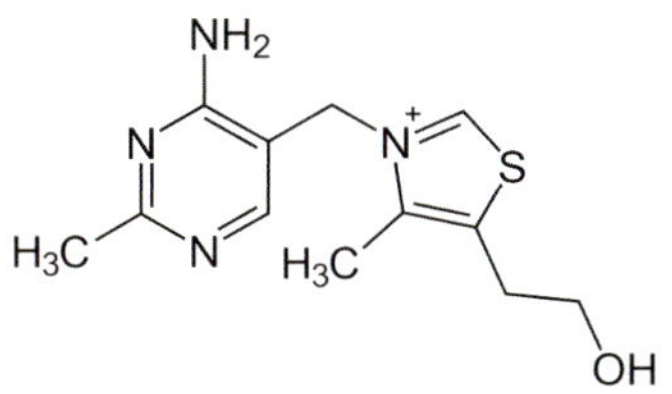

Thiamin Pyrophosphate

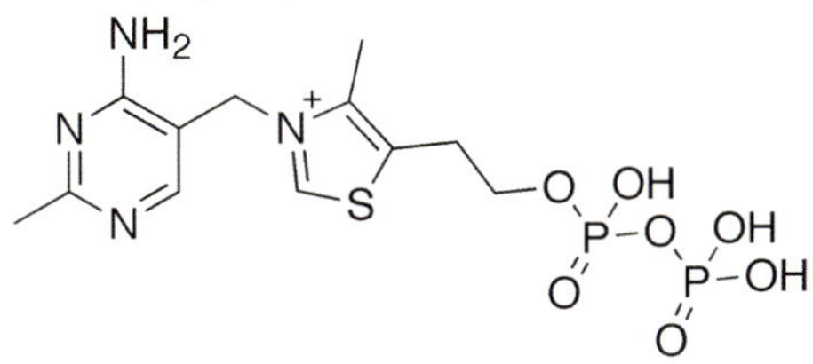

Natural and Supplemental Forms

Natural thiamin is either free-form (from plants) or in phosphorylated forms (from animals). Thiamin is also synthesized by certain gut bacteria. In all cases, thiamin must be dephosphorylated before being transported into the body as free-form thiamin, which is also the main transport form throughout the body. Supplement forms of thiamin are salt derivatives of free-form thiamine, most commonly thiamin HCl and thiamin mononitrate. We are unaware of any studies attempting to differentiate the benefits of the thiamin delivered through these forms, which essentially deliver a "bioequivalent" previtamin to the gut.

A lipophilic derivative of thiamin, called benfotiamine, has been used in some dietary supplements in the United States. The regulatory status of this new form of thiamin is uncertain and should not be considered a viable alternative for thiamin supplementation. Potential use of benfotiamine for other clinical therapies is beyond the scope of this review.

Potential for Toxicity

Thiamin has no known toxicity and an upper tolerable limit has not been determined by the IOM.

References:

- Thiamin Page of Linus Pauling Institute Website: http://lpi.oregonstate.edu/infocenter/vitamins/thiamin/.
- Wilcox CS. Do diuretics cause thiamine deficiency? *J Lab Clin Med.* 1999;134(3):192-193.
- Said HM. Intestinal absorption of water-soluble vitamins in health and disease. *Biochem J.* 2011 Aug 1;437(3):357-72.

Vitamin B_2/Riboflavin

Essential Nutrient Functions

Riboflavin, also known as vitamin B_2, is a water-soluble B vitamin. In the body, riboflavin is primarily utilized as an integral component of the coenzymes flavin adenine dinucleotide (FAD) and flavin mononucleotide (FMN). Coenzymes derived from riboflavin are termed flavocoenzymes, and enzymes that use a flavocoenzyme are called flavoproteins. These coenzymes act as electron carriers in a number of oxidation-reduction (redox) reactions involved in energy production and in numerous other metabolic pathways. Riboflavin-derived coenzymes are often used in metabolic processes that require vitamin B_6, folate, niacin and iron.

Intake Guidelines

Recommended Dietary Allowances (RDAs) for Riboflavin

Age	Males mg/day	Females mg/day	Pregnancy mg/day	Lactation mg/day
0-6 months	0.3 (AI)	0.3 (AI)		
6-12 months	0.4 (AI)	0.4 (AI)		
1-3 years	0.5	0.5		
4-8 years	0.6	0.6		
9-13 years	0.9	0.9		
14-18 years	1.3	1.0		
19+ years	1.3	1.1		
All ages			1.4	1.6

Unit(s) of Measure for Guidelines and Labeling

Riboflavin/Vitamin B_2 is reported by weight in mg of riboflavin.

General Levels of Deficiencies in the U.S.

The technical name for clinical riboflavin deficiency is ariboflavinosis. Riboflavin deficiency is rarely found in isolation in the U.S., though insufficient intake is more frequent in combination with deficiencies of other water-soluble vitamins. NHANES data from 2003 to 2006 show that the percent of Americans over the age of two with dietary intake of riboflavin below the EAR is less than 10% before fortification and supplementation.

Riboflavin

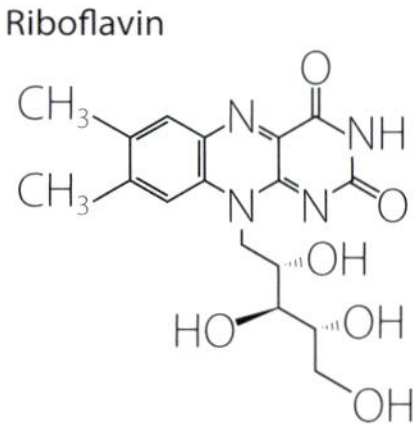

Flavin adenine dinucleotide (FAD)

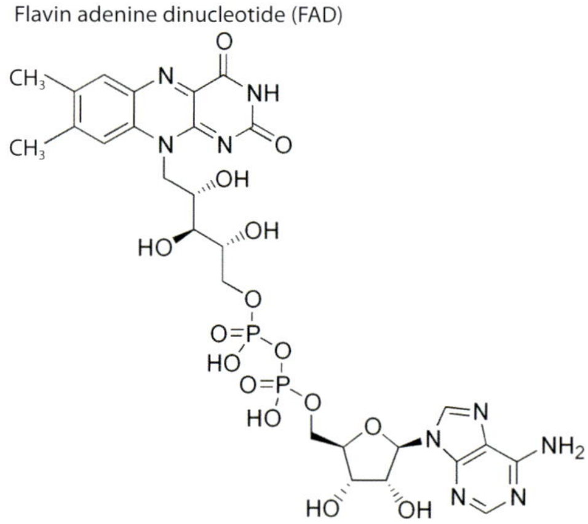

Natural and Supplemental Forms

Riboflavin is naturally found in foods as either free riboflavin or one of its coenzyme derivatives (FAD/FMN). The bioavailability of these compounds is similar, since each form is hydrolyzed to free riboflavin prior to transport into the body. Dietary supplements typically contain either the synthetic "bioidentical" riboflavin or the synthetic derivative called riboflavin monophosphate (riboflavin-5-phosphate, R5P). Riboflavin-5-phosphate is often marketed as an "activated" or natural form of riboflavin. As it turns out, this synthetic form, also a "bioidentical" form, must be dephosphorylated prior to transport into the body. This has been known since the mid 1960s (see references). We are unaware of any study that has attempted to compare the clinical benefits of supplementing free riboflavin with R5P; and unless R5P has an undocumented effect within the gastrointestinal lumen prior to being hydrolyzed to free riboflavin, no clinical difference would be anticipated. While no evidence suggests that R5P is an inferior form of the vitamin compared to free riboflavin, the additional manufacturing processes result in a raw material cost that is more than three times higher than normal riboflavin, an unnecessary cost to the supplement user.

Potential for Toxicity

There are no known toxic effects or adverse reactions related to riboflavin and the IOM lists no upper limit for riboflavin intake. Moderate to high-dose riboflavin therapy has been found to intensify urine color to a bright yellow (flavinuria), a harmless side effect.

References:

- Riboflavin Page of Linus Pauling Institute Website: http://lpi.oregonstate.edu/infocenter/vitamins/riboflavin/.
- Bates CJ. Bioavailability of riboflavin. *Eur J Clin Nutr.* 1997 Jan;51 Suppl 1:S38-42.
- Said HM. Intestinal absorption of water-soluble vitamins in health and disease. *Biochem J.* 2011 Aug 1;437(3):357-72.
- Jusko WJ, Levy G. Absorption, metabolism, and excretion of riboflavin-5'-phosphate in man. *J Pharm Sci.* 1967 Jan;56(1):58-62.

Vitamin B_3/Niacin

Essential Nutrient Functions

Niacin, or vitamin B_3, is a water-soluble vitamin that includes nicotinic acid and niacinamide, equivalent as "vitamins," but not for all therapies (see below). Niacinamide, or nicotinamide, is converted in the body to the coenzymes nicotinamide adenine dinucleotide (NAD) and nicotinamide adenine dinucleotide phosphate (NADP). These active coenzymes are used in a number of important redox-related metabolic reactions and other important functions within cells. Niacin is not technically an essential nutrient, as the body can produce niacinamide from the amino acid tryptophan, but it is *functionally* essential in most humans.

*Note: Even though the FDA has approved various products containing niacin as lipid-altering drugs, niacin products of similar doses and clinical benefit, even some sold as delayed-release, can be legally sold as dietary supplements as long as the manufacturers and distributors make no disease or drug claims.

Intake Guidelines

Recommended Dietary Allowances (RDAs) for Niacin

Age	Males mg NE*/day	Females mg NE/day	Pregnancy mg NE/day	Lactation mg NE/day
0-6 months	2 (AI)	2 (AI)		
6-12 months	4 (AI)	4 (AI)		
1-3 years	6	6		
4-8 years	8	8		
9-13 years	12	12		
14-18 years	16	14		
19+ years	16	14		
All ages			18	17

* AI - NE, niacin equivalent: 1 mg NE = 60 mg of tryptophan = 1 mg niacin

Unit(s) of Measure for Guidelines and Labeling

The IOM's RDA for niacin is listed as niacin equivalents (NE), measured in milligrams. For most dietary supplements, this is not an issue since 1 mg of either niacin or niacinamide is equal to 1 mg NE. However, foods containing tryptophan should additionally report 1 mg of NE for every 60 mg of tryptophan.

General Levels of Deficiencies in the U.S.

Niacin deficiency is well known as pellagra, though it is rarely diagnosed today in the U.S. NHANES data from 2003 to 2006 show the percent of Americans over the age of two with dietary intake of niacin, which includes NE from tryptophan intake, below the EAR is low—only 11%—and is nearly eliminated when considering intake from fortification and supplementation. Subjects with ESRD or those on dialysis may need additional niacin.

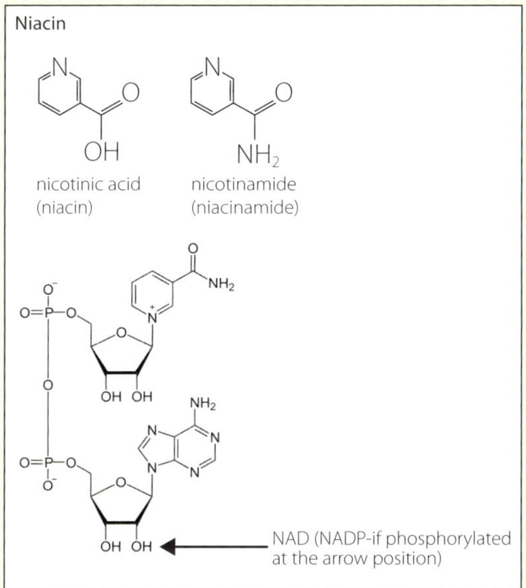

Natural and Supplemental Forms

Food niacin comes in the form of NAD/NADP or as a glycoside of nicotinic acid. In either case, intestinal enzymes must hydrolyze these food compounds to either free nicotinic acid or niacinamide prior to absorption, a pathway yet to be fully understood. As mentioned above, the majority of supplemental niacin uses either nicotinic acid or niacinamide/nicotinamide, both chemically synthesized "bioequivalent" compounds. A niacin salt formed with ascorbic acid, niacinamide ascorbate, is also available.

Low-dose niacin, for nutrient supplementation, is almost always used without modification; while high-dose niacin products, usually designed to modulate lipids, may be available as either unmodified, sometimes called crystalline or immediate-release niacin, or in extended-release delivery mechanisms to reduce the known flushing side effects of high-dose niacin therapy.

While not the subject of this review, the lipid-lowering effects of niacin are only known to be documented for nicotinic acid and are not associated with niacinamide/nicotinamide. Likewise, the compound known as inositol hexanicotinate (IHN), sometimes sold as "flush-free niacin," also demonstrates no clinically relevant lipid-altering effects, though many such claims have been made about this substance.

Potential for Toxicity

The tolerable upper limit of niacin is set at a threshold below the point when most individuals experience flushing, which is considered to be a benign, but a disturbing, side effect. Some subjects, however, experience a niacin-induced flushing effect at much lower doses and many multivitamin or "B-complex" vitamin products exceed the UL (conservatively set at 35 mg). In this case, niacinamide is more tolerable than nicotinic acid. High levels of niacin used for lipid-lowering can result in elevations of liver enzymes. This is less-common in immediate-release forms but can increase in the use of highly extended time-release forms, which are no longer available. Doses of 1,500 mg per day are more likely to cause an increase in liver enzymes than doses of 1,000 mg or less.

References:

- Niacin Page of Linus Pauling Institute Website: http://lpi.oregonstate.edu/infocenter/vitamins/niacin/.
- Said HM. Intestinal absorption of water-soluble vitamins in health and disease. *Biochem J.* 2011 Aug 1;437(3):357-72.
- MacKay D, Hathcock J, Guarneri E. Niacin: chemical forms, bioavailability, and health effects. *Nutr Rev.* 2012 Jun;70(6):357-66.
- Keenan JM. Wax-matrix extended-release niacin vs inositol hexanicotinate: a comparison of wax-matrix, extended-release niacin to inositol hexanicotinate "no-flush" niacin in persons with mild to moderate dyslipidemia. *J Clin Lipidol.* 2013 Jan-Feb;7(1):14-23.
- Rennick A, Kalakeche R, Seel L, Shepler B. Nicotinic acid and nicotinamide: a review of their use for hyperphosphatemia in dialysis patients. *Pharmacotherapy.* 2013 Jun;33(6):683-90.

Vitamin B_5/Pantothenic Acid

Essential Nutrient Functions

Vitamin B_5, or Pantothenic acid, is an essential nutrient for all forms of life. It is a precursor for the formation of coenzyme A (CoA), a vital coenzyme in numerous chemical reactions. CoA is required for chemical reactions that generate energy from food (fat, carbohydrates, and proteins), most notably in the acyl carrier for fatty acid synthesis.

Intake Guidelines

Adequate Intakes (AIs) for Pantothenic Acid

Age	Males mg/day	Females mg/day	Pregnancy mg/day	Lactation mg/day
0-6 months	1.7	1.7		
6-12 months	1.8	1.8		
1-3 years	2	2		
4-8 years	3	3		
9-13 years	4	4		
14-18 years	5	5		
19+ years	5	5		
All ages			6	7

Unit(s) of Measure for Guidelines and Labeling

Vitamin B_5/Pantothenic Acid is measured by weight in mg of pantothenic acid.

General Levels of Deficiencies in the U.S.

The occurrences of nonexperimental deficiencies in pantothenic acid are virtually unknown in the West today. The AI set for this nutrient is low and the food sources, though low in concentration, are diverse enough to adequately meet these levels. Functional insufficiencies may be realized in some individuals, especially those under metabolic and HPA-axis stress. Research in such relationships is mostly concentrated in Japanese subjects. Whether this represents a particular genetic or dietary phenomenon or merely a coincidence is unknown.

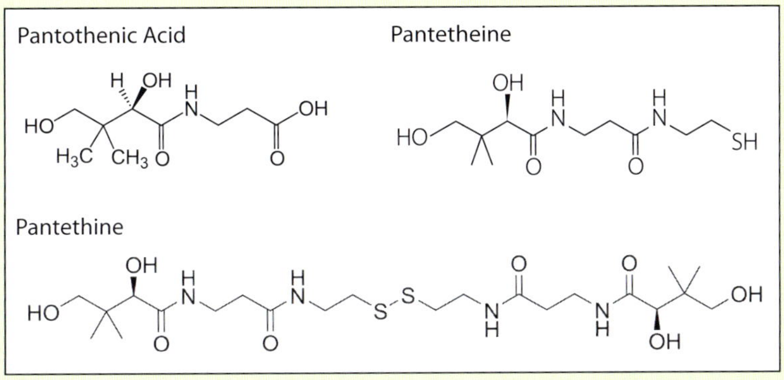

Natural and Supplemental Forms

Pantothenic acid in food is mostly found as coenzyme A, which must be converted to pantothenic acid in a multistep process in the human gut prior to intestinal transport. Commensal and some probiotic bacteria also produce pantothenic acid, though the amount of microbially derived pantothenic acid absorbed by humans is unknown.

Pantothenic acid is unstable. More stable supplement sources include pantothenol—a liquid form less common in the U.S.—and the familiar calcium salt, calcium-D-pantothenate, or D-calcium pantothenate. Because food-source CoA requires processing before being absorbed, calcium-D-pantothenate has approximately double the bioavailability as food-sourced pantothenic acid.

Pantethine is a disulfide dimer of the pantothenic acid-derivative pantetheine, and can be used as an alternative source for pantothenic acid. It is more commonly used in high doses (900 mg/day or more) for lipid modulation or fatty liver disease, a function of its metabolite cysteamine, not pantothenic acid.

Potential for Toxicity

Pantothenic acid and its derivatives are not known to be toxic and no tolerable upper limit has been set by the IOM. GI side effects have been reported for pantethine consumption greater than one gram and for calcium pantothenate exceeding 10 grams.

References:

- Pantothenic Acid Page of Linus Pauling Institute Website: http://lpi.oregonstate.edu/infocenter/vitamins/pa/.
- Tahiliani AG, Beinlich CJ. Pantothenic acid in health and disease. *Vitam Horm.* 1991;46:165-228.
- Jaroenporn S, Yamamoto T, Itabashi A, Nakamura K, Azumano I, Watanabe G, Taya K. Effects of pantothenic acid supplementation on adrenal steroid secretion from male rats. *Biol Pharm Bull.* 2008 Jun;31(6):1205-8.
- Schwabedal PE, Pietrzik K, Wittkowski W. Pantothenic acid deficiency as a factor contributing to the development of hypertension. *Cardiology.* 1985;72 Suppl 1:187-9.

Vitamin B_6

Essential Nutrient Functions

Vitamin B_6 is a water-soluble nutrient that generally describes three compound forms: pyridoxal (PL), pyridoxine (PN) and pyridoxamine (PM). Each of these compounds is a precursor to the eventual biologically active form pyridoxal 5'-phosphate (PLP or P5P), which is a coenzyme for more than 100 different enzymatic reactions in a number of metabolic capacities. Pyridoxamine 5'-phosphate (PMP) may also be a minor coenzyme in some enzyme reactions.

Intake Guidelines

Recommended Dietary Allowances (RDAs) for B_6

Age	Males mg/day	Females mg/day	Pregnancy mg/day	Lactation mg/day
0-6 months	0.1 (AI)	0.1 (AI)		
6-12 months	0.3 (AI)	0.3 (AI)		
1-3 years	0.5	0.5		
4-8 years	0.6	0.6		
9-13 years	1.0	1.0		
14-18 years	1.3	1.2		
19+ years	1.3-1.7	1.3-1.5		
All ages			1.9	2.0

Unit(s) of Measure for Guidelines and Labeling

Vitamin B_6 is measured by the weight in mg of pyridoxine or the molar equivalent of other compounds.

General Levels of Deficiencies in the U.S.

Vitamin B_6 deficiency is low in Western populations. Even so, NHANES data from 2003 to 2006 shows the percent of Americans over the age of two with dietary intake of vitamin B_6 below the EAR is 21%, which is reduced to less than 10% after fortification and supplementation. However, newer genomic-related studies show "healthy" individuals may experience metabolic perturbations related to a functional insufficiency of vitamin B_6. Unsupplemented vegans may have low blood levels of vitamin B_6, perhaps because many plant-sourced conjugates of vitamin B_6 are poorly absorbed.

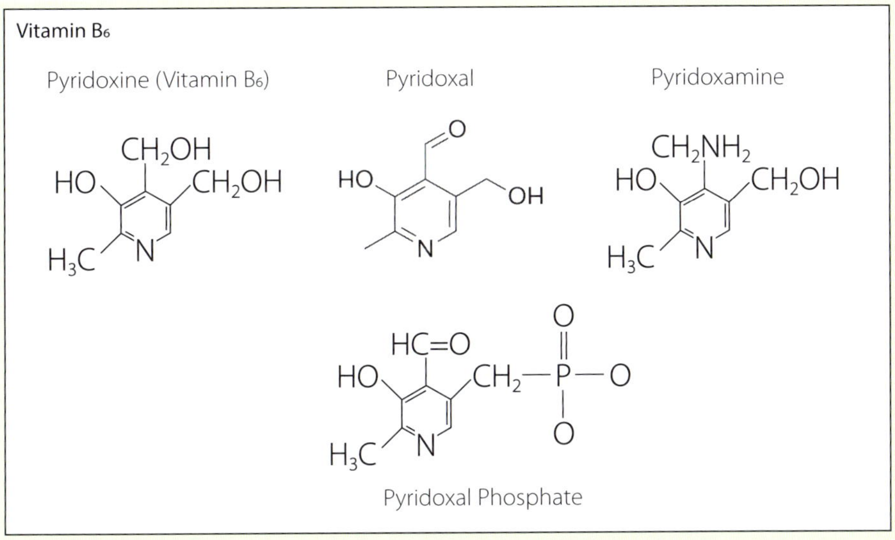

Natural and Supplemental Forms

Food sources of vitamin B_6 are found in all three forms—pyridoxine, pyridoxamine, pyridoxal—as well as in each of their phosphorylated and glucoside-conjugated forms. All phosphorylated compounds are hydrolyzed into their respective unphosphorylated forms prior to absorption, after which *in vivo* conversion allows each to act as vitamin precursors. Phosphorylation of the coenzyme form occurs as needed in the liver.

The primary vitamin B_6 ingredient used for food fortification and dietary supplements is the synthetic "bioequivalent" compound pyridoxine HCl. This compound has been shown to have higher bioavailability than food-source vitamin B_6, due to the reduced gastrointestinal hydrolysis of some (mostly plant) glucoside conjugates.

It is common for some manufacturers to use pyridoxal-5-phosphate (P5P) and market this ingredient as an "active" or "natural" form of supplemental B_6. While also being "bioequivalent," this ingredient is synthesized from pyridoxine HCl, which increases its cost by about seven times. When taken orally P5P must be dephosphorylated prior to absorption. Nonetheless, some clinicians believe, perhaps because serum vitamin B_6 levels are reported as pyridoxal phosphate (PLP), that oral P5P is more clinically appropriate. We know of no published studies that have attempted to show a clinical difference between pyridoxine HCl and P5P when used as supplements and, based on both the known need for dephosphorylation prior to absorption and added cost, P5P should not be viewed as superior to pyridoxine HCl—though it should be considered as clinically comparable with pyridoxine HCl when used in equal molar amounts.

Potential for Toxicity

Even though vitamin B_6 is water soluble, toxicity of this nutrient from supplements has been documented at high doses. The tolerable upper limit for vitamin B_6 is 100 mg/day in adults. (The IOM noted that, though several case reports show sensory neuropathy occurring at doses lower than 500 mg/day, studies in patients treated with vitamin B_6 at average dose of 200 mg/day for up to five years found no evidence of this effect). Several clinical trials using much higher doses have been published. These studies should be viewed as pharmacological, or orthomolecular, and are not related to supplemental or deficiency-correcting uses of vitamin B_6.

References:

- Vitamin B6 Page of Linus Pauling Institute Website: http://lpi.oregonstate.edu/infocenter/vitamins/vitaminB6/.
- Office of Dietary Supplements- National Institutes of Health- Health Professional Information. http://ods.od.nih.gov/factsheets/VitaminB6-HealthProfessional/.
- Said HM. Intestinal absorption of water-soluble vitamins in health and disease. *Biochem J.* 2011 Aug 1;437(3):357-72.
- Waldmann A, Dörr B, Koschizke JW, Leitzmann C, Hahn A. Dietary intake of vitamin B6 and concentration of vitamin B6 in blood samples of German vegans. *Public Health Nutr.* 2006 Sep;9(6):779-84.
- Gregory JF 3rd. Bioavailability of vitamin B-6. *Eur J Clin Nutr.* 1997 Jan;51 Suppl 1:S43-8.
- Gregory JF 3rd, Park Y, Lamers Y et al. Metabolomic analysis reveals extended metabolic consequences of marginal vitamin B-6 deficiency in healthy human subjects. *PLoS One.* 2013 Jun 11;8(6):e63544.

Vitamin B_7/Biotin

Essential Nutrient Functions

Biotin is a water-soluble vitamin generally classified as a B-complex vitamin. It is an essential micronutrient for humans, but only synthesized by bacteria, yeasts, molds, algae and a few plant species. Biotin's nutritive function is as a cofactor for five carboxylases involved in important metabolic reactions that include fatty acid metabolism, amino acid catabolism and gluconeogenesis. Recent research shows biotin is also involved with gene regulation via its involvement in histone modification. Since biotin deficiency, though rare, is known to diminish hair and nail strength, biotin is often used in products designed for hair and nails.

Intake Guidelines

Adequate Intakes (AIs) for Biotin

Age	Males mcg/day	Females mcg/day	Pregnancy mcg/day	Lactation mcg/day
0-6 months	5	5		
6-12 months	6	6		
1-3 years	8	8		
4-8 years	12	12		
9-13 years	20	20		
14-18 years	25	25		
19+	30	30		
All ages			30	35

Unit(s) of Measure for Guidelines and Labeling

Biotin is measured by weight in mcg.

General Levels of Deficiencies in the U.S.

Deficiency of biotin in the U.S. is low. Consuming high amounts of raw egg whites over a long period of time allows the undenatured avidin to bind biotin, preventing GI absorption, creating the potential for biotin deficiency. Cooking the eggs will prevent this. Lipoic acid has been noted in one animal study to inhibit a biotin-dependent carboxylase and shares a transporter with biotin. While lipoic acid has never been shown to hinder biotin metabolism in humans, some companies include a small amount of biotin in products containing high amounts of alpha-lipoic acid out of precaution.

Biotin

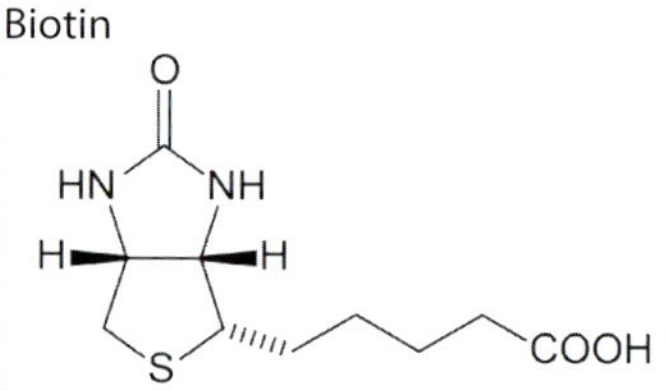

Natural and Supplemental Forms

Biotin is found in only a few foods, including cooked eggs, cooked liver, avocados and cooked salmon. Biotin is also made by some human gut bacteria and probiotic organisms. The amount of biotin produced by these gut microorganisms and absorbed by humans is difficult to measure. Finally, a synthesized "bioidentical" biotin is the primary source of biotin in food fortification and dietary supplements.

Potential for Toxicity
Biotin is not known to be toxic and the IOM has set no upper limit. The newly discovered ability of biotin to contribute to histone modification, an epigenetic influence of gene expression, warrants some precaution, but biotin's water-soluble character and its low abundance in foods and supplements makes any adverse event unlikely.

References:

- Biotin Page of Linus Pauling Institute Website: http://lpi.oregonstate.edu/infocenter/vitamins/biotin/.
- Hassan YI, Zempleni J. A novel, enigmatic histone modification: biotinylation of histones by holocarboxylase synthetase. *Nutr Rev.* 2008 Dec;66(12):721-5.
- Said HM. Cell and molecular aspects of human intestinal biotin absorption. *J Nutr.* 2009 Jan;139(1):158-62.
- Zempleni J, Hassan YI, Wijeratne SS. Biotin and biotinidase deficiency. *Expert Rev Endocrinol Metab.* 2008 Nov 1;3(6):715-724.
- Zempleni J, Mock DM. Biotin biochemistry and human requirements. *J Nutr Biochem.* 1999 Mar;10(3):128-38.
- Zempleni J, Trusty TA, Mock DM. Lipoic acid reduces the activities of biotin-dependent carboxylases in rat liver. *J Nutr.* 1997 Sep;127(9):1776-81.

Folate/Folic Acid/Vitamin B_9

Essential Nutrient Functions

Folate is the generic term for naturally occurring food folate and folic acid; the fully oxidized monoglutamate form of the vitamin used in dietary supplements and fortified foods. The only function of folate coenzymes in the body appears to be in mediating the transfer of one-carbon units (methyl-groups). Folate coenzymes act as acceptors and donors of one-carbon units in a variety of reactions critical to the metabolism of nucleic acids and amino acids, most notably in the conversion of homocysteine to methionine. Due to the relationship of widespread folate insufficiency with neural tube defects in early pregnancy, the U.S. instituted mandatory folic acid fortification of all enriched grain products in 1998.

Intake Guidelines

Recommended Dietary Allowances (RDAs) for Folate

Age	Males mcg/day	Females mcg/day	Pregnancy mcg/day	Lactation mcg/day
0-6 months	65 (AI)	65 (AI)		
6-12 months	80 (AI)	80 (AI)		
1-3 years	150	150		
4-8 years	200	200		
9-13 years	300	300		
14-18 years	400	400		
19+	400	400		
All ages			600	500

- One mcg of food folate provides one mcg of DFE
- One mcg of folic acid taken with meals or as fortified food provides 1.7 mcg of DFE
- One mcg of folic acid (supplement) taken on an empty stomach provides two mcg of DFE

Traditionally, the dietary folate requirement was defined as the amount needed to prevent a deficiency severe enough to cause symptoms like anemia. The most recent RDA (1998) was based primarily on the adequacy of red blood cell-folate concentrations at different levels of folate intake, as judged by the absence of abnormal hematological indicators.

When the Institute of Medicine set the new dietary recommendation for folate, they introduced a new unit, the Dietary Folate Equivalent (DFE). Use of the DFE reflects higher bioavailability of synthetic folic acid found in supplements and fortified foods compared to that of naturally occurring food folates.

Unit(s) of Measure for Guidelines and Labeling

As of 2018, food and supplement labels must use mcg of dietary folate equivalents (DFE), the IOM's measure of folate/folic acid for DRI calculations since 1998 (see page 19). DFEs are used because synthetic folic acid absorbs more readily than dietary folates (see page 75). When labeled using DFE, 1 mcg of a food-derived natural folate will be equivalent to 1 mcg DFE, while 1 mcg of folic acid is equivalent to 1.7 mcg DFE. Practitioners should note that under the DFE labeling format, only 235 mcg of folic acid is needed to reach the 100% DV of 400 mcg DFE (235 x 1.7). When folic acid is used in a supplement, the label must state the amount of DFE (and the % DV based on DFE) along with the actual amount of folic acid in mcg (in parentheses) for clarification and distinction. Since folinic acid and 5-MTHF, both synthetic folates, absorb similar to folic acid, they should be labeled with the same conversion factor (1.7 mcg DFE/mcg) and parenthetical mass declaration.

General Levels of Deficiencies in the U.S.

Without food fortification and supplementation of folic acid, deficiency of folate intake is high. NHANES data from 2003 to 2006 show the percent of Americans over the age of two with dietary intake of vitamin dietary folates below the EAR is nearly 90%, but after fortification this drops to only 10%. Even so, many studies suggest Americans have a functional deficiency in folate intake, evident in elevated plasma homocysteine (Hcy) levels. There is a robust debate about whether elevated Hcy, which can be treated with folate/folic acid therapy (usually with vitamin B_{12}) should be considered a modifiable risk factor for cardiovascular disease, osteoporosis and Alzheimer's disease; and whether it should be considered as a biological marker of folate status.

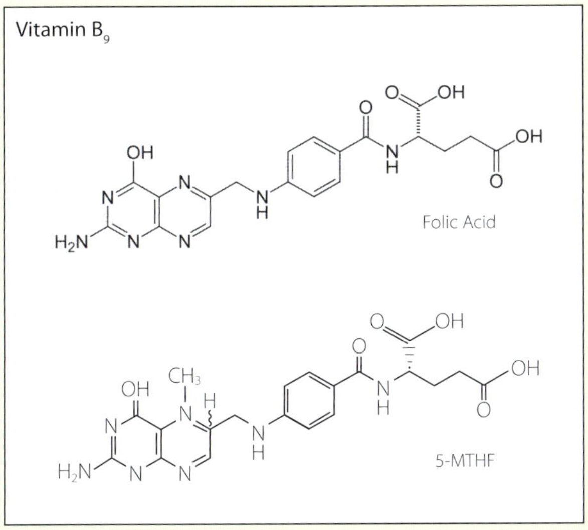

Natural and Supplemental Forms

Two sources of folate are available to the gut: a dietary source and a bacterial source from which the vitamin is generated by normal microbiota of the large intestine. Folates exist in mono and polyglutamate forms in diet. Dietary folate polyglutamates are first hydrolyzed to their monoglutamate forms by the action of folate hydrolase, then absorbed mainly in the proximal part of the small intestine via a specialized acidic pH-dependent carrier-mediated mechanism. The bioavailability of food folate is commonly estimated at 50% of folic acid bioavailability when establishing food recommendations, but this should be considered a rough estimate, as data on the bioavailability of food folate varies between 30% and 98%, depending on how the study is performed. Regardless, food-derived folates are rarely used in dietary supplement products.

Three basic forms of folate are frequently used in dietary supplements: folic acid, folinic acid (and derivatives) and 5-methyltetrahydrofolate (5-MTHF)—all derived synthetically. Folinic acid (e.g., calcium folinate) is a 5-formyl derivative of tetrahydrofolic acid (THF). Unlike other so-called "active" forms of vitamins, the 5-MTHF "bioidentical" form has clear but limited benefits over other folate forms. First, all folates must be hydrolyzed into monoglutamates, reduced and methylated prior to absorption (see figure), making 5-MTHF a readily absorbable folate; and second, a well-known genetic polymorphism in the final enzyme required to make 5-MTHF is found in a significant number of individuals, reducing their ability to make 5-MTHF.

That said, we should not overstate the clinical advantage of using 5-MTHF over folic acid; as clinical studies show only slight advantages in the general population, and only modest clinical advantages in individuals with the noted genetic predisposition for slow formation of methylfolates (folinic acid is rarely compared).

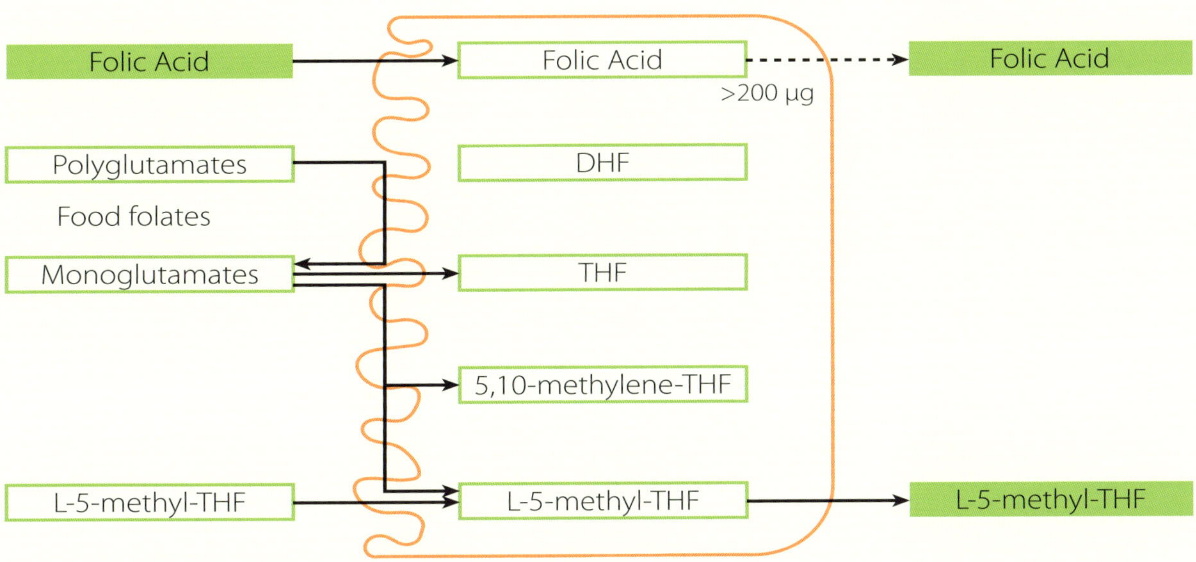

Intestinal folate absorption (from the brush border membrane through the mucosal cell via the portal vein into the peripheral circulation). DHF= dihydrofolate; THF= tetrahydrofolate. Adapted from Pietrzik et al.

One of the most well known single-nucleotide polymorphisms (SNP) in clinical discussion today is located in the gene that expresses a protein that helps to convert folic acid into its active biological molecule, 5-methyltetrahydrofolate. The protein is methylenetetrahydrofolate reductase, abbreviated as MTHFR. In sequencing the gene, researchers identified that some individuals had a cytosine (C) at base pair position 677 (the most common), and others had thymidine (T) at that position. This is often referred to as MTHFR C677T polymorphism, and causes an alanine-to-valine amino acid change at the 222 position of the protein. This small change in the protein results in less-efficient synthesis of active folate compounds—some estimates are 75% less efficient. About 45% of individuals in the U.S. are homozygous for the normal variant (677CC), but about 10% may be homozygous for the other variant (677TT) and others (~45%) heterozygous (677CT) with both gene variants. These heterozygous, and especially homozygous TT, individuals often have noticeably less-efficient methylation, accounting for higher risk for certain diseases and a higher need for folate supplementation.

Even so, clinical studies comparing the ability of folic acid and 5-MTHF supplementation to change serum folate levels or effect changes in homocysteine in both 677TT and 677CC subjects are mixed. Some studies show no statistical difference, or only slight benefit for 5-MTHF, while others show a strong statistical benefit for 5-MTHF supplementation, particularly in bioavailability studies. In a recent study comparing a single dose of either 400 mcg of folic acid or an equimolar amount of 5-MTHF (416 mcg) in women homozygous for either the CC or TT polymorphism, the 5-MTHF supplementation was able to increase plasma folate levels (AUC) by nearly twice that of folic acid. On the other hand, studies of supplementation for 16 or more weeks show only a small increase in the yet-unsaturated measures of folate status.

Beyond bioavailability and homocysteine-lowering, other issues are often discussed when comparing folic acid versus 5-MTHF supplementation. The first is that high-dose folic acid supplements result in an increase in serum levels of unmetabolized folic acid, apparently absorbed before its conversion to 5MTHF through passive absorption. While it is common for researchers to look for unmetabolized folic acid levels in the serum of folic acid-supplemented individuals, there is no clear evidence of a demonstrable negative consequence for these elevated levels. The second issue is high doses of folic acid can mask, not cause, vitamin B_{12} deficiency; supplementation with 5-MTHF appears to be less likely to have this consequence.

One last consideration must be given when deciding between folic acid and 5-MTHF supplementation, and that is cost. 5-MTHF salts—calcium or glucosamine salts are available—are up to 200 times more expensive compared to equimolar amounts of folic acid. Depending on the dose used, this difference can equate to a few dollars per day in the final retail cost of the product.

We recommend clinicians use 5-MTHF supplements, perhaps together in a B-complex product, in patients known to be homozygous (TT) for the MTHFR polymorphism. We also recommend supplementation of 5-MTHF, or 50:50 blends of folic acid:5-MTHF, for prenatal patients, those who are suspected of poor methylation and when using very-high-dose folate products. These suggestions should not be viewed as a recommendation to avoid folic acid in these subjects, as current data suggests neither lack of efficacy or harm when using folic acid in these subjects. There is, however, sufficient data and mechanisms to prefer 5-MTHF in these patient types. Folic acid is adequate for multivitamins intended for the average healthy population, especially where cost may hinder the use of necessary supplementation.

Potential for Toxicity

No adverse effects have been associated with the consumption of excess folate from foods. Concerns regarding safety are limited to synthetic folic acid intake, in regard to its ability to mask, not cause, vitamin B_{12} deficiency. Large doses of folic acid, typically more than five mg, given to an individual with an undiagnosed vitamin B_{12} deficiency could correct megaloblastic anemia without correcting the underlying vitamin B_{12} deficiency, leaving the individual at risk of developing irreversible neurologic damage. Products usually containing more than one mg of folic acid (or 5-MTHF) should be complemented with vitamin B_{12}. The tolerable upper limit for folic acid set by IOM is 1,000 mcg (one mg), often exceeded when used therapeutically.

References:

- Folic Acid Page of Linus Pauling Institute Website: http://lpi.oregonstate.edu/infocenter/vitamins/fa/.
- Office of Dietary Supplements- National Institutes of Health- Health Professional Information. http://ods.od.nih.gov/factsheets/Folate-HealthProfessional/.
- Said HM. Intestinal absorption of water-soluble vitamins in health and disease. *Biochem J.* 2011 Aug 1;437(3):357-72.
- Pietrzik K, Bailey L, Shane B. Folic acid and L-5-methyltetrahydrofolate: comparison of clinical pharmacokinetics and pharmacodynamics. *Clin Pharmacokinet*. 2010 Aug;49(8):535-48.
- Obeid R, Herrmann W. The emerging role of unmetabolized folic acid in human diseases: myth or reality? *Curr Drug Metab.* 2012 Oct;13(8):1184-95.
- Pietrzik K, Lamers Y, Brämswig S, Prinz-Langenohl R. Calculation of red blood cell folate steady state conditions and elimination kinetics after daily supplementation with various folate forms and doses in women of childbearing age. *Am J Clin Nutr.* 2007 Nov;86(5):1414-9.
- Green TJ, Liu Y, Dadgar S, Li W, Böhni R, Kitts DD. Wheat rolls fortified with microencapsulated L-5-methyltetrahydrofolic acid or equimolar folic acid increase blood folate concentrations to a similar extent in healthy men and women. *J Nutr.* 2013 Jun;143(6):867-71.
- Bostom AG, Shemin D et al. Controlled comparison of L-5-methyltetrahydrofolate versus folic acid for the treatment of hyperhomocysteinemia in hemodialysis patients. *Circulation.* 2000 Jun 20;101(24):2829-32.

Vitamin B_{12}/Cobalamin

Intake Guidelines

Recommended Dietary Allowances (RDAs) for Vitamin B_{12}

Age	Males mcg/day	Females mcg/day	Pregnancy mcg/day	Lactation mcg/day
0-6 months	0.4 (AI)	0.4 (AI)		
6-12 months	0.5 (AI)	0.5 (AI)		
1-3 years	0.9	0.9		
4-8 years	1.2	1.2		
9-13 years	1.8	1.8		
14-18 years	2.4	2.4		
19-50 years	2.4	2.4		
51+ years	2.4*	2.4*		
All ages			2.6	2.8

* Vitamin B12 intake should be from supplements or fortified foods due to the age-related increase in food bound malabsorption.

Essential Nutrient Functions

Vitamin B_{12} describes a small collection of large, complex organic molecules organized around a single metal ion: cobalt. These cobalt-containing vitamins are referred to as cobalamin. The biologically active forms of B_{12} include both methylcobalamin and 5-deoxyadenosyl cobalamin. Vitamin B_{12} functions as a cofactor for two key enzymes: methionine synthase as methylcobalamin and L-methylmalonyl-CoA mutase as 5-deoxyadenosyl cobalamin. Methionine synthase coverts homocysteine to methionine, providing a cellular precursor for the formation of the methyl donor S-adenosyl-methionine, or SAMe. L-methylmalonyl-CoA mutase converts L-methylmalonyl-CoA to succinyl-CoA, an essential biochemical reaction in fat and protein metabolism. Succinyl-CoA is also required for hemoglobin synthesis.

Unit(s) of Measure for Guidelines and Labeling

Vitamin B_{12} is measured by weight in mcg of cobalamin.

General Levels of Deficiencies in the U.S.

There is disagreement about whether intake measures adequately address the need for vitamin B_{12}. Using the EAR intake levels and subsequent RDA, NHANES data from 2003 to 2006 suggest few Americans fail to meet these intake guidelines. However, a systematic review of daily vitamin B_{12} loss, combined with poor food bioavailability, may reveal these RDA levels may still leave most Americans in a state of functional insufficiency.

Those most vulnerable to vitamin B_{12} deficiency are individuals with pernicious anemia, the elderly, strict vegetarians and those who regularly take proton pump inhibitors or other acid-blocking drugs. High doses of folic acid do not cause a vitamin B_{12} deficiency, but it can mask certain signs of vitamin B_{12} deficiency (B_{12} is often added to high dose folic acid supplements).

Vitamin B_{12}

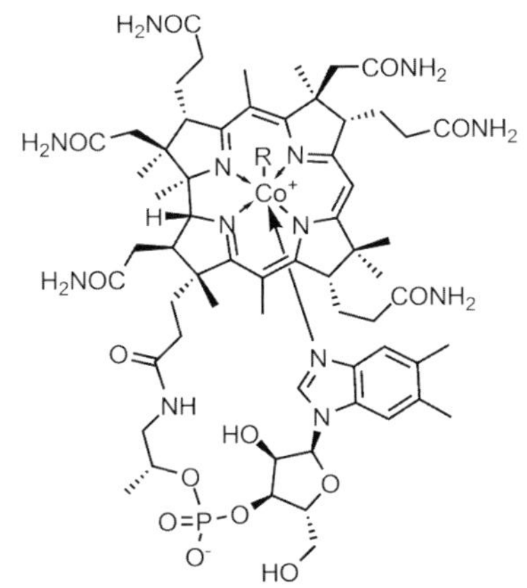

R = 5'-deoxyadenosyl, Me, OH, CN

Natural and Supplemental Forms

The absorption of vitamin B_{12} is more complex than any other vitamin. Food source cobalamins are found in three major forms—hydroxy, methyl, deoxyadenosyl—and one minor form: cyano. These are made exclusively by microorganisms, but accumulate in animals and are found in foods such as meats, fish, eggs and some dairy products. Food-source cobalamin must be released from its protein matrix, a process dependent on adequate stomach acid and pepsin. When released, free cobalamin attaches to proteins from the saliva (haptocorrin) and then, when reaching the higher pH of the small intestine, cobalamin finally combines with intrinsic factor (IF), a protein secreted from the parietal cells of the stomach. This cobalamin-IF complex then binds membrane receptors and is absorbed through endocytosis. The complex nature of oral vitamin B_{12} absorption has led to development of alternative delivery forms of vitamin B_{12} as cyanocobalamin: intramuscular injections, intranasal sprays or gels, and sublingual tablets. None qualify as dietary supplements and would be deemed drugs in the U.S.

Supplemental vitamin B_{12} is commonly available as cyanocobalamin, methylcobalamin or hydroxycobalamin, all "bioequivalent" compounds concentrated from yeast fermentation. Most available information on supplementation and fortification has been performed with cyanocobalamin, though there is no evidence to suggest any of the three forms would be treated differently by the body. Many clinicians prefer the use of methylcobalamin because it is more common in food sources; some prefer it in order to avoid the cyanide of cyanocobalamin, however, no data has suggested harm even with high-dose cyanocobalamin treatment. In this case, methylcobalamin is only slightly more expensive than cyanocobalamin, making it a suitable, if not preferable, form for supplementation.

Finally, studies have shown oral vitamin B_{12} at or near one mg will raise serum B_{12} levels to the same extent as intramuscular injections in studies with elderly, B_{12}-deficient subjects. It appears that when consumed at high doses, sufficient amounts of cobalamin can passively diffuse into the body without the need for adequate intrinsic factor. For this reason, we recommend clinicians consider oral supplements of one mg or more to be clinically equivalent to intramuscular, intranasal or sublingual vitamin B_{12} supplements.

Potential for Toxicity

Due to poor bioavailability of vitamin B_{12} and the lack of side effects from continuous high-dose therapies, there is no known toxicity to vitamin B_{12}. The IOM has not determined a tolerable upper limit for vitamin B_{12}.

References:

- Vitamin B12 Page of Linus Pauling Institute Website: http://lpi.oregonstate.edu/infocenter/vitamins/vitaminB12/.
- Office of Dietary Supplements- National Institutes of Health- Health Professional Information. http://ods.od.nih.gov/factsheets/VitaminB12-HealthProfessional/.
- Said HM. Intestinal absorption of water-soluble vitamins in health and disease. *Biochem J.* 2011 Aug 1;437(3):357-72.
- Elmadfa I, Singer I. Vitamin B-12 and homocysteine status among vegetarians: a global perspective. *Am J Clin Nutr.* 2009 May;89(5):1693S-1698S.
- Allen LH. How common is vitamin B-12 deficiency? *Am J Clin Nutr.* 2009 Feb;89(2):693S-6S.
- Doets EL, In 't Veld PH, Szczecińska A et al. Systematic review on daily vitamin B12 losses and bioavailability for deriving recommendations on vitamin B12 intake with the factorial approach. *Ann Nutr Metab.* 2013;62(4):311-22.
- Vidal-Alaball J, Butler CC et al. Oral vitamin B12 versus intramuscular vitamin B12 for vitamin B12 deficiency. *Cochrane Database Syst Rev.* 2005 Jul 20;(3):CD004655.

Vitamin C

Essential Nutrient Functions

Vitamin C, also known as ascorbic acid, is a water-soluble vitamin naturally present in some foods (naturally and fortified) and available as a dietary supplement. Humans, unlike most animals, are unable to synthesize vitamin C endogenously, making it an essential dietary component. Vitamin C is the primary water-soluble, nonenzymatic antioxidant in plasma and tissues. Vitamin C also participates in redox recycling of other important antioxidants; for example, vitamin C is known to regenerate vitamin E from its oxidized form.

Intake Guidelines

Recommended Dietary Allowances (RDAs) for Vitamin C

Age	Males mg/day	Females mg/day	Pregnancy mg/day	Lactation mg/day
0-6 months	40 (AI)	40 (AI)		
6-12 months	50 (AI)	50 (AI)		
1-3 years	15	15		
4-8 years	25	25		
9-13 years	45	45		
14-18 years	75	65	80	115
19+	90	75	85	120
Smokers	125	110		

In the U.S., the RDA for vitamin C was revised in 2000 upward from the previous recommendation of 60 mg daily for men and women. The RDA is based on the amount of vitamin C intake necessary to maintain neutrophil concentration with minimal urinary excretion of ascorbic acid, presumed to provide sufficient antioxidant protection. The recommended intake for smokers is 35 mg/day higher than for nonsmokers, because smokers are under increased oxidative stress from the toxins in cigarette smoke and generally have lower blood levels of vitamin C. The Linus Pauling Institute recommends a vitamin C intake of at least 400 mg daily for adult men and women.

Unit(s) of Measure for Guidelines and Labeling

Vitamin C is measured by weight of ascorbic acid, ascorbate or dehydroascorbate.

General Levels of Deficiencies in the U.S.

As common as vitamin C is in both food and supplement forms, it is surprising that NHANES data from 2003 to 2006 show the percent of Americans over the age of two with dietary intake of vitamin C below the EAR is more than 45%; and near 35% after considering both fortification and supplementation. Though rare, scurvy is still present in developed countries in individuals with extremely poor diets.

Vitamin C

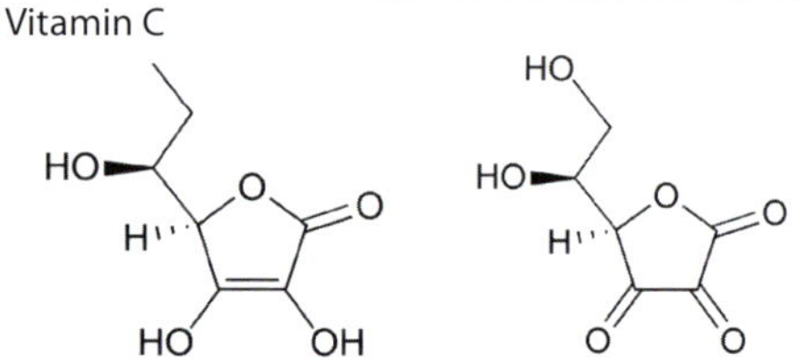

Ascorbic Acid   Dehydroascorbic Acid

Natural and Supplemental Forms

Natural vitamin C is found as either ascorbic acid or dehydroascorbic acid, or their anion forms. The most common natural-sourced vitamin C used in supplements comes from rose hips and acerola fruit. Supplemental vitamin C is commonly in the form of L-ascorbic acid, usually synthesized from corn-derived L-sorbose, or in one of many ascorbate salts, along with calcium, sodium, magnesium, potassium, palmitic acid, etc.

According to the Linus Pauling Institute, considered one of the leading experts in vitamin C research, *"natural and synthetic L-ascorbic acid are chemically identical, and there are no known differences in their biological activity. A study of 12 males (six smokers and six nonsmokers) found bioavailability of synthetic ascorbic acid (powder administered in water) to be slightly superior to that of orange juice, based on blood levels of ascorbic acid, and not different based on ascorbic acid in leukocytes (white blood cells).*

A study in 68 male nonsmokers found that ascorbic acid consumed in cooked broccoli, orange juice, orange slices and as synthetic ascorbic acid tablets are equally bioavailable, as measured by plasma ascorbic acid levels."

Likewise, various mineral ascorbates claim to have superior bioavailability. One in particular, Ester-C®, is popular as a dietary supplement. Ester-C® contains mainly calcium ascorbate, but also has small amounts of the vitamin C metabolites dehydroascorbic acid (oxidized ascorbic acid), calcium threonate, and trace levels of xylonate and lyxonate. The manufacturer states the metabolites, especially threonate, increase bioavailability of the product's vitamin C. They indicate they have performed a study in humans demonstrating increased bioavailability of vitamin C in Ester-C®. This study has not been published in a peer-reviewed journal. A small published study of vitamin C bioavailability in eight women and one man found no difference between Ester-C® and commercially available ascorbic acid tablets with respect to the absorption and urinary excretion of vitamin C.

Finally, there is debate about supplementing vitamin C with added flavonoids (e.g., quercetin, rutin, etc.). While data is mixed as to the ability of added flavonoids to increase the bioavailability of ascorbic acid, we believe this practice is without harm as dietary flavonoids have many other documented benefits in humans, and the added flavonoid signals are contextually appropriate for vitamin C delivery.

Potential for Toxicity

Vitamin C is considered non-toxic, but has unwanted side effects in most people when consumed in high amounts. However, the dose that brings about these side effects (temporary diarrhea/GI disturbance) is different in each individual and is considered part of some "alternative" therapies (see Linus Pauling Institute website for extensive discussion). In any case, the IOM has published the tolerable upper limit for vitamin C at 2,000 mg (two g) per day.

References:

- Vitamin C Page of Linus Pauling Institute Website: http://lpi.oregonstate.edu/infocenter/vitamins/vitaminC/.
- Office of Dietary Supplements- National Institutes of Health- Health Professional Information. http://ods.od.nih.gov/factsheets/VitaminC-HealthProfessional/.
- Velandia B, Centor RM, McConnell V, Shah M. Scurvy is still present in developed countries. *J Gen Intern Med.* 2008 Aug;23(8):1281-4.
- Mangels, A.R. et al. The bioavailability to humans of ascorbic acid from oranges, orange juice, and cooked broccoli is similar to that of synthetic ascorbic acid. *Journal of Nutrition.* 1993; volume 123: pages 1054-1061.
- Gregory, J.F. Ascorbic acid bioavailability in foods and supplements. *Nutrition Reviews.* 1993; volume 51: pages 301-309.
- Johnston, C.S. & Luo, B. Comparison of the absorption and excretion of three commercially available sources of vitamin C. *Journal of the American Dietetic Association.* 1994; volume 94: pages 779-781.
- Hollman PC, Katan MB. Bioavailability and health effects of dietary flavonols in man. *Arch Toxicol Suppl.* 1998;20:237-48.

Vitamin D

Essential Nutrient Functions

Vitamin D is a fat-soluble precursor compound that can be converted in the body to its active, hormone-like nutrient 1,25 dihydroxyvitamin D. Vitamin D acts primarily via regulation of gene expression (genomics) facilitated by the action of the vitamin D receptor, a nuclear transcription factor (see page 22 for more details). Vitamin D is not strictly an essential "vitamin," in that humans are capable of producing the active nutrient when appropriate amounts of sunlight contact the skin.

Intake Guidelines

Recommended Dietary Allowances (RDAs) for Vitamin D

Age	Males mcg/day (IU/day)	Females mcg/day (IU/day)	Pregnancy mcg/day (IU/day)	Lactation mcg/day (IU/day)
0-6 months	10 mcg (400 IU) (AI)	10 mcg (400 IU) (AI)		
6-12 months	10 mcg (400 IU) (AI)	10 mcg (400 IU) (AI)		
1-3 years	15 mcg (600 IU)	15 mcg (600 IU)		
4-8 years	15 mcg (600 IU)	15 mcg (600 IU)		
9-13 years	15 mcg (600 IU)	15 mcg (600 IU)		
14-18 years	15 mcg (600 IU)	15 mcg (600 IU)		
Adults 19-50	15 mcg (600 IU)	15 mcg (600 IU)		
Adults 51-70	15 mcg (600 IU)	15 mcg (600 IU)		
Adults 71+	20 mcg (800 IU)	20 mcg (800 IU)		
All ages			15 mcg (600 IU)	15 mcg (600 IU)

Our discussion of IOM's new guidelines can be found on Page 84

Unit(s) of Measure for Guidelines and Labeling

Vitamin D levels are reported in International Units (IU) or mcg. To convert mcg of vitamin D_3 into IUs, multiply by 40 (one mcg = 40 IU). Dietary supplement and food labels prior to 2018 were only required to report vitamin D in IUs. Since 2018, labels must report using mcg, while including the IU equivalent in parentheses is voluntary.

General Levels of Deficiencies in the U.S.

The past few decades have revolutionized our understanding of the importance of this nutrient and raised the awareness of the prevalence and consequences of global vitamin D deficiency. In the U.S., outside of fish, fish-liver oil and fortified foods (e.g., milk), vitamin D must be obtained through sunlight or dietary supplements. NHANES data from 2003 to 2006 show the percent of Americans over the age of two with dietary intake of vitamin D below the EAR is nearly 100%. Meaning, unless subjects are getting enough regular sunlight or supplementing vitamin D, they will be low in vitamin D. Those with dark skin or who avoid skin exposure to sunlight are also at risk for vitamin D deficiency. In addition, obesity increases the need for vitamin D supplementation, so the number of individuals with functional insufficiencies regardless of their vitamin D intake grows with the obesity epidemic. See the extended monograph on page 84 for a discussion of serum vitamin D levels in the context of determining individual need for supplementation.

Vitamin D

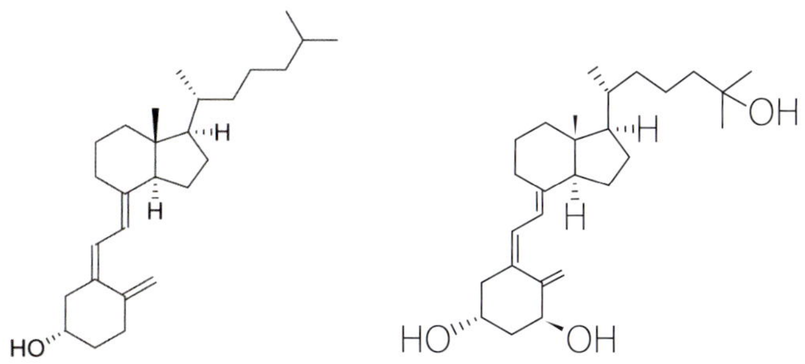

Vitamin D_3 (Cholecalciferol) 1,25-dihydroxyvitamin D

Natural and Supplemental Forms

The only reliable and 100%-natural form of vitamin D for humans comes through direct conversion from sunlight exposure or the consumption of oily fish such as sardines, mackerel and salmon. Vitamin D used for supplementation or fortification is mostly from "bioidentical" vitamin D_3, which comes from the conversion of cholesterol derivatives found in sheep wool lanolin. This process and source, which requires exposure to the same light (UVB) that helps our skin make vitamin D_3, is a concern for strict vegan individuals. The other source of vitamin D, used in pharmaceutical products and some supplements, is ergocalciferol, also known as vitamin D_2. This compound comes from UV light-exposed ergosterol (mostly from yeast) and was used in pharmaceutical preparations for decades before the more commonly used vitamin D_3. A review of the chemistry and clinical outcomes of these two compounds suggests vitamin D_3 is preferable as a supplemental nutrient.

Potential for Toxicity

Hypervitaminosis D is rare, but technically possible with long-term, very-high daily vitamin D supplementation. For instance, while 50,000 IU (1250 mcg) has been documented as a safe once-weekly supplement, this amount has not been documented to be safe when used daily for long periods. The tolerable upper intake level set by the IOM is 100 mcg (4000 IU), a number that we believe is too conservative and based on poor science (please read further on the following pages). Serum 25(OH)D levels above 100 ng/ml should be considered a sign of oversupplementation of vitamin D_3.

References:

- Vitamin D Page of Linus Pauling Institute Website: http://lpi.oregonstate.edu/infocenter/vitamins/vitaminD/.
- Office of Dietary Supplements- National Institutes of Health- Health Professional Information. http://ods.od.nih.gov/factsheets/VitaminD-HealthProfessional/.
- Wang L, Song Y et al. Circulating 25-hydroxy-vitamin D and risk of cardiovascular disease: a meta-analysis of prospective studies. *Circ Cardiovasc Qual Outcomes.* 2012 Nov;5(6):819-29.
- Pike JW, Meyer MB. Fundamentals of vitamin D hormone-regulated gene expression. *J Steroid Biochem Mol Biol.* 2013 Nov 12. pii: S0960-0760(13)00234-3.
- Houghton LA, Vieth R. The case against ergocalciferol (vitamin D_2) as a vitamin supplement. *Am J Clin Nutr.* 2006 Oct;84(4):694-7.

Target Levels and Optimal Dosing of Vitamin D

Research supporting vitamin D supplementation has increased dramatically over the past decade and has significantly revitalized interest in this important nutrient. While in the past, vitamin D was mainly recognized for its role in bone health, recent epidemiological and randomized-controlled trials have uncovered relationships between low levels of vitamin D and a number of chronic conditions, including muscle pain and weakness, autoimmune diseases such as type 1 diabetes, colorectal cancer, cardiovascular disease, inflammatory bowel disease, and multiple sclerosis. These significant and widespread findings have prompted new controversy in defining "optimal" serum levels of vitamin D, as well as the doses needed to achieve them. This discussion will review key conclusions of the recent Institute of Medicine (IOM) report on vitamin D and address the question of optimal dosing of vitamin D for the prevention of chronic disease.

Dietary reference intakes (DRIs) for vitamins established by the IOM are intended to serve as a guide for good nutrition and to provide the basis for nutrient guidelines in the U.S. and Canada. In the case of vitamin D, the process of establishing recommendations for intake levels is more complex for several reasons. Unlike other vitamins, serum levels of vitamin D are the result of both dietary intake, mainly through fatty fish, eggs, beef and supplements, and synthesis of the nutrient within the skin after exposure to UVB sunlight. Both factors vary from person to person, though sun exposure is the source of 90 – 95% of vitamin D for the majority of the population not consuming supplements.[1] Like dietary intake, exposure to the sun is variable and often significantly reduced as a result of increased sunscreen use and more time spent indoors, adding to the complexity of formulating recommendations for intake.

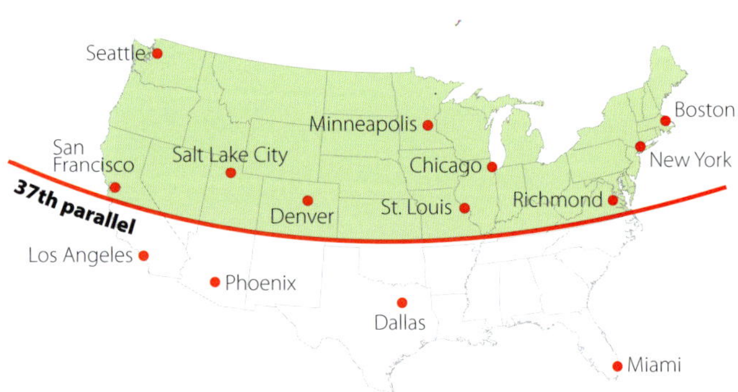

Figure A: 37th Parallel in U.S.- Often considered the line, above which, it is difficult to form vitamin D from sunlight exposure.

Note: Except during the summer months, the skin makes little if any vitamin D from sun exposure at latitudes above 37 degrees north (in the United States, the shaded region in the map) or below 37 degrees south of the equator. People who live in these areas are at relatively greater risk for vitamin D deficiency[2]

In light of emerging data, the recently issued IOM report[3] on vitamin D recommends increasing the DRI for vitamin D intake for all age groups as follows:

- Infants: double intake to 400 IU (10 mcg)
- Ages one – 50: triple intake to 600 IU (15 mcg)
- Ages 51 – 70: double intake to 600 IU (15 mcg)
- Ages 71+: increase intake by 33%, up to 800 IU (20 mcg)

According to the IOM report, average total dietary intake of vitamin D is well below the median requirement. However, the report also claims that a majority of Americans and Canadians have adequate levels of vitamin D, with average blood levels above the target level of 20 ng/mL (50 nmol/L), the level deemed necessary by the IOM for the general population based on bone-health studies. In addition, the IOM report highlights "emerging evidence that too much [vitamin D]... may be harmful," and warns that once intake of vitamin D surpasses the upper limit (UL) of 4,000 IUs per day, the risk for harm begins to increase, with very high levels known to cause kidney and tissue damage.

Response to the IOM report

The changes made to the recommended intake of vitamin D by the IOM are conservative, and have come as a surprise to many researchers and physicians who have questioned the relevance of these new DRIs in the clinical setting. While increases in the intake guidelines for vitamin D may have a beneficial effect overall, they do not reflect the large body of evidence that demonstrates a need for intake to be *at least* 2,000 IU/day for the prevention of chronic diseases in adults. Part of this discrepancy is because the committee only considered studies on vitamin D and bone health, and neglected to include research on other chronic conditions such as colorectal cancer, citing conflicting data. The report also neglected to mention large segments of the population with an inadequate vitamin D status, such as minority populations, despite data from the National Health and Nutritional Examination Surveys (NHANES) that examined over 15,390 participants and found that serum levels of 25(OH)D were below recommended levels for a large portion of the general adult population.

The IOM committee also raised concerns about vitamin D toxicity; however, the number of reports on such occurrences is small, while reports of deficiency have reached epidemic numbers. The kidney's ability to limit production of calcitriol, the active form of vitamin D, is a tightly controlled mechanism, thus concern about toxicity may be disproportionate compared to evidence for risk of deficiency.

Laboratory values

The IOM report emphasized current measurements, or cutoff points, of sufficiency and deficiency of 25(OH)D in use by laboratories have not been set using rigorous scientific studies. They suggest that since no central authority has determined which cut-off points to use, reports of deficiency may be skewed and numbers overestimated. In fact, laboratory reference-ranges for serum 25(OH)D levels have long been based on average values from populations of healthy individuals. It is the recent research, suggesting health-based cutoff values be aimed at preventing secondary hyperparathyroidism and bone loss, that pushed for the numbers to be increased.[4] Furthermore, recent evaluations have detected an improvement in the clinical measurement of vitamin D; it is projected the availability of reference materials from the National Institute of Standards and Technology will further improve confidence in these measurements.[5] However, it is important to note values deemed sufficient by major laboratories differ from those recommended in the latest research.

Target serum levels

The IOM report references data that suggest sun exposure contributes meaningful amounts of vitamin D to North Americans, indicating a majority of the population is meeting its needs for vitamin D. In addition to geographical limits on sun exposure experienced by many North Americans, this conclusion is based on a low target-serum level of 20 ng/ml (50 nmol/L; to convert from ng/mL to nmol/l, multiply by 2.5), shown in recent studies to be insufficient for the prevention of chronic vitamin D-associated diseases. However, there is increasing agreement among vitamin D researchers that values less than approximately 30 – 32 ng/mL (75 – 80 nmol/l) should be classified as "low," making low vitamin D status common worldwide.[5] Interestingly, even the now-higher levels recommended by the IOM seem to be insufficient for bone health. Two 2009 meta-analyses of double-blind, randomized, controlled trials have found 20 ng/ml (50 nmol/l) to be insufficient for fracture or fall reduction based on achieved 25(OH)D levels in the treatment groups.[6,7] Moreover, the 2010 position-paper of the International Osteoporosis Foundation (IOF) has recommended a threshold of 30 ng/ml (75 nmol/l) for optimal fall and fracture reduction, and a dietary intake of 800 to 1,000 IU of vitamin D per day for seniors age 60 years and older.[8]

While benefits of serum concentrations higher than 20 ng/ml (50 nmol/l) on endpoints other than bone health have not been documented by randomized trials, the evidence for benefit is quite strong for certain conditions, especially colorectal cancer.[9] Studies from areas of epidemiology, and molecular and cellular biology have shown increasing support for serum concentrations of 25(OH)D higher than 28 ng/ml (70 nmol/L) as being both natural and beneficial to human health.[10,11] A report from the Office of Dietary Supplements of the National Institutes of Health has further concluded there is not enough evidence to recommend a specific upper limit of serum 25(OH)D that would indicate vitamin D sufficiency.

Optimal dosages

Many U.S. experts consider 30 ng/mL (75 nmol/L) 25(OH)D to be an optimal serum level of vitamin D, such as Michael Holick, one of the world's leading researchers on vitamin D, who agrees that 30 ng/mL (75 nmol/L) "is required to maximize vitamin D's beneficial effects for health." When using this functional target of 28 – 30 ng/mL (70 – 75 nmol/L), an intake of 600 IU (the new adult DRI) is insufficient for most to achieve such levels and the question arises as to what dose of vitamin D is needed to attain this higher target in most patients. Based on the suggestion that one mcg or 40 IU per day increases 25(OH)D serum levels by an average of 0.4 ng/mL (one nmol/L)[10,12] lower intakes in the range of 200 – 600 IU (5 – 15 mcg) per day would not increase serum vitamin D levels in a sufficient manner.[13-15]

According to a 2008 review,

"Supplementation with 1,000 IU per day [of cholecalciferol] will usually result in about a 10 ng/mL elevation of serum 25(OH)D when given over 3 – 4 months. Therefore, a

normal-weight, healthy adult with an initial level of 10 ng/mL would generally require about 2,000 IU per day to achieve a level of 30 ng/mL in the absence of cutaneous UVB exposure. However, its kinetics are not linear; 1,000 IU per day will substantially raise low baseline levels, but a similar dose will not increase higher baseline levels by a similar increment (that is, 2,000 IU per day may not raise 30 ng/mL to 50 ng/mL). In the absence of significant UVB exposure, input from diet and supplements of approximately 1,000 IU (25 mcg) per day for every 15 kg of body weight may be needed, i.e. an obese 150-kg adult may require up to 10,000 IU per day to achieve a 25(OH) D level of 50 ng/mL."[16]

A recent study from the *American Journal of Clinical Nutrition*[17] examined what the optimal dose of vitamin D would need to be in order to raise serum 25(OH)D levels to greater than 30 ng/mL (75 nmol/L) without exceeding 88ng/mL (220 nmol/L). The six-month, double-blind, randomized, placebo-controlled trial enrolled 138 healthy men (n=26) and women (n=112) ages 18 – 65; initial doses of vitamin D were determined from baseline status. Individuals with a 25(OH)D baseline concentration between 20 – 32 ng/mL (50 – 80 nmol/L) were given 50 μg/day of vitamin D_3 (2,000 IU) and those with a baseline concentration below 20 ng/mL (50 nmol/L) were given 100 μg/day of vitamin D_3 (4,000 IU). The patients were followed at eight-week intervals and the dose was increased or decreased in 50 μg or 20 μg increments after each visit. The mean daily dose given was 86 μg/day (3,440 IU) of vitamin D_3. After optimization through computer modeling, an optimal daily dose of 115 μg/day (4,600 IU) of supplemental vitamin D_3 was found to be necessary for most patients in order to maintain serum 25(OH)D levels between the range of 30 – 88 ng/mL (75 – 220 nmol/L). When the observations from this study were projected onto the population of the third National Health and Nutrition Examination Survey (NHANES III), an optimal dose of 3,800 IU of vitamin D per day was found to be necessary for those above a baseline reading of 22 ng/ml (55 nmol/L), and a dose of 5,000 IU for those below the baseline.

In the case of severe vitamin D deficiency,[18] some studies have suggested loading doses of 50,000 IU once weekly for two to three months or three-times weekly for one month, with added doses of 800 – 2000 IU per day regardless of dosing pattern, to prevent recurrent deficiency. One study that looked at daily, weekly and monthly protocols of vitamin D_3 supplementation with an outcome measure of 25(OH)D found all three patterns of dosing and supplementation equally beneficial.[19] The dosing approach should be selected based on patient adherence and should take into account personal health goals, ethnic background, age, geographic location and season.

Vitamin D_2 or D_3

Studies on rickets prevention in the 1930s led to the long-term assumption that vitamin D_2 and D_3 are equally effective in humans.[20] However, previous results were often skewed by the stability of preparations used in the studies, and there is a lack of consistent and objective evidence that the two forms of the vitamin are equivalent with regards to increasing 25(OH)D levels.[20] Since the serum half-life of D_3 is longer, it is the preferred form if administered less than once weekly.[18] A growing number of studies over the past decade have also found evidence D_3 increases serum 25(OH)D levels more efficiently than D_2.[20,21] One group found the increase in blood levels with vitamin D_3 to be 70% greater (1.7 times) than the increase provided by D_2. In addition, a 2010 study found after 12 weeks of weekly supplementation with 50,000 IU of vitamin D in 33 adults, levels increased significantly more in the D_3 group than in the D_2 group, with D_3 being 87% more potent in raising serum concentrations, and with two-to-three-fold greater tissue storage than D_2.[12,22]

The Vitamin K Question

Vitamin K has also been increasingly linked to bone health in recent years and has spurred a new interest among clinicians in the supplementation of the vitamin together with vitamin D and calcium in many bone-health support protocols.[23] A growing number of epidemiological studies have highlighted a key role of vitamin K in optimizing bone heath.[24] Low vitamin K intake and low plasma levels of the vitamin have repeatedly been associated with low bone-mineral density as well as increased osteoporotic fractures in postmenopausal women;[25-28] however, other randomized controlled trials have shown mixed results.[23,29] Newer research has found vitamin D and K work synergistically to support bone health.[30,31,32] One study suggests high doses of vitamin D may increase the demand for vitamin K. This model implies the administration of doses of vitamin D beyond the upper limit could cause a functional deficiency of vitamin K, based upon the role of Vitamin D in upregulating the expression of Gla proteins, while osteocalcin activation depends on vitamin K-mediated carboxylation.[33] Such literature suggests vitamin K be supplemented together with vitamin D, though no conclusive randomized controlled trials to date support this hypothesis.[34] Despite this lack of evidence, the synergistic relationship of vitamins K and D warrants monitoring serum K or uncarboxylated osteocalcin levels, and supplementing dosages of vitamin K as necessary.

Conclusion

While the IOM has done well to recognize the need for increased vitamin D consumption by all Americans, optimal vitamin D levels will likely not be achieved (for all of vitamin D's benefits) with the new recommendations. We advocate a target goal of 30 ng/mL for all patients and suggest a serum level of 40 – 70 ng/mL may be needed in various vitamin D-related chronic health conditions. The following are recommendations for assessing serum levels and recommending vitamin D_3 dosages for different age groups.

A. Serum 25-OH Vitamin D Levels

	ng/mL	nmol/L
Deficiency	<15	25 to 37
Insufficiency	15 to 30	37 to 75
Minimum target	30	75
Therapeutic*	40-70	100 to 175
Upper limit	100	250
Excessive	>100	>250

*May be considered "optimal" in patients with specific vitamin D-mediated chronic disease conditions. Evidence is lacking for specific recommendations. The Vitamin D Council recommends a target level of 50-80 ng/mL, year-round.

B. Recommended Daily Doses of Vitamin D_3[35,36]

	1 & younger	1 & older	Adults	71 & older	Blood Testing
The Point Institute*	Not more than 25 mcg (1000 IU)	25 mcg (1,000 IU)	95-125 mcg (3,800-5,000 IU)	95-125 mcg (3,800-5,000 IU)	Every 6 months
IOM-DRI	10 mcg (400 IU)	15 mcg (600 IU)	15 mcg (600 IU)	20 mcg (800 IU)	
Dr. Michael Holick	25 mcg (1,000 IU)	25 mcg (1,000 IU)	50-75 mcg (2,000-3,000 IU)	50-75 mcg (2,000-3,000 IU)	
Vitamin D Council	25 mcg (1,000 IU)	25 mcg (1000 IU) per 25 lbs	125 mcg (5,000 IU)	125 mcg (5000 IU)	Every 2-3 months

Dose should be monitored by testing and adjusted based on sunlight exposure

Other points to remember:

- Serum vitamin D testing should be for 25-OH not 1,25 OH vitamin D
- When supplementing vitamin D, choose D_3 over D_2
- Add vitamin K as necessary; if possible, monitor blood levels
- Obesity increases the need for vitamin D supplementation; weight loss may reduce need for vitamin D supplementation

References

1. Holick MF. The vitamin D epidemic and its health consequences. *J Nutr.* Nov 2005;135(11):2739S-2748S.
2. http://www.health.harvard.edu/newsweek/time-for-more-vitamin-d.htm.
3. IOM. http://www.iom.edu/Reports/2010/Dietary-Reference-Intakes-for-Calcium-and-Vitamin-D/Report-Brief.aspx?page=2.
4. http://lpi.oregonstate.edu/infocenter/vitamins/vitaminD/.
5. Binkley N, Ramamurthy R, Krueger D. Low vitamin D status: definition, prevalence, consequences, and correction. *Endocrinol Metab Clin North Am.* Jun 2010;39(2):287-301, table of contents.
6. Bischoff-Ferrari HA, Willett WC, Wong JB, et al. Prevention of nonvertebral fractures with oral vitamin D and dose dependency: a meta-analysis of randomized controlled trials. *Arch Intern Med.* Mar 23 2009;169(6):551-561.
7. Bischoff-Ferrari HA, Dawson-Hughes B, Staehelin HB, et al. Fall prevention with supplemental and active forms of vitamin D: a meta-analysis of randomised controlled trials. *BMJ.* 2009;339:b3692.
8. Dawson-Hughes B, Mithal A, Bonjour JP, et al. IOF position statement: vitamin D recommendations for older adults. *Osteoporos Int.* Jul 2010;21(7):1151-1154.
9. Giovannucci E. Epidemiological evidence for vitamin D and colorectal cancer. J *Bone Miner Res.* Dec 2007;22 Suppl 2:V81-85.
10. Vieth R. Why the optimal requirement for Vitamin D3 is probably much higher than what is officially recommended for adults. J *Steroid Biochem Mol Biol.* May 2004;89-90(1-5):575-579.
11. Mosekilde L. Vitamin D requirement and setting recommendation levels: long-term perspectives. *Nutr Rev.* Oct 2008;66(10 Suppl 2):S170-177.
12. R.P. Heany KMD, T.C. Chen, M.F. Holick, M.J. Barger-Lux. Human serum 25-hydroxycholecalciferol response to extended oral dosing with cholecalciferol. *Am J Clin Nutr.* 2003;77:204-210.
13. FM Gloth III JT, SS Sherman, BW Hollis. Is the recommended daily allowance for Vitamin D too low for the homebound elderly? *J. Am. Geriatr. Soc.* 1991;39:137-141.
14. H. Glerup KM, L. Poulsen, et al. Hypovitaminosis D myopathy without biochemical signs of osteomalacic bone involvement. *Calcif Tissue Int.* 2000;66(419-424).
15. R. Vieth DC, GA Hawker, HM Trang, LA Rubin. Wintertime Vitamin D insufficiency is common in young Canadian women and their vitamin D intake does not prevent it. *Eur. J Clin Nut.* 2001;55(1091-1097).
16. Cannell JJ, Hollis BW. Use of vitamin D in clinical practice. *Altern Med Rev.* Mar 2008;13(1):6-20.
17. Aloia JF, Patel M, Dimaano R, et al. Vitamin D intake to attain a desired serum 25-hydroxyvitamin D concentration. *Am J Clin Nutr.* Jun 2008;87(6):1952-1958.
18. Kennel KA, Drake MT, Hurley DL. Vitamin D deficiency in adults: when to test and how to treat. *Mayo Clin Proc.* Aug 2010;85(8):752-757.
19. Ish-Shalom S, Segal E, Salganik T, Raz B, Bromberg IL, Vieth R. Comparison of daily, weekly, and monthly vitamin D3 in ethanol dosing protocols for two months in elderly hip fracture patients. *J Clin Endocrinol Metab.* Sep 2008;93(9):3430-3435.
20. Trang HM, Cole DE, Rubin LA, Pierratos A, Siu S, Vieth R. Evidence that vitamin D3 increases serum 25-hydroxyvitamin D more efficiently than does vitamin D2. *Am J Clin Nutr.* Oct 1998;68(4):854-858.

21. Daroux M, Shenouda M et al. Vitamin D2 versus vitamin D3 supplementation in hemodialysis patients: a comparative pilot study. *J Nephrol*. 2013 Jan-Feb;26(1):152-7

22. Heaney RP, Recker RR, Grote J, Horst RL, Armas LA. Vitamin D3 Is More Potent Than Vitamin D2 in Humans. *J Clin Endocrinol Metab*. Dec 22 2010.

23. Cheung AM, Tile L, Lee Y, et al. Vitamin K supplementation in postmenopausal women with osteopenia (ECKO trial): a randomized controlled trial. *PLoS Med.* Oct 14 2008;5(10):e196.

24. Lanham-New SA. Importance of calcium, vitamin D and vitamin K for osteoporosis prevention and treatment. *Proceedings of the Nutrition Society*. 2008;67(02).

25. Feskanich D, Weber P, Willett WC, Rockett H, Booth SL, Colditz GA. Vitamin K intake and hip fractures in women: a prospective study. *Am J.Clin.Nutr.* 1999;69(1):74-79.

26. Hodges SJ AK, Vergnaud P, Obrant K, Delmas PD. Circulating levels of vitamins K1 and K2 decreased in elderly women with hip fracture. J *Bone Miner Res*. 1993;8:1241–1245.

27. Hodges SJ PM, Stamp TC, Catterall A, Shearer MJ, et al. Depressed levels of circulating menaquinones in patients with osteoporotic fractures of the spine and femoral neck. *Bone* 1991;12:387-389.

28. Bitensky L HJ, Catterall A, Hodges SJ, Pilkington MJ, et al. Circulating vitamin K levels in patients with fractures. *J Bone Joint Surg BR*. 1988;70:663–664.

29. Purwosunu Y, Rachman IA, Reksoprodjo S, Sekizawa A. Vitamin K2 treatment for postmenopausal osteoporosis in Indonesia. *Journal of Obstetrics and Gynaecology Research*. 2006;32(2):230-234.

30. Bolton-Smith C, McMurdo ME, Paterson CR, et al. Two-year randomized controlled trial of vitamin K1 (phylloquinone) and vitamin D3 plus calcium on the bone health of older women. *J Bone Miner.Res.* 2007;22(4):509-519.

31. Iwamoto J, Takeda T, Ichimura S. Treatment with vitamin D3 and/or vitamin K2 for postmenopausal osteoporosis. *Keio J Med.* Sep 2003;52(3):147-150.

32. Braam LA, Knapen MH, Geusens P, et al. Vitamin K1 supplementation retards bone loss in postmenopausal women between 50 and 60 years of age. *Calcif Tissue Int.* Jul 2003;73(1):21-26.

33. Pizzorno L. Vitamin D and Vitamin K Team Up to Lower CVD Risk: Part II. http://www.lmreview.com/articles/view/vitamin-d-and-vitamin-k-team-up-to-lower-cvd-risk-part-II/#fn-44-72.

34. Masterjohn C. Vitamin D toxicity redefined: Vitamin K and the molecular mechanism. *Medical Hypotheses.* 2007;68(5):1026-1034.

35. Holick MF. Vitamin D Deficiency. *New Engl. J. Med.* 2007;357:266-281.

36. Council VD. http://www.vitamindcouncil.org/.

Vitamin E

Essential Nutrient Functions

Vitamin E and its related compounds are key fat-soluble antioxidants. These compounds, known as tocopherols and tocotrienols, are responsible for a number of biological functions; but only one compound, alpha-tocopherol, is deemed a vitamin.

Intake Guidelines

Recommended Dietary Allowances (RDAs) for Vitamin E

Age	Males mg/day *(IU/day)	Females mg/day *(IU/day)	Pregnancy mg/day *(IU/day)	Lactation mg/day *(IU/day)
0-6 months (AI)	4 mg (6 IU)	4 mg (6 IU)		
6-12 months (AI)	5 mg (7.5 IU)	5 mg (7.5 IU)		
1-3 years	6 mg (9 IU)	6 mg (9 IU)		
4-8 years	7 mg (10.5 IU)	7 mg (10.5 IU)		
9-13 years	11 mg (16.5 IU)	11 mg (16.5 IU)		
14-18 years	15 mg (22.5 IU)	15 mg (22.5 IU)		
Adults 19+	15 mg (22.5 IU)	15 mg (22.5 IU)		
All ages			15 mg (22.5 IU)	19 mg (28.5 IU)

*Calculated as d-alpha-tocopherol. 1mg=1.49 IU.

Unit(s) of Measure for Guidelines and Labeling

Vitamin E can be measured and reported in milligrams or International Units (IU). After 2018, food and dietary supplement labels must report vitamin E as mg of alpha-tocopherol. When a synthetic (all-racemic) form of vitamin E is used in a supplement, it is considered to have one half of the potency (i.e., 2 mg of all-racemic= 1 mg of natural tocopherol) for labeling purposes. The IU equivalent of vitamin E may be absent from the label after 2018.

General Levels of Deficiencies in the U.S.

True vitamin E deficiency is rarely diagnosed in the United States. However, insufficient intake of vitamin E is widespread. NHANES data from 2003 to 2006 show that the percent of Americans over the age of two with dietary intake of vitamin E below the EAR is 90%, and above 60% when all supplemented vitamin E is included.

Vitamin E

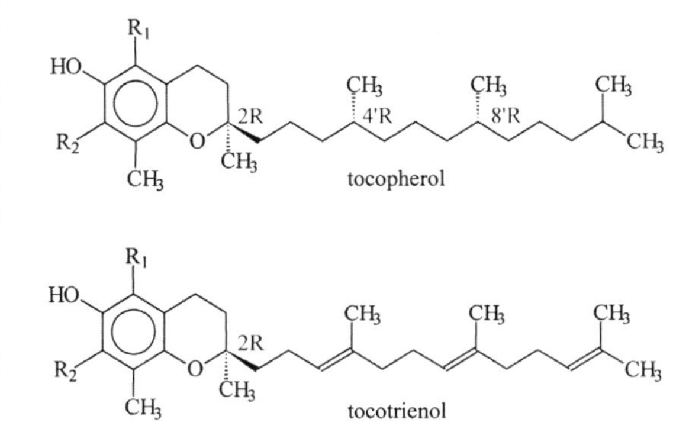

R_1	R_2	
CH_3	CH_3	α
CH_3	H	β
H	CH_3	γ
H	H	δ

Natural and Supplemental Forms

Describing the multiple forms of natural and synthetic vitamin E can be confusing. The reason is that while the alpha-form of tocopherol is the only form defined as having vitamin E activity, there are seven other compounds in the vitamin E family that may have varying levels of biological activity. The eight forms of "vitamin E" are alpha, beta, gamma and delta tocopherol; and alpha, beta, gamma and delta tocotrienol. The four forms differ in the arrangement of methyl-groups around the chromanol ring; while each of the four tocotrienol molecules contain three double-bonds within the aliphatic side chain.

Mixed tocopherols vs. alpha-tocopherol

Even though alpha-tocopherol is the only form used to officially calculate vitamin E, it is not the most abundant food source of tocopherol in the U.S.; in fact, because of the high consumption of soybean and corn oil, gamma-tocopherol is consumed in much higher amounts than alpha-tocopherol. However, in the rat resorption-gestation test (the test that defined the vitamin's activity), gamma-tocopherol only has about 10% of the measure of vitamin E activity The question researchers are currently asking is what role each of the other (non-alpha) forms of tocopherol provide nutritionally, and what level of supplementation of these compounds is warranted.

There is a growing body of evidence that different forms of tocopherols can act in physiologically different ways when consumed by humans. This suggests vitamin E might be better supplemented as a mix of the various forms, usually labeled as "mixed tocopherols." Others argue that since gamma-tocopherol is abundant in the diet, alpha-tocopherol supplementation alone is sufficient. However, some data suggest supplementation with alpha-tocopherol alone can *hinder* dietary gamma-tocopherol bioavailability, increasing the case for the use of mixed tocopherols. In any case, only the alpha-tocopherol portion of the ingredient can be listed as vitamin E; the weight of other tocopherols must be listed, in mg, below the line separating items with and without a DV in the Supplement Facts box.

Natural vs. synthetic

The tocopherol molecules above have three different chiral centers: position two, four and eight along the aliphatic side chain. These positions are critical in understanding the difference between natural and synthetic vitamin E. In natural vitamin E, all three chiral carbons are in the "R" position (as noted in the figure above). Natural vitamin E, then, is sometimes referred to as RRR-alpha-tocopherol. On the other hand, synthetic vitamin E is an equal mixture of eight different isomers based on the combination (R or S) of these three chiral positions (RSR, RSS, etc.). Together these are called d,l alpha-tocopherol or all-racemic alpha-tocopherol. Because these other isomers have less to no vitamin E activity, synthetic vitamin E has much less activity, by weight, than natural vitamin E, derived from soybean, corn and other commercial oils. While the difference in activity is considered when calculating the IU for these isomers, the presence of these nonactive isomers may result in the diminished effect seen in many clinical trials using synthetic vitamin E, especially when using mg rather than IU dosing.

Liquid vs. powder vitamin E

Vitamin E, both natural and synthetic, can be delivered in the liquid "alcohol" form- listed as tocopherol, or as an ester complex with succinic acid (succinate) or acetic acid (acetate). These complexes might be listed as tocopheryl or sometimes still as tocopherol. According to Maret Traber of the Linus Pauling Institute, tocopherol esters are more resistant to oxidation during storage than unesterified tocopherols. When taken orally, the succinate or acetate moiety is removed from alpha-tocopherol in the intestine, and the bioavailability of alpha-tocopherol from alpha-tocopheryl succinate and alpha-tocopheryl acetate is equivalent to that of free alpha-tocopherol. The accepted biological activities, expressed in IU/mg, of the most common forms of vitamin E are given in the adjacent table.

Form	IU/mg
dl-alpha-tocopheryl acetate	1.00
dl-alpha-tocopherol	1.10
d-alpha-tocopheryl acetate	1.36
d-alpha-tocopherol	1.49

Potential for Toxicity

Vitamin E is fairly nontoxic but high doses are considered to increase the risk of impaired blood clotting. The upper limit set by the IOM is 1,000 mg/day (~1,500 IU of natural or 1,100 IU of synthetic vitamin E). Many surgeons restrict vitamin E therapy prior to surgery out of an abundance of caution.

References:

- Opinion on mixed tocopherols, tocotrienol tocopherol and tocotrienols as sources for vitamin E added as a nutritional substance in food supplements. *The EFSA Journal* (2008) 640, 1-34.
- Vitamin E Page of Linus Pauling Institute Website: http://lpi.oregonstate.edu/infocenter/vitamins/vitaminE/.
- Office of Dietary Supplements- National Institutes of Health- Health Professional Information. http://ods.od.nih.gov/factsheets/VitaminE-HealthProfessional/.
- Bieri JG, McKenna MC. Expressing dietary values for fat-soluble vitamins: changes in concepts and terminology. *Am J Clin Nutr.* 1981 Feb;34(2):289-95.
- Reiter E, Jiang Q, Christen S. Anti-inflammatory properties of alpha- and gamma-tocopherol. *Mol Aspects Med.* 2007 Oct-Dec;28(5-6):668-91.
- Cook-Mills JM. Isoforms of Vitamin E Differentially Regulate PKC α and Inflammation: A Review. J *Clin Cell Immunol.* 2013 Mar 14;4(137).
- Wolf G. How an increased intake of alpha-tocopherol can suppress the bioavailability of gamma-tocopherol. *Nutr Rev.* 2006 Jun;64(6):295-9.

Vitamin K

Essential Nutrient Functions

Vitamin K is the name given to several similar fat-soluble nutrients known as vitamin K_1 and vitamin K_2. The "K" is derived from the German word "koagulation," related its first major known function. Vitamin K functions as a cofactor for enzymes that catalyze carboxylation of the amino acid glutamic acid, resulting in its conversion to gamma-carboxyglutamic acid. This vitamin K-dependent carboxylation is critical to the calcium-binding function of those proteins. Vitamin K's role in blood coagulating proteins is well known, but it is also critical to calcium movement in bones (osteocalcin) and important tissues, including arterial wall calcium (matrix GLA protein).

Intake Guidelines

Adequate Intakes (AIs) for Vitamin K

Age	Males mcg/day	Females mcg/day	Pregnancy mcg/day	Lactation mcg/day
0-6 months	2.0	2.0		
6-12 months	2.5	2.5		
1-3 years	30	30		
4-8 years	55	55		
9-13 years	60	60		
14-18 years	75	75	75	75
Adults 19+	120	90	90	90

The Institute of Medicine established the adequate intake (AI) level for vitamin K in the U.S. based on consumption levels of healthy individuals. The AI for infants was based on estimated intake of vitamin K from breast milk.

Unit(s) of Measure for Guidelines and Labeling

Vitamin K values are for vitamin K_1 (phylloquinone), found in natural food sources and supplements, but do not include vitamin K_2 (menaquinone), the form synthesized by bacteria in the human intestine and available in some supplements. Generally, values are those derived by high-performance liquid chromatography and are reported in mcg.

General Levels of Deficiencies in the U.S.

Based on estimated nutrient intake, deficiency of vitamin K is relatively low in the U.S. NHANES data from 2003 to 2006 show the percent of Americans over the age of two with dietary intake of vitamin K below the EAR is about 30%, which remains mostly unchanged when considering fortification and supplementation. More recently, the measure of under-carboxylated osteocalcin (ucOC) is being explored as a measure of adequate activity of vitamin K, suggesting higher intake, especially of vitamin K_2, may be needed to supply the necessary nonclotting effects of vitamin K.

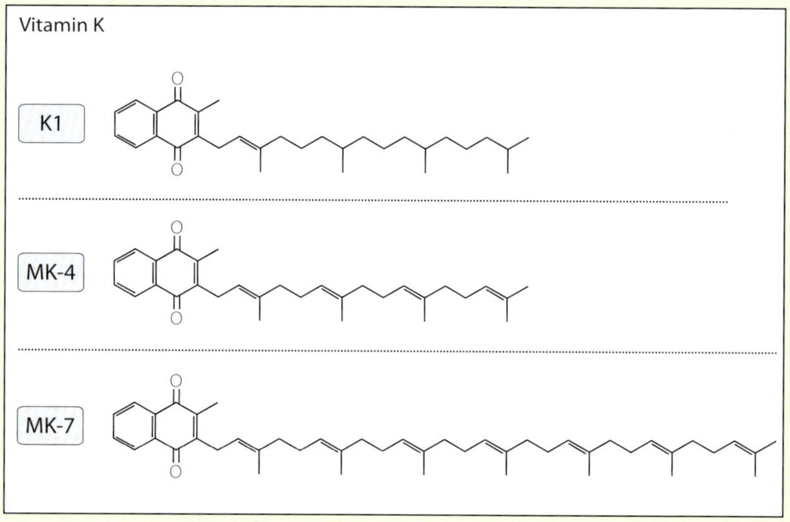

Natural and Supplemental Forms

There are several forms of vitamin K with similar biological activity. Vitamin K_1 (phylloquinone) is the form we encounter in plants—highest in raw kale, Swiss chard, spinach and cooked broccoli. The vitamin K_1 found in most supplements is a synthetic "bioidentical" compound produced by organic synthesis. Vitamin K_2 describes not one compound but several compounds, called menoquinones, names based on the number of five-carbon units in their side chain. These compounds are made naturally in animals by gut bacteria and can also result from bacterial fermentation of some foods, most notably the fermented soy product natto. Following absorption, vitamin K_2 is distributed to the liver, in which MK-6 through MK-13 comprise 90 % of total vitamin K composition. Only 10% of the hepatic vitamin K stores consist of vitamin K_1.

Two dietary supplement ingredients are currently available as vitamin K_2: MK-7 and MK-4 (see figure for structures). Commercial sources of MK-7 come from natto fermentation or organic synthesis, while commercial sources of MK-4 are prepared by organic synthesis and almost exclusively used in Japan. It is critical for clinicians to understand the difference between these two forms of vitamin K_2, as their effective doses are dramatically different. Because of greater bioavailability and bioactivity of MK-7 over MK-4, clinically relevant doses are different by orders of magnitude: ~45 **mg**/day of MK-4 and only 45 – 180 **mcg** for MK-7. For comparison, many therapeutic uses of vitamin K_1 are typically near one mg/day. Therapeutic uses aside, supplementation of vitamin K should mimic food sources by combining both vitamin K_1 and the MK-7 version of vitamin K_2. Vitamin K_3, menadione, a purely synthetic analog, is not available as a dietary supplement and, due to toxicity, is no longer recommended or available.

Potential for Toxicity

The concerns for toxicity or adverse events related to vitamin K stem from its well-known effects on coumadin therapy, which essentially works as a vitamin K antagonist. These fears have led many to wrongly conclude high-doses of vitamin K will trigger blood coagulation/clots in healthy individuals not treated with coumadin. The IOM has set no upper limit for vitamin K intake.

References:

- Vitamin K Page of Linus Pauling Institute Website: http://lpi.oregonstate.edu/infocenter/vitamins/vitaminK/.
- Theuwissen E, Magdeleyns EJ et al. Vitamin K status in healthy volunteers. *Food Funct.* 2013 Dec 2.
- Nimptsch K, Rohrmann S, Nieters A, Linseisen J. Serum undercarboxylated osteocalcin as biomarker of vitamin K intake and risk of prostate cancer: a nested case-control study in the Heidelberg cohort of the European prospective investigation into cancer and nutrition. *Cancer Epidemiol Biomarkers Prev.* 2009 Jan;18(1):49-56.
- Beulens JW, Booth SL et al. The role of menaquinones (vitamin K_2) in human health. *Br J Nutr.* 2013 Oct;110(8):1357-68.
- Sato T, Schurgers LJ, Uenishi K. Comparison of menaquinone-4 and menaquinone-7 bioavailability in healthy women. *Nutr J.* 2012 Nov 12;11:93.

Supplementing Minerals

Compared to the variety of organic compounds that make up the vitamin world, essential dietary minerals are fairly simple molecules. Basically, there are a select number of inorganic "metals," or mineral elements, known to be essential in our diet (neither plants nor animals can synthesize minerals, but both can act as bioaccumulators). Often they are divided by their necessary intake amount: macrominerals, or major elements, and microminerals, or trace elements. While the lines between these two can be drawn differently, major elements typically include: calcium, magnesium, phosphorus, potassium, sodium, chloride and sulfur; trace elements include: zinc, copper, manganese, iron, selenium, iodine, chromium, cobalt and molybdenum, though debates swirl about the need for fluoride, chromium, vanadium, arsenic, boron and a few others.

In either case, minerals remain essentially unchanged as they cycle from the soil, into plants and animals, and then back to the soil or water systems. The mineral might at one point be a metallic ore, an ion in solution, or found in an organic complex or salt. Minerals can remain stationary in the earth for millennia or they can be transported through wind, rain, ground water and volcanic activity, or by intentional human intervention. In fact, man's ability to manipulate metals is the hallmark of human technology. From the Bronze Age through the Iron Age and all the way to the Space Age, mankind has been exploiting the use of metals/minerals in an attempt to improve their lives.

As they pertain to biological systems, the mineral content of soils has been extensively studied in relation to both wild fauna/flora and agricultural outcomes. The testing and replenishing of soil minerals is a hallmark of agricultural practice today, built on decades of research linking the need for certain amounts and ratios of vital minerals for plant growth and disease prevention. Likewise, livestock health has been tied to the soils they graze on and/or the minerals in their feed. Mineral supplementation within animal feed or through mineral blocks is common worldwide when raising livestock.

As with the discovery and understanding of vitamins, the nutritional impact of minerals on human health has been tied to known consequences of intake deficiencies or toxicities, though the consequences of mineral deficiencies are often more subtle. In fact, unlike many well-known diseases associated with vitamin deficiencies (e.g., scurvy, rickets, beriberi), most mineral deficiencies are simply named by their low blood levels (e.g., hypocalcemia, hypokalemia, etc.).

As the following monographs will show, some minerals, like chromium, have limited and specific known functions in the body, and others, like calcium, magnesium and zinc, serve a range of functions. Minerals can serve as enzyme cofactors for an array of important physiological reactions; they can help cells create important ionic gradients along membranes to allow for membrane depolarization (e.g., nerve conductivity, mast cell degranulation, etc.), and they can function as key structural components within the body (e.g., DNA, bones, hemoglobin).

Food-derived Minerals vs. Supplements

As with the "natural" vs. "synthetic" debate for vitamins, a similar set of arguments often characterizes the mineral world. However, unlike organic vitamin molecules, minerals cannot be synthesized per se; though they are almost always modified (and different) when delivered through food fortification and supplementation (with a few exceptions). Humans naturally consume minerals mostly from eating plants and animals; and drinking ground water. The low-concentrations of dissolved minerals in water are primarily in their ionic form (e.g., Ca^{++}), while food forms of minerals (especially those from plants) are mostly bound within complexes of proteins or other organic compounds.

On the other hand, minerals used for food

fortification and supplementation are typically purified mineral salts or organic complexes; mostly created by reacting concentrated mineral sources with other ingredients. For instance, calcium carbonate is a naturally occurring salt found in limestone, chalk, coral and seashells, and can be used directly in supplements or reacted with an organic acid (ascorbic acid, citric acid); and precipitated to make a new calcium salt (calcium ascorbate, calcium citrate). These mineral salts differ in many characteristics—percent of mineral content, solubility, pH, bioavailability—differences that may affect their clinical effectiveness. Complicating matters further, the guideline recommendations for mineral intake do not distinguish the source of the mineral, whether food type or supplement salt, nor are they standardized to the mineral bioavailability from different sources.

Unreacted Blends and True Reacted Minerals

When commercial sources of supplemental mineral compounds are created by reacting two ingredients, such as magnesium oxide and ascorbic acid, a new compound is formed upon precipitation: magnesium ascorbate. It is not uncommon for ingredient manufacturers to simply blend these two ingredients as dry powders, while still labeling the mixture (incorrectly) as magnesium ascorbate. The problem is the unreacted blend, a much cheaper final product, does not have the properties of the truly reacted new compound (pH, solubility, bioavailability, etc.). Unfortunately, since good manufacturing practices are more concerned about the accuracy of the elemental mineral claim, little focus in product testing is placed on distinguishing the non-mineral components.

Why does this matter? As many of the mineral monographs will show, the bioavailabilities of some mineral compounds are quite different from one another. A particular example is the vast difference between the bioavailability of equivalent levels of magnesium found as magnesium oxide and magnesium ascorbate. Magnesium ascorbate has a lower mineral content, but a truly reacted compound allows for much higher magnesium bioavailability compared to magnesium oxide. However, when the high mineral content of magnesium oxide is diluted by blending, rather than reacting, with ascorbic acid, this poorly absorbable form is made worse by merely diluting the mineral content.

Companies with knowledgeable quality control laboratory personnel and appropriate methods and procedures should be able to distinguish a mineral blend from a truly reacted compound. In many cases, purchasing USP mineral compounds is the best guarantee when it comes to reacted mineral salts and organic complexes, with the exception of the highly recommended amino acid chelates, which have no USP monographs (see below).

Chelated Minerals

Another area of confusion is the definition of a mineral chelate. Technically, a chelate is defined as an organic chemical that forms two or more coordinated bonds with a central metal ion (chelate comes from the latin for "claw"). There is, however, no regulatory specification of a mineral chelate. While it is true some minerals can form chelates with organic acids such as citric acid (citrates), malic acid (malate), gluconic acid (gluconate) etc., these must be reacted in a specific way, and ratio, to form compounds that act like chelates when consumed orally. Though many of these are excellent sources of the mineral they contain, these types of compounds should be viewed as ionic salts and not chelates when found in dietary supplement products.

An abundant amount of research, primarily performed by Albion Laboratories, has been done to produce amino acid chelates that maintain their integrity throughout the digestive process. Most of these minerals are chelated to glycine in a 1:2 ratio (e.g., magnesium bisglycinate), though lysine and arginine are sometimes used. Amino acid chelates can, if manufactured properly, enable absorption of the attached mineral through the pathway normally used for amino acids, allowing for the release of the mineral once in the tissues. By avoiding the standard transport mechanisms for ionic minerals, amino acid mineral chelates also avoid much of the natural competition between mineral absorption observed when high levels of mineral salts are used. These amino acid chelates are also associated with less GI discomfort. These amino acid chelated compounds can be combined with salts or organic complexes to maximize the different pathways for mineral absorption, especially when high doses of calcium or magnesium are warranted for therapeutic reasons.

Elemental Claim

Prior to 1997, minerals could be described on product labels based on the total weight of each compound. This meant a person would need to estimate the amount of the mineral itself, a task that could be done only if they knew the percentage of the mineral of that particular compound. For instance, 1,000 mg of calcium carbonate might deliver 360 – 400 mg of calcium; while 1,000 mg of a reacted calcium citrate would only deliver 200 mg. Since 1998, all minerals with a DV must be listed on a Supplement Facts panel by their elemental claim, followed by their compound source in parenthesis. Thus, calcium (as carbonate) 360 mg, or calcium (as citrate) 200 mg, would be the way to label the 1,000 mg equivalents of these two products. Mineral ingredients with no DV might still be listed by their traditional compound claims; mostly related to their therapeutic, not nutritional, use (e.g., strontium citrate or vanadyl sufate).

The following monographs, like the previous vitamin monographs, will only cover issues related to supplemental minerals (not their potential for therapeutic interventions).

Mineral Monographs

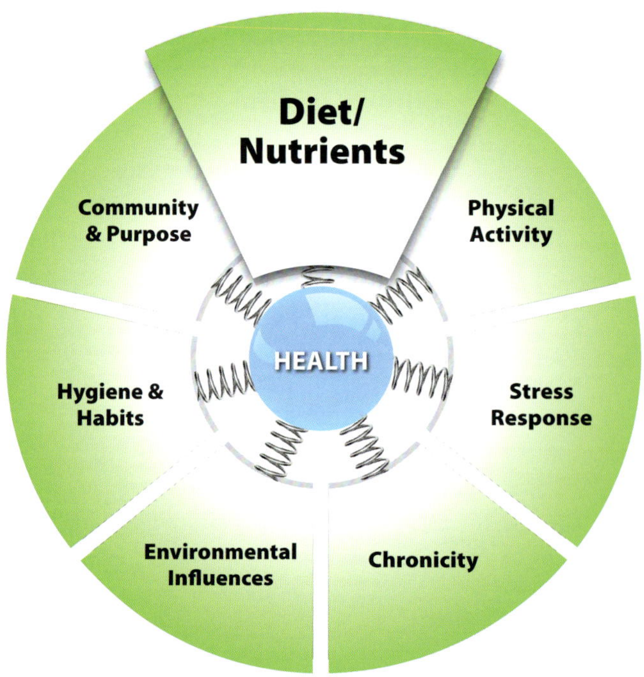

20
Ca
Calcium
40.078

Calcium

20
Ca
Calcium
40.078

Essential Mineral Functions

Calcium is the most abundant mineral in the human body, nearly all of it found in our skeletal system. Calcium is a critical secondary messenger within cells and key to relaxation and contraction of both smooth and skeletal muscle. Bone calcium is found in hydroxyapatite crystals with phosphorus and acts as a reservoir to help keep serum and tissue calcium concentrations within a narrow range.

Intake Guidelines

Recommended Dietary Allowances (RDAs) for Calcium

Age	Males mg/day	Females mg/day	Pregnancy mg/day	Lactation mg/day
0-6 months	200 (AI)	200 (AI)		
6-12 months	260 (AI)	260 (AI)		
1-3 years	700	700		
4-8 years	1,000	1,000		
9-13 years	1,300	1,300		
14-18 years	1,300	1,300	1,300	1,300
Adults 19-50	1,000	1,000	1,000	1,000
Adults 51-70	1,000	1,200		
Adults 71+	1,200	1,200		

* Updated recommendations for calcium intake based on the optimization of bone health were released by the Institute of Medicine in 2010 and differ in age and gender.

General Levels of Deficiencies in the U.S.

Insufficient intake of calcium is common in the U.S. NHANES data from 2003 – 2006 show the percent of Americans over the age of two with dietary intake of calcium below the EAR is more than 50%; reduced to just under 40% when fortification and supplementation intake are included.

Natural and Supplemental Forms

Food calcium is found primarily in dairy products and green leafy vegetables. While calcium rich plants in the brassica family (broccoli, bok choy, cabbage, mustard, and turnip greens) contain calcium equal in bioavailability as that in milk, some food components have been found to inhibit the absorption of calcium. Oxalic acid, also known as oxalate, is the most potent inhibitor of calcium absorption and is found at high concentrations in spinach and rhubarb, and at somewhat lower concentrations in sweet potatoes and dried beans. Phytic acid is a less potent inhibitor of calcium absorption than oxalate. Yeasts possess an enzyme (phytase) that breaks down phytic acid in grains during fermentation, lowering the phytic acid content of breads and other fermented foods. Only concentrated sources of phytate, such as wheat bran or dried beans, substantially reduce calcium absorption.

There are many different forms of calcium used in dietary supplements and OTC drugs. The primary compound forms (and their approximate % calcium) include: calcium carbonate (36%), calcium orotate (11%), calcium citrate (24%), calcium citrate-malate (20%), calcium ascorbate (9%), calcium aspartate (20%), calcium hydroxyapetite (37%), tricalcium phosphate (34%), calcium lactate (18%), dicalcium malate (29%) and calcium amino acid chelates (bisglycinate-18%).

Unfortunately, systematic comparisons between all, or even most, of the major forms of calcium (in vitamin D-sufficient subjects) have not been performed. The majority of calcium supplementation studies to date have been done with calcium carbonate, the most concentrated and cheapest form of calcium. Because of this, there have been many studies comparing various forms of calcium to the bioavailability of calcium carbonate. In a 1987 *New England Journal of Medicine* publication, 500 mg of calcium from milk and several salts (acetate, gluconate, lactate, citrate, and carbonate) were deemed to absorb similarly (27 – 39%) in healthy, fasting, young subjects. While some studies did show a higher bioavailability for calcium citrate, when adjusting for cost, there was little measurable clinical advantage in relation to the subject's calcium status. Complicating these and other studies on the various forms of calcium are known differences of calcium absorption between subjects, unknown factors that can block calcium absorption, and known downregulation of calcium absorption that occurs when calcium doses increase. For this reason, many guidelines suggest that doses above 500 mg of calcium in salt forms in a **single dose** are likely to be of little added value.

With regard to salts and organic complexes (non-amino acid chelates), we generally recommend those that provide organic compounds within the citric acid cycle (citrate, malate) or other potential beneficial activities (ascorbate) over carbonate when using salts. While there is little in the way of documented data to confirm the additional benefits, these bioavailable forms, combined with the forms mentioned below, allow for the delivery of calcium and other organic compounds.

There are several forms of supplemental calcium that are really calcium/phosphorus complexes: tricalcium phosphate and calcium hydroxyapatite (durapetite). The benefit of these forms is there appears to be some relationship between phosphorus intake and calcium utilization within bone in animal studies. Both bone forms of hydroxyapatite (from bovine) and mineral forms have been used in dietary supplements; though bone-form hydroxyapatite ingredients have fallen out of favor and both forms have been known to have elevated lead levels.

One of the more popular forms of calcium is an amino acid chelate form, or bisglycinate. The bioavailability of this form is much greater than other salt forms of calcium on an empty stomach (and typically more tolerable), though it provides a lower mineral payload.

We suggest a clinician advise patients to consume as much calcium from dietary sources as possible. Those who avoid dairy and are unable to ensure adequate daily intake of calcium should consider supplemental calcium sources. Combining calcium sources from calcium salts, organic salts/chelates, amino acid chelates and phosphate complexes is a way to maximize calcium absorption while reducing the likelihood of negative interactions with other minerals or food-absorption inhibitors. Supplemental calcium should be consumed with vitamin D (400 IU or more). Clinicians should also consider additional vitamin K_2 (MK-7, 45 mcg or more) with calcium supplementation.

Potential for Toxicity

Very high levels of supplemental calcium can lead to hypercalcemia, rarely seen with dietary calcium alone. Clinicians should consider calcium from multiple supplemental sources and ask patients about other undisclosed supplemental calcium, including OTC and pharmaceutical products containing calcium. While some studies have suggested an increased risk for kidney stones in subjects consuming therapeutic doses of calcium for osteoporosis (most studies used calcium carbonate), systematic reviews of these studies indicate the risk for kidney stones is not significantly elevated during appropriate calcium supplementation. The tolerable upper limit for calcium intake is set between two to three grams per day for adults; there is no therapeutic use that would warrant exceeding this dose.

References:

- Calcium Page of Linus Pauling Institute Website: http://lpi.oregonstate.edu/infocenter/minerals/calcium/.
- Office of Dietary Supplements- National Institutes of Health- Health Professional Information. http://ods.od.nih.gov/factsheets/Calcium-HealthProfessional.
- Fulgoni VL 3rd, Keast DR, Bailey RL, Dwyer J. Foods, fortificants, and supplements: Where do Americans get their nutrients? *J Nutr.* 2011 Oct;141(10):1847-54.
- Sheikh MS, Santa Ana CA, Nicar MJ, Schiller LR, Fordtran JS. Gastrointestinal absorption of calcium from milk and calcium salts. *N Engl J Med.* 1987 Aug 27;317(9):532-6.
- Heaney RP, Dowell MS, Bierman J, Hale CA, Bendich A. Absorbability and cost effectiveness in calcium supplementation. *J Am Coll Nutr.* 2001 Jun;20(3):239-46.
- Fishbein L. Multiple sources of dietary calcium—some aspects of its essentiality. *Regul Toxicol Pharmacol.* 2004 Apr;39(2):67-80.
- Shapiro R, Heaney RP. Co-dependence of calcium and phosphorus for growth and bone development under conditions of varying deficiency. *Bone.* 2003 May;32(5):532-40.
- Candelas G, Martinez-Lopez JA, Rosario MP, Carmona L, Loza E. Calcium supplementation and kidney stone risk in osteoporosis: a systematic literature review. *Clin Exp Rheumatol.* 2012 Nov-Dec;30(6):954-61.

24
Cr
Chromium
51.996

Chromium

24
Cr
Chromium
51.996

Essential Mineral Functions

The role of chromium as an absolutely essential nutrient is not universally agreed upon. The discovery of a protein called Low-Molecular Weight Chromium Binding Substance (LMWCr or chromodulin) appears to mediate chromium's ability to increase the autophosphorylation of the insulin receptor in the presence of insulin; enhancing insulin's signaling effects.

Intake Guidelines

Adequate Intakes (AIs) for Chromium

Age	Males mcg/day	Females mcg/day	Pregnancy mcg/day	Lactation mcg/day
0-6 months	0.2	0.2		
6-12 months	5.5	5.5		
1-3 years	11	11		
4-8 years	15	15		
9-13 years	25	21		
14-18 years	35	24	29	44
Adults 19-50	35	25	30	45
Adults 51+	30	20		

* There is not enough information on chromium requirements to set a recommended dietary allowance (RDA); the IOM has set an adequate intake level (AI) based on chromium content in normal diets.

General Levels of Deficiencies in the U.S.

The level of chromium intake and need for basic nutrient functions is not well understood. Rarely is frank chromium deficiency ever seen. The supplementation of chromium at levels well above AI (400 – 1,000 mcg) has been used in clinical trials to modulate glucose/insulin sensitivity in diabetic and overweight subjects with mixed results. Chromium appears to have much more impact on postprandial levels of insulin and glucose than on fasting levels of each.

Natural and Supplemental Forms

Food sources of chromium are not well characterized or consistently measured. In the late 1950s, a chromium-containing molecule derived from yeast was characterized and named "Glucose Tolerance Factor." The organic forms of chromium, especially those containing nicotinic acid, are attempts to mimic GTF. The supplemental forms of chromium (with their percent Cr) include organic compounds such as chromium picolinate (12%), chromium nicotinate(s) (10%) and amino acid chelates (bisglycinate-2.5%).

Chromium is poorly absorbed from most forms of supplemental chromium. Studies comparing different forms in animals and humans have concluded chromium bioavailability in humans is higher than in rats, but is inconsistent in human subjects based on the form used. Chromium picolinate, as a proprietary compound, has the largest number of clinical trials compared to other forms. Results of these trials have all shown increased levels of chromium after intake, the repletion effect, though clinical results have been mixed. Isolated adverse events (kidney toxicity) have been reported in some trials using chromium picolinate at therapeutic doses (>400 mcg/day).

Polynicotinate forms and amino acid chelates of chromium are also available as proprietary/branded ingredients. While some animal data suggests physiological differences may exist between these forms over picolinate salts (favoring nicotinate forms), head-to-head comparisons for nutrient repletion in humans have not revealed a significant difference.

Potential for Toxicity

The toxicity of chromium is related to the hexavalent Cr (VI) form of the metal used in making metallic components, which can be highly toxic to human tissues. The trivalent form of chromium Cr (III) is the form found in foods and supplements and appears to have no known level of toxicity. The IOM has set no upper tolerable limit for chromium. Adverse events mentioned for therapeutic doses of chromium picolinate are likely due to the patients weakened system or a reaction to the picolinic acid and unrelated to the chromium itself.

References:

- Chromium Page of Linus Pauling Institute Website: http://lpi.oregonstate.edu/infocenter/minerals/chromium.
- Office of Dietary Supplements- National Institutes of Health- Health Professional Information. http://ods.od.nih.gov/factsheets/Chromium-HealthProfessional.
- Chen Y, Watson HM, Gao J, Sinha SH, Cassady CJ, Vincent JB. Characterization of the organic component of low-molecular-weight chromium-binding substance and its binding of chromium. *J Nutr.* 2011 Jul;141(7):1225-32.
- Onakpoya I, Posadzki P, Ernst E. Chromium supplementation in overweight and obesity: a systematic review and meta-analysis of randomized clinical trials. *Obes Rev.* 2013 Jun;14(6):496-507.
- Wang ZQ, Cefalu WT. Current concepts about chromium supplementation in type 2 diabetes and insulin resistance. *Curr Diab Rep.* 2010 Apr;10(2):145-51.
- Laschinsky N, Kottwitz K, Freund B, Dresow B, Fischer R, Nielsen P. Bioavailability of chromium(III)-supplements in rats and humans. *Biometals.* 2012 Oct;25(5):1051-60.
- Jain SK, Rains JL, Croad JL. Effect of chromium niacinate and chromium picolinate supplementation on lipid peroxidation, TNF-alpha, IL-6, CRP, glycated hemoglobin, triglycerides, and cholesterol levels in blood of streptozotocin-treated diabetic rats. *Free Radic Biol Med.* 2007 Oct 15;43(8):1124-31.

29
Cu
Copper
63.546

Copper

29
Cu
Copper
63.546

Essential Mineral Functions

Copper is an essential trace mineral for both humans and animals. Found predominantly in the cupric (2+) form, copper can also transition to its cuprous (1+) form. Its ability to accept and donate electrons makes it a helpful cofactor for key redox enzymes, sometimes called cuproenzymes. Multi-copper oxidases are critical for appropriate iron metabolism.

Intake Guidelines

Recommended Dietary Allowances (RDAs) for Copper

Age	Males mcg/day	Females mcg/day	Pregnancy mcg/day	Lactation mcg/day
0-6 months	200 (AI)	200 (AI)		
6-12 months	220 (AI)	220 (AI)		
1-3 years	340	340		
4-8 years	440	440		
9-13 years	700	700		
14-18 years	890	890		
Adults 19+	900	900		
All ages			1,000	1,300

* According to the IOM, a variety of indicators were used to establish the RDA for copper, including plasma copper concentration, serum ceruloplasmin activity, superoxide dismutase activity in red blood cells and platelet copper concentration. The RDA for copper reflects the results of depletion-repletion studies and is based on the prevention of deficiency.

General Levels of Deficiencies in the U.S.

Estimates of deficient copper intake in the U.S. are low. NHANES data from 2003 – 2006 show the percent of Americans over the age of two with dietary intake of dietary copper below the EAR is less than 5%. Chronic daily zinc supplementation (>50 mg/day) can result in low copper absorption. Copper supplementation should be added when high-dose zinc supplementation is implemented.

Natural and Supplemental Forms

Copper is found in a wide variety of foods and is high in organ meats, shellfish, nuts and seeds. Some wheat-bran cereals and whole-grain products are also good sources of copper. Supplemental copper (with percent Cu) is found as cupric oxide (75%), copper chloride (45%), copper lysinate (10%), copper gluconate (14%), copper sulfate (39%) and as an amino acid chelate (10%).

Potential for Toxicity

Copper toxicity is rare and the IOM has set the upper limit at 10 mg/day for adults. Since there are no well-known clinical reasons to give more than a few mg of copper per day—even these studies are limited in efficacy—doses above the upper limit should not be used unless following a protocol known to be safe and effective.

References:

- Copper Page of Linus Pauling Institute Website: http://lpi.oregonstate.edu/infocenter/minerals/copper/.
- Vashchenko G, MacGillivray RT. Multi-copper oxidases and human iron metabolism. *Nutrients.* 2013 Jun 27;5(7):2289-313.
- Food and Nutrition Board, Institute of Medicine. Copper. Dietary reference intakes for vitamin A, vitamin K, boron, chromium, copper, iodine, iron, manganese, molybdenum, nickel, silicon, vanadium, and zinc. Washington, D.C.: National Academy Press; 2001:224-257. (National Academy Press)
- Fulgoni VL 3rd, Keast DR, Bailey RL, Dwyer J. Foods, fortificants, and supplements: Where do Americans get their nutrients? *J Nutr.* 2011 Oct;141(10):1847-54.

53
I
Iodine
126.904

Iodine

53
I
Iodine
126.904

Essential Mineral Functions

Iodine is a trace element required for the production of human thyroid hormones triiodothyronine (T_3) and thyroxine (T_4), and, therefore, is essential for normal thyroid function. Our understanding of iodine beyond its role in thyroid-hormone is much less understood, though growing evidence suggests iodine may have a direct effect on immune health and breast health.

Intake Guidelines

Recommended Dietary Allowances (RDAs) for Iodine

Age	Males mcg/day	Females mcg/day	Pregnancy mcg/day	Lactation mcg/day
0-6 months	110 (AI)	110 (AI)		
6-12 months	130 (AI)	130 (AI)		
1-3 years	90	90		
4-8 years	90	90		
9-13 years	120	120		
14-18 years	150	150		
Adults 19+	150	150		
All ages			220	290

* The recommended amounts by IOM are calculated using several methods, including the measurement of iodine accumulation in the thyroid glands of individuals with normal thyroid function.

General Levels of Deficiencies in the U.S.

While iodine deficiency is a global concern, frank deficiency of iodine appears to be uncommon in the U.S. due to the ubiquitous use of iodized table salt; sea salt and kosher salt contain no appreciable level of iodine. Nonetheless, insufficient iodine intake is considered to play a role in the widely undiagnosed subclinical hypothyroid conditions of millions of Americans. Individuals who avoid seafood and iodized salt may have low iodine in their diet. Certain vegetables are known to contain goitrogens, compounds that interfere with iodine/thyroid function (cabbage, broccoli, cauliflower and Brussels sprouts). Clinically, it is rare to observe a goitrogenic effect due to overconsumption of these vegetables even with low iodine intake.

Natural and Supplemental Forms

Food sources of iodine are mainly from seaweed, milk, iodized salt, and some fish and shellfish sources. Nearly all supplemental iodine comes from potassium iodide (75%) or concentrated (and sometimes standardized) kelp or other sea vegetables. Iodine absorption from seaweed/kelp ingredients is quite bioavailable and is suitable for most applications of iodine supplementation; although manufacturers must monitor for unwanted contaminants (e.g., heavy metals) when using these sources.

Potential for Toxicity

Therapeutic uses of iodine/iodide for thyroid or other conditions usually contain levels of iodine well above those needed for minimal nutrient deficiencies and sometimes above IOM's upper limit of 1,100 mcg (1.1 mg) per day in adults. Clinicians should not routinely use iodine doses above the upper limit unless they are following a specific protocol known to be safe and effective.

References:

- Iodine Page of Linus Pauling Institute Website: http://lpi.oregonstate.edu/infocenter/minerals/iodine
- Office of Dietary Supplements- National Institutes of Health- Health Professional Information. http://ods.od.nih.gov/factsheets/Iodine-HealthProfessional.
- Pearce EN, Andersson M, Zimmermann MB. Global iodine nutrition: Where do we stand in 2013? *Thyroid.* 2013 May;23(5):523-8.
- Cooper DS, Ridgway EC. Thoughts on prevention of thyroid disease in the United States. *Thyroid.* 2002 Oct;12(10):925-9.
- Aquaron R, Delange F, Marchal P, Lognoné V, Ninane L. Bioavailability of seaweed iodine in human beings. *Cell Mol Biol* (Noisy-le-grand). 2002 Jul;48(5):563-9.

26 **Fe** Iron 55.847

Iron

26 **Fe** Iron 55.847

Essential Mineral Functions

Iron is one of the most abundant metals in the earth and is used for both human technology and physiology. There are over 100 different enzymes and proteins that use iron as a cofactor, mostly for its ability to bind oxygen. Over two-thirds of the body's store of iron is attached to hemoglobin. Iron metabolism and transfer throughout the body is tightly regulated, as free iron is toxic to cells and tissue.

Intake Guidelines

Recommended Dietary Allowances (RDAs) for Iron

Age	Males mg/day	Females mg/day	Pregnancy mg/day	Lactation mg/day
0-6 months	0.27 (AI)	0.27 (AI)		
6-12 months	11	11		
1-3 years	7	7		
4-8 years	10	10		
9-13 years	8	8		
14-18 years	11	15	27	10
Adults 19-50	8	18	27	9
Adults 51+	8	8		

* The RDA for iron is based on the prevention of iron deficiency and maintenance of adequate iron stores in individuals eating a mixed diet.

General Levels of Deficiencies in the U.S.

Iron deficiency is one of the most common nutrient deficiencies in the world and more common in the U.S. than most people think. NHANES data from 2003 – 2006 show the percent of Americans over the age of two with dietary intake of dietary iron below the EAR is just over 20%; but this only tells part of the story. Insufficient stores of iron and specific need for more iron create a functional insufficiency in many individuals. Those who might need more iron intake include: pregnant women; preterm and low-birth-weight infants; teenage girls; women of childbearing age, especially those with heavy menstrual losses; people with renal failure, especially those undergoing routine dialysis; people with gastrointestinal disorders who do not absorb iron normally, such as Crohn's and Celiac; gastric-bypass patients; individuals engaged in regular intense exercise; obese subjects and vegetarians.

Natural and Supplemental Forms

Unfortified food sources of iron come either as heme iron (from hemoglobin and myoglobin found in meat, fish and poultry) or non-heme iron (plants, dairy and most iron supplements). Heme iron has higher bioavailability than non-heme iron and, unlike non-heme iron sources, is not influenced by the factors that diminish its absorption—most notably the phytic acid present in legumes, grains, and rice. Small amounts of phytic acid (five to 10 mg) can reduce non-heme iron absorption by 50%. Ascorbic acid or organic acids (citric, malic, tartaric, lactic) can enhance the absorption of non-heme iron (food or supplements).

Iron supplements are common as both prescription products and dietary supplements. The most common forms of iron used (with their percent iron) are: ferrous fumerate (33%), ferrous sulfate (monohydrate 33%, heptahydrate 22%), ferrous gluconate (12%), ferrous oxide (77%) and ferrous amino acid chelate (bisglycinate, 20%). Several studies have looked at the relative safety, side-effect profile and bioavailability of these forms, all of which are non-heme iron compounds. Since iron bioavailability is highly regulated by a person's iron status, only subtle differences in iron bioavailability have been demonstrated in clinical trials, favoring bisglycinate chelates. Recently, Milman et al. showed that 25 mg of elemental iron from ferrous bisglycinate chelate was just as effective in maintaining iron status during the second and third trimester of pregnancy as 50 mg of elemental iron from ferrous sulfate. The bisglyinate chelate form was also associated with fewer gastrointestinal side effects.

Potential for Toxicity

Accidental overdose of iron-containing products is the single largest cause of poisoning fatalities in children under six years old. For this reason, products containing appreciable amounts of iron are required to have childproof packaging and the following warning on the package: *WARNING: Accidental overdose of iron-containing products is a leading cause of fatal poisoning in children under 6. Keep this product out of reach of children. In case of accidental overdose, call a doctor or poison control center immediately.*

Clinicians should remind those taking iron supplements to remember to close the childproof packaging and keep these products away from children. The use of iron above the upper tolerable limit set by the IOM (45 mg/day) should only be considered when following a protocol known to be appropriate and safe for the patient. Also, since high iron stores may play a role as a pro-oxidant, increasing the risk for atherosclerosis and cancer (this is still debated), many clinicians may want to avoid iron supplementation in men, postmenopausal women, and populations not known to have a risk for iron deficiency. Most companies distributing multivitamins for professional use have iron-free options to choose from.

References:

- Iron Page of Linus Pauling Institute Website: http://lpi.oregonstate.edu/infocenter/minerals/iron/.
- Office of Dietary Supplements- National Institutes of Health- Health Professional Information. http://ods.od.nih.gov/factsheets/Iron-HealthProfessional.
- Tussing-Humphreys L, Pusatcioglu C, Nemeth E, Braunschweig C. Rethinking iron regulation and assessment in iron deficiency, anemia of chronic disease, and obesity: introducing hepcidin. *J Acad Nutr Diet.* 2012 Mar;112(3):391-400.
- Bovell-Benjamin AC, Viteri FE, Allen LH. Iron absorption from ferrous bisglycinate and ferric trisglycinate in whole maize is regulated by iron status. *Am J Clin Nutr.* 2000 Jun;71(6):1563-9.
- Fulgoni VL 3rd, Keast DR, Bailey RL, Dwyer J. Foods, fortificants, and supplements: Where do Americans get their nutrients? *J Nutr.* 2011 Oct;141(10):1847-54.
- Milman N, Jønsson L, Dyre P, Pedersen PL, Larsen LG. Ferrous bisglycinate 25 mg iron is as effective as ferrous sulfate 50 mg iron in the prophylaxis of iron deficiency and anemia during pregnancy in a randomized trial. *J Perinat Med.* 2013 Oct 24:1-10.
- Ferrari P, Nicolini A, Manca ML, Rossi G, Anselmi L, Conte M, Carpi A, Bonino F. Treatment of mild non-chemotherapy-induced iron deficiency anemia in cancer patients: comparison between oral ferrous bisglycinate chelate and ferrous sulfate. *Biomed Pharmacother.* 2012 Sep;66(6):414-8.

12
Mg
Magnesium
24.305

Magnesium

12
Mg
Magnesium
24.305

Essential Mineral Functions

Magnesium is one of the most abundant and important minerals in the body. There are over 300 different enzymatic reactions that rely upon magnesium as a cofactor. ATP, a vital energy molecule in the body, functions as a magnesium complex.

Intake Guidelines

Recommended Dietary Allowances (RDAs) for Magnesium

Age	Males mg/day	Females mg/day	Pregnancy mg/day	Lactation mg/day
0-6 months	30 (AI)	30 (AI)		
6-12 months	75 (AI)	75 (AI)		
1-3 years	80	80		
4-8 years	130	130		
9-13 years	240	240		
14-18 years	410	360	400	360
Adults 19-30	400	310	350	310
Adults 31+	420	320	360	320

* RDA levels are based on magnesium balance studies (intake vs. loss), not physiological need.

General Levels of Deficiencies in the U.S.

Low intake of magnesium is the most common mineral deficiency in the U.S. NHANES data from 2003 – 2006 show the percent of Americans over the age of two with dietary intake of dietary magnesium below the EAR is nearly 60%, only reduced to just under 45% when fortification and supplementation intake are included. Conditions or situations that may increase the need for magnesium include: Crohn's disease, chronic diarrhea, renal disease, use of diuretics and high-dose zinc supplementation (regular use above 50 mg/day).

Natural and Supplemental Forms

Food magnesium is high in nuts (almonds, cashews, and peanuts), cooked spinach and beans (black, soy, edamame), and some cereal grains. Unlike calcium, there is little public awareness of the sources and general deficiency of magnesium intake.

Because the demand for magnesium supplementation is high, there are many different forms available. The primary compound used (and their approximate percent magnesium) include: magnesium oxide (60%), magnesium chloride (25%), magnesium carbonate (25%), magnesium citrate (16%), magnesium ascorbate (18%), magnesium lactate (12%), magnesium aspartate (20%), magnesium threonate (7%) and magnesium amino acid chelate (glycinate -10%).

Head-to-head comparisons of each form of magnesium in human subjects have not been performed. A recent study performed in rats using 10 different forms of magnesium salts showed organic salts absorb slightly better than inorganic salts, ranging from 50 – 70% available. In humans, magnesium oxide is one of the most commonly used magnesium sources in retail supplements, despite being shown to have a very low bioavailability (~4% in some studies); while other inorganic and organic salts have substantially higher bioavailability. Generally, organic salts and chelates, including amino acid chelates, have higher bioavailability over inorganic salts and much higher than magnesium oxide. Other than bioavailability and changes in serum magnesium, virtually no clinically based outcomes have been tested comparing different forms of magnesium in humans.

Recent animal studies using magnesium threonate have suggested higher cerebral spinal fluid magnesium levels compared to magnesium chloride, as well as enhanced learning and memory compared to magnesium citrate. These animal studies also suggest independent activities associated with both higher magnesium levels and threonate levels. These studies have not yet been repeated in humans and may be offset (practically) by the very low (7%) content of magnesium.

Like our recommendation for calcium, magnesium supplementation intended to deliver high amounts of magnesium (~150 mg or more) should be done with a combination of highly bioavailable forms as organic salts and chelates, especially magnesium glycinate chelates.

Potential for Toxicity

Excessive intake of magnesium is usually self-limiting as excessive doses typically induce diarrhea, a therapeutic goal of many magnesium-based laxatives. While the IOM recognizes higher levels of magnesium may be applicable for certain patients under the care of a healthcare professional, the upper limit for adults is set at 350 mg/day of supplemental (not total dietary) magnesium. The dose that causes a laxative effect is typically much lower for magnesium oxide than for the organic and amino acid chelates, though individual variability is significant.

References:

- Magnesium Page of Linus Pauling Institute Website: http://lpi.oregonstate.edu/infocenter/minerals/magnesium/.
- Office of Dietary Supplements- National Institutes of Health- Health Professional Information. http://ods.od.nih.gov/factsheets/Magnesium-HealthProfessional.
- Fulgoni VL 3rd, Keast DR, Bailey RL, Dwyer J. Foods, fortificants, and supplements: Where do Americans get their nutrients? *J Nutr.* 2011 Oct;141(10):1847-54.
- Coudray C, Rambeau M et al. Study of magnesium bioavailability from ten organic and inorganic Mg salts in Mg-depleted rats using a stable isotope approach. *Magnes Res.* 2005 Dec;18(4):215-23.
- Firoz M, Graber M. Bioavailability of US commercial magnesium preparations. *Magnes Res.* 2001 Dec;14(4):257-62.
- Slutsky I, Abumaria N et al. Enhancement of learning and memory by elevating brain magnesium. *Neuron.* 2010 Jan 28;65(2):165-77.

25
Mn
Manganese
54.938

Manganese

25 Mn Manganese 54.938

Essential Mineral Functions

Manganese is an important mineral cofactor for a number of key metabolic enzymes, most notably for superoxide dismutase (MnSOD), a critical antioxidant enzyme within mitochondria. Manganese is also important for wound healing, bone formation and glucose metabolism.

Intake Guidelines

Adequate Intakes (AIs) for Manganese

Age	Males mg/day	Females mg/day	Pregnancy mg/day	Lactation mg/day
0-6 months	0.003	0.003		
6-12 months	0.6	0.6		
1-3 years	1.2	1.2		
4-8 years	1.5	1.5		
9-13 years	1.9	1.6		
14-18 years	2.2	1.6		
Adults 19+	2.3	1.8		
All ages			2.0	2.6

* The IOM based the AI on average dietary intakes of manganese determined by the Total Diet Study, an annual survey of the mineral content of representative American diets.

General Levels of Deficiencies in the U.S.

Frank manganese deficiency has not been documented in humans eating natural diets. Both mechanistic and human data suggest diabetic and osteoporotic subjects may have lower manganese levels compared to control populations. Supplementing these subjects within the AI range may be warranted, but there is limited data to suggest manganese supplementation will change clinical outcomes in these subjects.

Natural and Supplemental Forms

Food sources of manganese include whole grains, nuts, leafy vegetables and teas. Supplemental sources (and percent Mn) include: manganese sulfate (36%), manganese gluconate (11%), manganese ascorbate (20%), manganese oxide (72%) and amino acid chelate (glycinate -16%) forms. Some studies suggest that manganese bioavailability can be reduced when consumed with iron, calcium and magnesium supplements; though bioavailability of different forms of manganese has not been well studied in human subjects.

Potential for Toxicity

Incidences of manganese toxicity are mostly related to inhalation of manganese dust (welders, smelters) and unrelated to ingesting manganese in foods or supplements. Some cases of toxicity in children have been traced to high manganese levels in drinking water. We do not suggest clinicians recommend supplementing manganese above the tolerable upper limit (11 mg/day) unless they are following a protocol known to be safe and effective.

References:

- Manganese Page of Linus Pauling Institute Website: http://lpi.oregonstate.edu/infocenter/minerals/manganese.
- Food and Nutrition Board, Institute of Medicine. Manganese. Dietary reference intakes for vitamin A, vitamin K, boron, chromium, copper, iodine, iron, manganese, molybdenum, nickel, silicon, vanadium, and zinc. Washington, D.C.: National Academy Press; 2001:394-419. (National Academy Press).
- Keen CL, Zidenberg-Cherr S. Manganese. In: Ziegler EE, Filer LJ, eds. Present Knowledge in Nutrition. 7th ed. Washington D.C.: ILSI Press; 1996:334-343.
- Greger JL. Dietary standards for manganese: overlap between nutritional and toxicological studies. *J Nutr.* 1998 Feb;128(2 Suppl):368S-371S.

42
Mo
Molybdenum
95.94

Molybdenum

42
Mo
Molybdenum
95.94

Essential Mineral Functions

Molybdenum is a necessary mineral incorporated into an organic-molybdenum cofactor (called Moco; see figure) for at least four different human enzymes: sulfite oxidase, xanthine oxidase, aldehyde oxidase, and mitochondrial amidoxime reducing component. All known functions of molybdenum in humans are related to this cofactor function in these enzymes (molybdenum is important for nitrogen fixation in numerous bacterial species, secondarily related to human health).

Intake Guidelines

Recommended Dietary Allowances (RDAs) for Molybdenum

Age	Males mcg/day	Females mcg/day	Pregnancy mcg/day	Lactation mcg/day
0-6 months	2 (AI)	2 (AI)		
6-12 months	3 (AI)	3 (AI)		
1-3 years	17	17		
4-8 years	22	22		
9-13 years	34	34		
14-18 years	43	43		
Adults 19+	45	45		
All ages			50	50

* The recommended dietary allowance (RDA) for molybdenum is based on the results of nutritional balance studies conducted in eight healthy young men under controlled laboratory conditions.

General Levels of Deficiencies in the U.S.

While inborn errors are known for the synthesis of Mo-cofactor (Moco), these are not related to deficient intake of molybdenum. In fact, dietary intake deficiencies are virtually unknown. Average molybdenum intake in the U.S. is estimated to be well above the RDA.

Molybdenum cofactor (Moco)

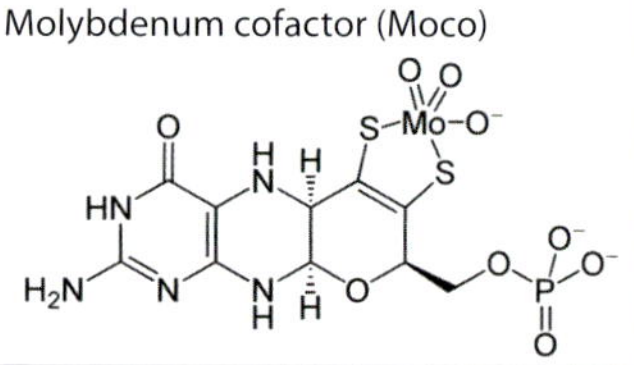

Natural and Supplemental Forms

Food sources of molybdenum include legumes, such as beans, lentils and peas, grain products and nuts. Supplement sources (with percent Mo) include molybdenum citrate (22%), ammonium molybdate (57%), sodium molybdate (46%) and amino acid chelate forms (glycinate-2.5%). The form most widely used for supplementation in the U.S. is the molybdenum glycinate chelate.

Potential for Toxicity

Molybdenum toxicity is rare, but can occur at very high doses (1.5 mg/day or higher). The IOM has set the tolerable upper intake levels at 2000 mcg (2 mg), more than 40 times higher than the RDA. Since there are no human clinical trials suggesting safe and effective uses of molybdenum near or above the UL, doses much closer to the RDA should be used for molybdenum supplementation.

References:

- Molybdenum Page of Linus Pauling Institute Website: http://lpi.oregonstate.edu/infocenter/minerals/molybdenum.
- Schwarz G, Belaidi AA. Molybdenum in human health and disease. *Met Ions Life Sci.* 2013;13:415-50.
- Turnlund JR, Keyes WR, Peiffer GL. Molybdenum absorption, excretion, and retention studied with stable isotopes in young men at five intakes of dietary molybdenum. *Am J Clin Nutr.* 1995;62(4):790-796.
- Bayram E, Topcu Y et al. Molybdenum cofactor deficiency: review of 12 cases (MoCD and review). *Eur J Paediatr Neurol.* 2013 Jan;17(1):1-6.
- Food and Nutrition Board, Institute of Medicine. Molybdenum. In: Dietary reference intakes for vitamin A, vitamin K, boron, chromium, copper, iodine, iron, manganese, molybdenum, nickel, silicon, vanadium, and zinc. Washington, D.C.: National Academy Press; 2001:420-441. (National Academy Press).

15
P
Phosphorus
30.974

Phosphorus

15
P
Phosphorus
30.974

Essential Mineral Functions

Phosphorus, mostly in the form of phosphate, is an essential mineral for nearly every cell function in the body. Phosphate components are integral to the structure of DNA, ATP, phospholipids and the calcium-phosphate hydroxyapatite that makes up bone—where over 80% of the phosphate in our bodies reside. The addition and subtraction of phosphate moieties (by kinases/phosphorylases and phosphatases/dephosphorylases, respectively) is one of the most important secondary signaling pathways used within cells. Phosphates also act in concert with other minerals and organic acids to maintain our body's pH buffering system.

Intake Guidelines

Recommended Dietary Allowances (RDAs) for Phosphorus

Age	Males mg/day	Females mg/day	Pregnancy mg/day	Lactation mg/day
0-6 months	100 (AI)	100 (AI)		
6-12 months	275 (AI)	275 (AI)		
1-3 years	460	460		
4-8 years	500	500		
9-13 years	1,250	1,250		
14-18 years	1,250	1,250	1,250	1,250
Adults 19+	700	700	700	700

* The RDA for phosphorus is based on the maintenance of normal serum phosphate levels in adults, believed to represent adequate phosphorus intake to meet cellular and bone formation needs.

General Levels of Deficiencies in the U.S.

Phosphorus is found in nearly all foods and frank deficiency is nearly unknown in the U.S. NHANES data from 2003 – 2006 show the percent of Americans over the age of two with dietary intake of dietary phosphorus below the EAR is around 5%. Patients who suffer from anorexia, alcoholism, or have had a recent episode of diabetic ketoacidosis may have hypophosphatemia. Low phosphate levels are also known to occur in subjects using aluminum-containing antacids.

Natural and Supplemental Forms

Dietary supplements often contain phosphorus in various forms (with different percent phosphorus): potassium phosphate (17%), sodium phosphate (21%), calcium-phosphate complexes (dicalcium phosphate, 22%), hydroxyapatite (17%), etc. Multivitamin supplements rarely have or need RDA levels of phosphorus, as the average individual does not generally need phosphorus supplementation.

Potential for Toxicity

Generally, phosphorus is nontoxic. The common exception to this is when kidney function is compromised and phosphorus levels increase, allowing for unregulated calcium deposition in tissues, especially the kidneys. The tolerable upper limit is lower in subjects older than 70 y (3 grams/day) because it is assumed they have slightly less kidney function than younger subjects (UL of 4 grams/day). The National Kidney Foundation makes the following phosphorus recommendations (based on evidence or their professional opinion) for those with chronic kidney disease:

- Dietary phosphorus should be restricted to 800 to 1,000 mg/day (adjusted for dietary protein needs) when the serum phosphorus levels are elevated (>4.6 mg/dL [1.49 mmol/L]) at Stages 3 and 4 of CKD, (OPINION) and >5.5 mg/dL (1.78 mmol/L) in those with kidney failure (Stage 5). (EVIDENCE)
- Dietary phosphorus should be restricted to 800 to 1,000 mg/day (adjusted to dietary protein needs) when the plasma levels of intact PTH are elevated above target range of the CKD stage. (EVIDENCE)
- The serum phosphorus levels should be monitored every month following the initiation of dietary phosphorus restriction. (OPINION)

References:

- Phosphorus Page of Linus Pauling Institute Website: http://lpi.oregonstate.edu/infocenter/minerals/phosphorus.
- Food and Nutrition Board, Institute of Medicine. Phosphorus. Dietary Reference Intakes: Calcium, Phosphorus, Magnesium, Vitamin D, and Fluoride. Washington D.C.: National Academy Press; 1997:146-189. (National Academy Press).
- Fulgoni VL 3rd, Keast DR, Bailey RL, Dwyer J. Foods, fortificants, and supplements: Where do Americans get their nutrients? *J Nutr.* 2011 Oct;141(10):1847-54.
- National Kidney Foundation Website, CLINICAL PRACTICE GUIDELINES (4): http://www.kidney.org/professionals/kdoqi/guidelines_bone/guide4.htm.
- Cupisti A, Kalantar-Zadeh K. Management of natural and added dietary phosphorus burden in kidney disease. *Semin Nephrol.* 2013 Mar;33(2):180-90.

19
K
Potassium
39.098

Potassium

19
K
Potassium
39.098

Essential Mineral Functions

Potassium is an important mineral that acts to regulate electrolyte balance and cellular membrane electrical potential in concert with sodium. The concentration of potassium in the cell and sodium outside the cell allows for key electrochemical gradient activities, such as the sodium-potassium ATPase.

Intake Guidelines

Adequate Intakes (AIs) for Potassium

Age	Males mg/day	Females mg/day	Pregnancy mg/day	Lactation mg/day
0-6 months	400	400		
6-12 months	700	700		
1-3 years	3,000	3,000		
4-8 years	3,800	3,800		
9-13 years	4,500	4,500		
14-18 years	4,700	4,700		
Adults 19+	4,700	4,700		
Adults 14-50			4,700	5,100

* AI levels are measured in mg of potassium, but clinicians are often familiar with measuring potassium in milliequivelents (mEq) or millimoles (mmol), which for potassium happen to be the same. To convert mg of potassium to mEq, simply divide by 39.1 (the atomic weight of potassium). For example: 100 mg of potassium would be 2.55 mEq; conversely 5 mEq would be (multiply by 39.1) equal to 195.5 mg of potassium. The Institute of Medicine established an adequate intake level (AI) for potassium based on intake levels found to lower blood pressure, reduce salt sensitivity and minimize the risk of kidney stones.

General Levels of Deficiencies in the U.S.

In the general population, low potassium levels (hypokalemia) are rarely due to insufficient dietary intake of potassium. Hypokalemia is usually found where potassium excretion or metabolism is compromised by one of the following: use of potassium-wasting diuretics (e.g., thiazide diuretics or furosemide), alcoholism, severe vomiting or diarrhea, overuse or abuse of laxatives, anorexia nervosa or bulimia, magnesium depletion or congestive heart failure (CHF).

Natural and Supplemental Forms

A variety of fruits, nuts and vegetables contain potassium, providing enough for the average individual. The use of potassium in dietary supplements is usually reserved for specific applications (see conditions associated with potassium deficiency above) and is often limited to less than 99 mg of potassium per serving to prevent hyperkalemia. Some common sources of potassium (with percent K) include potassium aspartate (20%), potassium chloride (52%), potassium citrate (38%), potassium carbonate (56%), potassium gluconate (15%), potassium iodide (23%) and potassium glycinate complex (18%); potassium forms only weak chelates/complexes with amino acids.

Potential for Toxicity

Excess intake of potassium is not known to cause toxicity in healthy individuals with normal kidney function and the IOM has set no tolerable upper limit. Individuals with poor kidney function or on one of the following drugs may experience hyperkalemia when using supplemental potassium sources: potassium-sparing agents (spironolactone, triamterene, amiloride), angiotensin converting enzyme (ACE) inhibitors (captopril, enalapril, fosinopril), NSAIDs (indomethacin, ibuprofen, ketorolac), heparin, digitalis, beta-blockers, alpha-blockers, and angiotensin receptor blockers (ARBs- losartan, valsartan, irbesartan, candesartan).

References:

- Potassium Page of Linus Pauling Institute Website: http://lpi.oregonstate.edu/infocenter/minerals/potassium.
- Food and Nutrition Board, Institute of Medicine. Potassium. Dietary Reference Intakes for Water, Potassium, Sodium, Chloride, and Sulfate. Washington, D. C.: National Academies Press; 2005:186-268. (National Academies Press).
- Cohn JN, Kowey PR, Whelton PK, Prisant LM. New guidelines for potassium replacement in clinical practice: a contemporary review by the National Council on Potassium in Clinical Practice. *Arch Intern Med.* 2000 Sep 11;160(16):2429-36.

34
Se
Selenium
78.09

Selenium

34
Se
Selenium
78.09

Essential Mineral Functions

Selenium is a required cofactor for more than 20 different proteins/enzymes (selenoproteins). The most well known selenoproteins are glutathione peroxidases, thioredoxin reductase and iodothyronine deiodinases, needed for the conversion of T4 to T3.

Intake Guidelines

Recommended Dietary Allowances (RDAs) for Selenium

Age	Males mcg/day	Females mcg/day	Pregnancy mcg/day	Lactation mcg/day
0-6 months	15 (AI)	15 (AI)		
6-12 months	20 (AI)	20 (AI)		
1-3 years	20	20		
4-8 years	30	30		
9-13 years	40	40		
14-18 years	55	55	60	70
Adults 19+	55	55	60	70

* The RDA is based on the amount of dietary selenium required to maximize activity of the antioxidant enzyme glutathione peroxidase in plasma.

General Levels of Deficiencies in the U.S.

Average intake of selenium is about twice the current RDA. Numerous chronic diseases are theorized to be associated with insufficient selenium-related functions, conditions for which some justification may be warranted for selenium supplementation as an intervention/therapy.

Natural and Supplemental Forms

Food sources are found in meats and seafood, and especially high in Brazil nuts (two Brazil nuts are apparently biologically equivalent to 100 mcg of selenomethionine supplementation). Dietary supplement sources (with their percent Se) are usually inorganic salts: sodium selenite (45%), sodium selenate (41%); or organic complexes: selenium aspartate (2%), selenocysteine (47%), selenomethionine (40%) or selenium glycinate complex (1%); selenium forms only weak chelates/complexes with amino acids. Selenium-enriched yeast is used for animal (mostly horses) and, sometimes, human supplementation. Made correctly, this brewer's yeast fermentation should yield 50% or more of the selenium as selenomethionine; however, no standards are required for this product and many manufacturers merely blend harvested yeast with inorganic selenium.

Potential for Toxicity

Acute selenium toxicity is only known to occur in rare situations, however chronic selenium toxicity can occur with high daily consumption of selenium in foods or supplements. The Institute of Medicine has set the tolerable upper intake level (UL) for selenium at 400 mcg/day in adults based on the prevention of hair and nail brittleness and loss, early signs of chronic selenium toxicity.

References:

- Selenium Page of Linus Pauling Institute Website: http://lpi.oregonstate.edu/infocenter/minerals/selenium.
- Food and Nutrition Board, Institute of Medicine. Selenium. Dietary reference intakes for vitamin C, vitamin E, selenium, and carotenoids. Washington D.C.: National Academy Press; 2000:284-324. (National Academy Press).
- Finley JW. Bioavailability of selenium from foods. *Nutr Rev.* 2006 Mar;64(3):146-51.
- Thomson CD, Chisholm A, McLachlan SK, Campbell JM. Brazil nuts: an effective way to improve selenium status. *Am J Clin Nutr.* 2008 Feb;87(2):379-84.
- Rayman MP. The use of high-selenium yeast to raise selenium status: how does it measure up? *Br J Nutr.* 2004 Oct;92(4):557-73.

30
Zn
Zinc
65.39

Zinc

30
Zn
Zinc
65.39

Essential Mineral Functions

Zinc acts as a cofactor for nearly 300 different enzymes that perform a wide range of metabolically important functions in most tissues. Zinc is also critical for maintaining the structural integrity of important zinc-finger, DNA-binding domains of transcription factors that regulate gene expression.

Intake Guidelines

Recommended Dietary Allowances (RDAs) for Zinc

Age	Males mg/day	Females mg/day	Pregnancy mg/day	Lactation mg/day
0-6 months	2 (AI)	2 (AI)		
6-12 months	3	3		
1-3 years	3	3		
4-8 years	5	5		
9-13 years	8	8		
14-18 years	11	9	12	13
Adults 19+	11	8	11	12

* A reliable indicator of zinc nutritional status is not readily available; therefore the RDA for zinc is based on several indicators of zinc nutritional status and represents the daily intake likely to prevent deficiency in nearly all individuals in a specific age and gender group.

General Levels of Deficiencies in the U.S.

It is now recognized that zinc insufficiency (marginal deficiency) is a global phenomenon. However, NHANES data from 2003 – 2006 show the percent of Americans over the age of two with intake of dietary zinc below the EAR is around 15% before fortification and supplementation, which then drops to 8%. Those vulnerable to zinc insufficiency include: children and adolescents, especially premature and low-birth-weight infants; pregnant and lactating women; the elderly; anorexic subjects; those with persistent or acute diarrhea; subjects with Celiac; short bowel; Crohn's; ulcerative colitis or chronic renal disease; alcoholics and strict vegetarians.

Natural and Supplemental Forms

Food sources of zinc are primarily found in meat, dairy and some seafood—oysters are very high in zinc—though some nuts and legumes provide smaller amounts for vegetarians. Phytic acid can greatly impede food-sourced zinc absorption. Dietary supplement forms of zinc (with their percent Zn) include: zinc ascorbate (10%), zinc carbonate (52%), zinc aspartate (30%), zinc citrate (34%), zinc gluconate (12%), zinc oxide (80%), zinc picolinate (20%) and zinc undecylenate (14%) (usually to deliver undecylenic acid for its antifungal properties), zinc carnosine (21%) and zinc amino acid chelate (bisglycinate, 20%).

Head-to-head bioavailability of various zinc compounds is limited. In 1987, a study using 50 mg of zinc (from citrate, gluconate and picolinate rotation without washout) showed no difference in serum zinc levels but higher hair, urine and RBC levels of zinc were associated with the zinc picolinate. No further studies have been done to test the efficacy of zinc picolinate bioavailability since that time. A more recent study (Gandia et al.) using 15 mg of zinc (bisglycinate or gluconate) in 12 female volunteers (crossover design) showed a significantly higher absorption when consuming the bisglycinate form. The other advantage of the bisglycinate chelate is this form is neither greatly influenced by, nor a contributor to, changes in bioavailability related to copper or iron.

Potential for Toxicity

Acute toxicity of zinc is rare and often related to inhaled metallic zinc, not supplements. The tolerable upper limit for zinc set by the IOM is 40 mg per day in adults. For general supplemental purposes, this level should not be exceeded. However, the use of zinc supplementation above the upper limit for specific therapeutic uses has been shown to be safe and (often) effective. Long-term zinc usage above 40 mg/day should be done in the context of a protocol known to be safe and effective. The use of copper supplements should be considered as some studies have shown that high-dose zinc can reduce copper status.

References:

- Zinc Page of Linus Pauling Institute Website: http://lpi.oregonstate.edu/infocenter/minerals/zinc.
- Food and Nutrition Board, Institute of Medicine. Zinc. Dietary reference intakes for vitamin A, vitamin K, arsenic, boron, chromium, copper, iodine, iron, manganese, molybdenum, nickel, silicon, vanadium, and zinc. Washington, D.C.: National Academy Press; 2001:442-501. (National Academy Press).
- Fulgoni VL 3rd, Keast DR, Bailey RL, Dwyer J. Foods, fortificants, and supplements: Where do Americans get their nutrients? *J Nutr*. 2011 Oct;141(10):1847-54.
- King JC. Does zinc absorption reflect zinc status? *Int J Vitam Nutr Res*. 2010 Oct;80(4-5):300-6.
- Foster M, Chu A, Petocz P, Samman S. Effect of vegetarian diets on zinc status: a systematic review and meta-analysis of studies in humans. J *Sci Food Agric*. 2013 Aug 15;93(10):2362-71.
- Barrie SA, Wright JV, Pizzorno JE, Kutter E, Barron PC. Comparative absorption of zinc picolinate, zinc citrate and zinc gluconate in humans. *Agents Actions*. 1987 Jun;21(1-2):223-8.
- Gandia P, Bour D et al. A bioavailability study comparing two oral formulations containing zinc (Zn bis-glycinate vs. Zn gluconate) after a single administration to twelve healthy female volunteers. *Int J Vitam Nutr Res*. 2007 Jul;77(4):243-8.

Functionally Essential Nutrients

There are a few nutrients that, while not absolutely essential, should be considered functionally essential in many patients where regular supplementation may be warranted. These nutrients can be made by humans but are often insufficiently synthesized due to reduced precursor consumptions, reduced levels of the vitamin and mineral cofactors needed by the enzymes that produce them, genetic predisposition, or other functional metabolic conditions.

These nutrients include long-chain omega-3 and omega-6 fatty acids (covered on pages 43-47), choline, inositol, carnitine, coenzyme Q_{10} and lipoic acid. Some of these ingredients may find their way into multivitamins, especially choline, but more often these are used in specialty products designed for specific needs. Most of these nutrients have also been successfully used, usually at higher than supplemental doses, for specific therapeutic interventions. These therapeutic uses will not be covered in the following monographs unless specifically related to conditions that deplete the nutrient itself (i.e., statin-induced CoQ_{10} depletion).

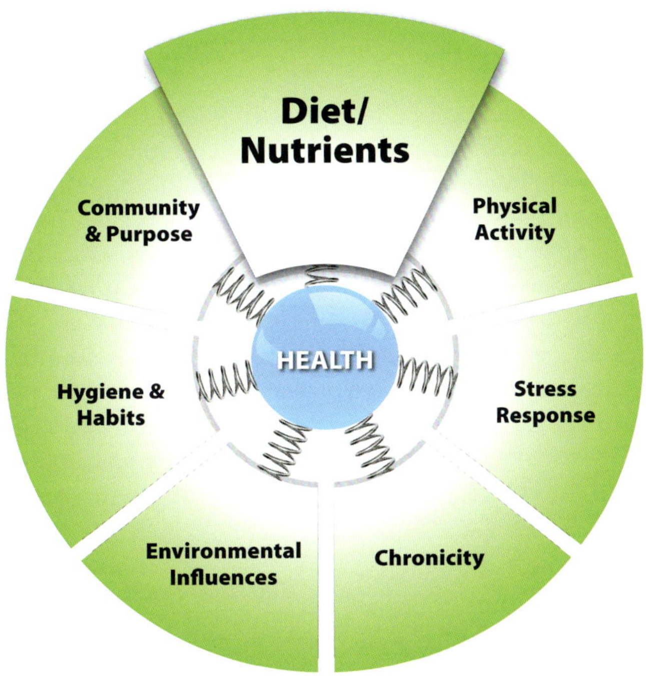

Choline

Choline is a vital component of two important phospholipids, phophatidylcholine and sphingomyelin. These phospholipids are important components of cell membranes and also precursors to secondary messengers within cells. Choline is also the precursor to acetylcholine, a critical neurotransmitter for memory and basic muscle contraction. Choline can also be metabolized into betaine (trimethylglycine), a molecule used for some methylation reactions (e.g., converting homocysteine to methionine).

Intake Guidelines

Adequate Intakes (AIs) for Choline

Age	Males mg/day	Females mg/day	Pregnancy mg/day	Lactation mg/day
0-6 months	125	125		
6-12 months	150	150		
1-3 years	200	200		
4-8 years	250	250		
9-13 years	375	375		
14-18 years	550	400		
Adults 19+	550	425		
All ages			450	550

Deficiency of choline in the diet has been linked to nonalcoholic fatty liver disease, atherosclerosis, and, potentially, neurological and memory disorders. During pregnancy, choline deficiency increases the risk for fetal neural tube defects. NHANES data collected from 2003 to 2004 suggest choline intake in the majority of Americans is well below the AI, putting many at risk for conditions related to insufficient choline intake.

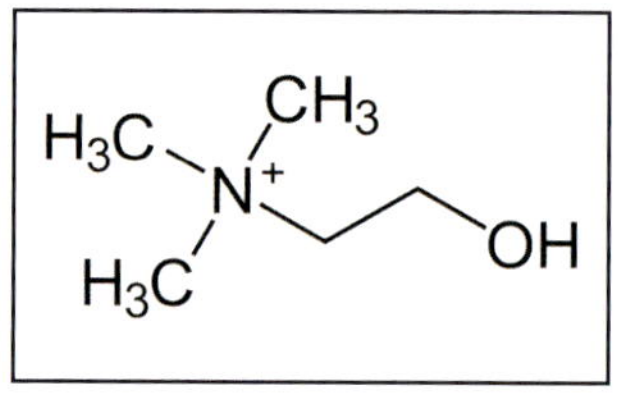

In addition, several nutrigenetic and epigenetic phenomena are known to increase the need for choline intake. Studies performed on subjects intentionally fed a low-choline diet identified several single nucleotide polymorphisms (SNP) and changes in DNA methylation in genes (or promoter sequences of genes) involved in choline or folate metabolism that affected the efficiency of choline metabolism. Choline insufficiency may also be compounded by the popular recommendation to consume fewer eggs, one of the most common dietary sources of choline in the American diet.

Besides eggs, food sources of choline include beef liver (highest), wheat germ, cooked beef and cod, and cooked cruciferous vegetables (broccoli and Brussels sprouts). Choline found in dietary supplements is usually in the salt forms of choline bitartrate or choline chloride (often only a liquid), products derived from the synthetic conversion of tartaric acid. Lecithin (phosphotidylcholine, PC) is another popular supplement providing choline, but pure lecithin/PC is only about 13% choline by weight, compared to the more commonly used choline bitartrate, which is 40% choline—many commercially available lecithins are blends of PC with other phospholipids from soy, lowering the choline content even further.

We suggest consuming choline within a varied diet, as only small amounts of choline will be found in multivitamin supplements. Prudent consumption of eggs, along with the other major sources of choline, can be easily incorporated into a Mediterranean or Paleo-Med diet. Unusually high doses are rare, and unnecessary, and the IOM has set a tolerable upper limit at 3.5 gm/day in adults. Excessive conversion to trimethylamine will cause a fish-like body odor when choline consumption is too high.

References

- Choline Page- Linus Pauling Institute website: http://lpi.oregonstate.edu/infocenter/othernuts/choline
- Zeisel SH, da Costa KA. Choline: an essential nutrient for public health. *Nutr Rev.* 2009 Nov;67(11):615-23.
- Jensen, H.; Batres-Marques; Carriquiry, A.; Schalinske, K. Choline in the diets of the U.S,. Population: NHANES, 2003–2004; Presented at the National Nutrient Data Bank Conference; 2007.
- Zeisel SH. Nutritional genomics: defining the dietary requirement and effects of choline. *J Nutr.* 2011 Mar;141(3):531-4.

Inositol

Inositol (cyclohexane-1,2,3,4,5,6-hexol) occurs in nature primarily in its myo-inositol conformation (see figure). Like choline, inositol was often classified as a B-complex nutrient, although it is not an essential nutrient because it can be synthesized in humans from glucose-6-phosphate. Inositol is a precursor to several important cell-signaling molecules called inositol phosphates (IP6-AKA phytic acid, IP3 etc.) and the lipid-signaling molecule family, phosphoinositol phosphates (e.g., Phosphatidylinositol 3-phosphate: PI(3)P).

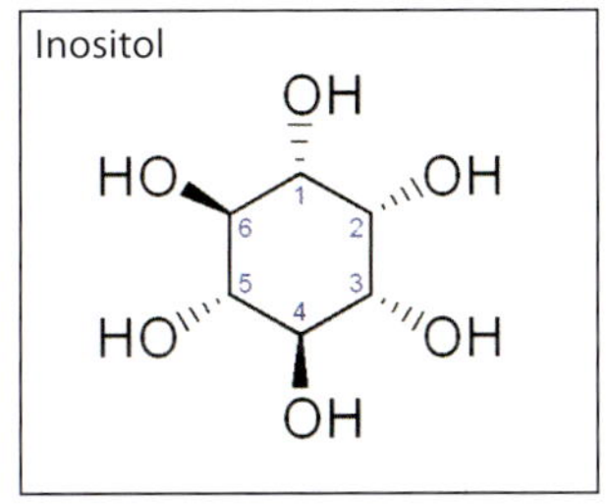

There is no DRI for inositol and deficiency diseases related to inositol are not described, although from animal model experiments, prenatal myo-inositol deficiency is thought to be play a role in fetal galactosemia. Inositol is found in most foods, but is particularly high in citrus fruits and juices, cantaloupe, legumes and nuts. (Clements and Darnell list several hundred food sources of myo-inositol).

Therapeutic supplementation of myo-inositol or inositol (unknown isomer) has been studied in humans at a range of dosages, up to 28 grams. Multivitamin or B-complex supplements containing a few hundred mg of inositol or myo-inositol are very common. These supplemental forms are derived from phytic acid (IP6), usually sourced from rice bran. The use of inositol hexaniacinate (or nicotinate) as a form of flush-free niacin is discouraged; they are ineffective for lipid-lowering and provide a lower percent of inositol than other available forms. Using high doses of myo-inositol or IP6 should only be done when following a protocol known to be safe and effective.

References:

- A detailed account of inositol chemistry can be found at http://en.wikipedia.org/wiki/Inositol.
- Berry GT. Is prenatal myo-inositol deficiency a mechanism of CNS injury in galactosemia? *J Inherit Metab Dis.* 2011 Apr;34(2):345-55.
- Clements RS Jr, Darnell B. Myo-inositol content of common foods: development of a high-myo-inositol diet. *Am J Clin Nutr.* 1980 Sep;33(9):1954-67.

Carnitine

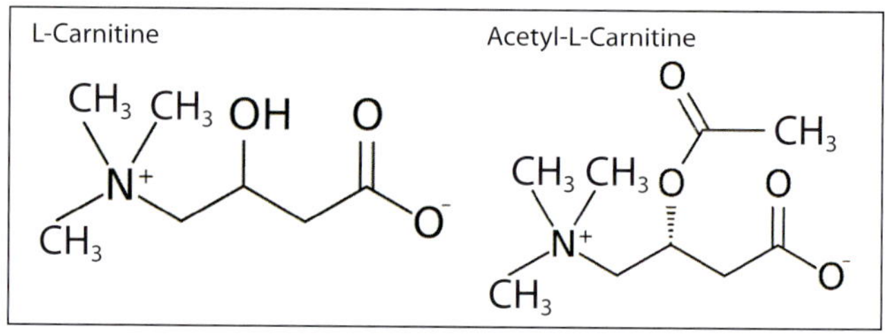

Humans can synthesize carnitine (β-hydroxy-β-N-trimethylaminobutyric acid or L-carnitine) from the amino acids lysine and methionine, primarily in the kidney and liver. Biosynthesis of carnitine requires adequate levels of lysine and methionine, as well as vitamin and mineral cofactors such as iron, vitamin B_6, niacin and, perhaps, vitamin C.

Carnitine accumulates in tissues needing energy from fatty acids (skeletal muscle, cardiac muscle and testes) where carnitine acts to help shuttle acyl-coA across the mitochondrial membrane, so it can be used for cellular energy through β-oxidation (see figure).

There is much debate about the likelihood of carnitine deficiency in humans and the need to routinely supplement with L-carnitine. Genetic disorders in the protein that transports carnitine can lead to primary carnitine deficiency, but frank carnitine deficiencies are rare. The nucleoside analogues used in the treatment of HIV infection, including zidovudine (AZT), didanosine (ddI), zalcitabine (ddC), and stavudine (d4T), may produce a secondary L-carnitine deficiency.

Dietary sources of carnitine, originally named for its presence in meat, are mostly found in animal meat. Highest levels are from beef, modest levels from pork, and the lowest in chicken. Other sources include dairy products, fish, avocados and tempeh. With such limited amount of carnitine found in a vegetarian's diet, many studies have looked into the endogenous synthesis, absorption capacity and muscle levels of carnitine in vegetarian subjects. Although vegetarians appear to have a higher absorption and retention of carnitine than those consuming

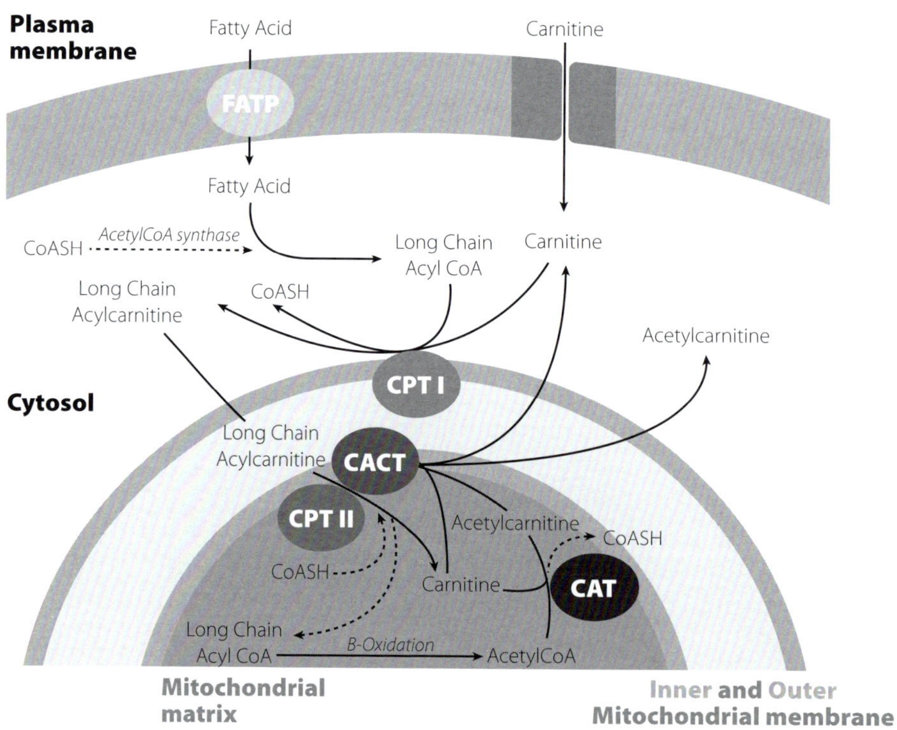

Carnitine is actively transported into the cytosol to participate in the shuttling of activated long chain fatty acids into the mitochondria where β-oxidation takes place. Carnitine palmitoyltransferase I (CPTI), Carnitine palmitoyltransferase II (CPTII), Carnitine-acylcarnitine translocase (CACT), Carnitine-acetyl transferase (CAT). Adapted from Flanagan et al.

higher carnitine through meat-containing diets, carnitine levels are generally 20 – 30% lower in strict vegetarians. More importantly, Stephens et al. have shown that vegetarians have a lowered capacity to move carnitine into muscle tissue, partly due to down-regulation of the protein that transports carnitine into muscle tissue. The consequence of this lower muscle carnitine in strict vegetarians is yet to be explored, but after 11 years of a strict vegetarian diet, one male subject was able to normalize muscle carnitine levels after six months on an omnivorous diet.

Supplemental L-carnitine is available as pure L-carnitine (liquid), L-carnitine salts (tartrate, fumerate) and carnitine esters (acetyl-carnitine, propionyl-L-carnitine). The carnitine portion of these commercially available products is produced by bacterial fermentation and not from an animal source. Limited head-to-head studies have been done to compare bioavailability or clinical outcomes for each of these substances. In pigs, L-carnitine tartrate has the highest absorption, similar to liquid L-carnitine, compared to other salts, all of which were better than the ester forms. In humans, the absorption and pharmacokinetics of L-carnitine and its salts compared to acetyl-carnitine appear to be very similar and, at least for nutrient supplementation purposes, should be considered equivalent. Some subtle therapeutic differences have been noted in various clinical outcomes between these two carnitine forms, comparisons that are beyond the scope of this monograph.

High doses of supplemental carnitine (2-3 grams and above) can lead to some gastrointestinal complaints and a fish-like body odor. Doses higher than two grams/day should be used only when following a protocol known to be safe and effective for the patient being managed.

References

- Carnitine Page of Linus Pauling Institute Website: http://lpi.oregonstate.edu/infocenter/othernuts/carnitine.
- Office of Dietary Supplements- National Institutes of Health- Health Professional Information. http://ods.od.nih.gov/factsheets/Carnitine-HealthProfessional.
- Flanagan JL, Simmons PA, Vehige J, Willcox MD, Garrett Q. Role of carnitine in disease. *Nutr Metab (Lond).* 2010 Apr 16;7:30.
- Lombard KA, Olson AL, Nelson SE, Rebouche CJ. Carnitine status of lactoovovegetarians and strict vegetarian adults and children. *Am J Clin Nutr.* 1989 Aug;50(2):301-6.
- Rebouche CJ, Chenard CA. Metabolic fate of dietary carnitine in human adults: identification and quantification of urinary and fecal metabolites. *J Nutr*. 1991 Apr;121(4):539-46.
- Stephens FB, Marimuthu K et al. Vegetarians have a reduced skeletal muscle carnitine transport capacity. *Am J Clin Nutr.* 2011 Sep;94(3):938-44.
- Rebouche CJ. Kinetics, pharmacokinetics, and regulation of L-carnitine and acetyl-L-carnitine metabolism. *Ann N Y Acad Sci*. 2004 Nov;1033:30-41.

Coenzyme Q$_{10}$

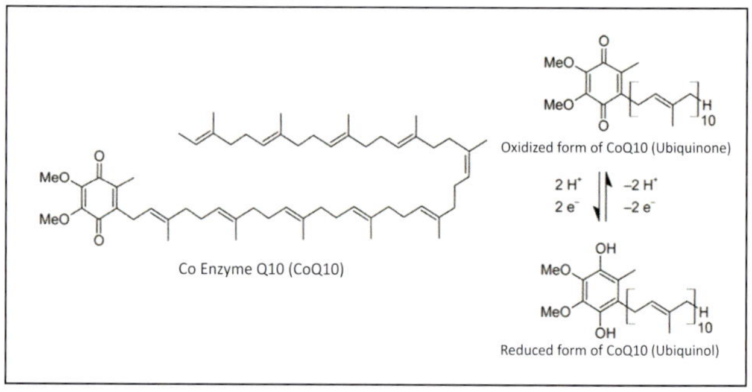

Coenzyme Q$_{10}$ (CoQ$_{10}$) is a fat-soluble compound within the ubiquinone family, containing a benzoquinone head group and 10 isoprenyl units (each five carbons long, see figure). CoQ$_{10}$ is naturally found in both the oxidized (ubiquinone) and reduced (ubiquinol forms) in the body and is one of many fat-soluble coenzymes that help to shuttle electrons within the inner membrane of the mitochondria (known as the electron transport chain), critical for the formation of ATP. CoQ$_{10}$ also appears to act as a cellular/mitochondrial antioxidant molecule. Humans synthesize CoQ$_{10}$ via a complex biochemical pathway involving over a dozen different enzymes. Endogenous synthesis, along with small dietary amounts of CoQ$_{10}$, appear to be adequate to prevent overt deficiencies of CoQ$_{10}$ in the average healthy individual.

Food sources of CoQ$_{10}$ are nearly all derived from animal products: beef, pork, chicken or fish; although other sources include soybean and canola oils, roasted nuts and seeds (peanuts, sesame, pistachio), and boiled broccoli or cauliflower. Food source CoQ$_{10}$ is difficult to predict as food preparation can diminish or enhance CoQ$_{10}$ content and bioavailability. For omnivorous individuals, daily CoQ$_{10}$ consumption is around three to six mg/day; vegetarians are known to have lower serum CoQ$_{10}$ levels owing to a lower consumption of CoQ$_{10}$ containing foods. Even so, with the exception of rare genetic conditions, CoQ$_{10}$ deficiencies are not described in the general population.

Regardless, because of the overwhelming amount of research looking into antioxidant and genomic mechanisms of CoQ$_{10}$, and growing discussions of how mitochondrial function and oxidation contribute to the aging process, along with many positive clinical trials for chronic disease outcomes (at higher doses), daily CoQ$_{10}$ supplementation is common here in the United States. In addition, the evidence is strong that CoQ$_{10}$ levels are depleted in subjects taking statin medications (including active red yeast rice-RYR products), while CoQ$_{10}$ supplementation can reverse this depletion and even some of the statin-induced changes to heart/muscle function. Because of these data and the many other potential benefits—and few, if any, side effects—we suggest that CoQ$_{10}$ (at least 100 mg of an absorption-improved form) be recommended to all patients taking prescription statin drugs. (While RYR products containing active monocolin K also deplete CoQ$_{10}$ [case report and animal studies], these products are not legal to sell as dietary supplements in the United States.)

CoQ$_{10}$ used in dietary supplements is produced by bacterial fermentation and purified into a crystalline powder that is poorly absorbed due to its lack of water-solubility. Small amounts of powdered, unmodified CoQ$_{10}$ are often added to multivitamins (tablets, capsules or powders) that have virtually no bioavailability and no benefit. Over the past few decades, CoQ$_{10}$ manufacturers have devised and patented numerous ways to increase the bioavailability of CoQ$_{10}$ supplements, primarily by helping it maintain solubility through the digestive process. This process usually involves combining the CoQ$_{10}$ with other lipid-soluble components, mixing with surfactants to make it more water-soluble, changing the size of the particles or combining the CoQ$_{10}$ with compounds that allow it to absorb, forming liposomes, microspheres, nanoparticles, nanoemulsions and self-emulsifying systems. In general, these methods have improved overall absorption by about three times, compared to dry, unmodified powder; although some have been more successful than others.

A full-scale review of all current CoQ$_{10}$ products, and marketing claims based on absorption, is beyond the scope of this monograph. The information is complicated by the fact that many of the studies were performed with different doses, subject types and study lengths; and often remain unpublished for public scrutiny. More relevant is nearly all of these studies are single-dose, noncrossover studies that are difficult to interpret, since the CoQ$_{10}$

absorption variability between individuals is unpredictable. Finally, and perhaps most importantly, many of these highly absorbable forms contain very low doses of CoQ_{10} at a very high cost, rarely meeting the cost-to-benefit ratio gained by the improved bioavailability.

Ubiquinol vs. Ubiquinone

As with many antioxidant molecules, CoQ_{10} can be isolated in either the reduced form (ubiquinol) or the oxidized form (ubiquinone). When ubiquinol first became commercially available in 2006, many clinicians assumed this reduced form would be a better therapeutic option, even though it was much more expensive. We now know ubiquinone (CoQ_{10}-oxidized form) is absorbed and converted almost completely to ubiquinol in the enterocytes. Since the number of human studies using ubiquinol is so few and virtually none of these studies measure outcomes comparing ubiquinol supplementation to the more studied, and much less expensive, CoQ_{10}-ubiquinone, we cannot recommend the use of ubiquinol for routine supplementation. Clinicians may choose to use ubiquinol in isolated cases where published clinical trials warrant such use. Both forms are considered safe at supplemental and therapeutic doses, although ubiquinol is considerably more expensive; it is not uncommon to see 300 mg of ubiquinone priced lower than 100 mg of ubiquinol.

References:

- CoQ_{10} Page-Linus Pauling Institute webpage: http://lpi.oregonstate.edu/infocenter/othernuts/coq10
- Pravst I, Zmitek K, Zmitek J. Coenzyme Q_{10} contents in foods and fortification strategies. *Crit Rev Food Sci Nutr.* 2010 Apr;50(4):269-80.
- Linnane AW, Zhang C et al. Human aging and global function of coenzyme Q_{10}. *Ann NY Acad Sci.* 2002 Apr;959:396-411.
- Littlefield N, Beckstrand RL, Luthy KE. Statins' effect on plasma levels of Coenzyme Q_{10} and improvement in myopathy with supplementation. *J Am Assoc Nurse Pract.* 2014 Feb;26(2):85-90.
- Vercelli L, Mongini T, Olivero N, Rodolico C, Musumeci O, Palmucci L. Chinese red rice depletes muscle coenzyme Q_{10} and maintains muscle damage after discontinuation of statin treatment. *J Am Geriatr Soc.* 2006 Apr;54(4):718-20.
- Yang HT, Lin SH, Huang SY, Chou HJ. Acute administration of red yeast rice (Monascus purpureus) depletes tissue coenzyme Q(10) levels in ICR mice. *Br J Nutr.* 2005 Jan;93(1):131-5.
- Beg S, Javed S, Kohli K. Bioavailability enhancement of coenzyme Q_{10}: an extensive review of patents. *Recent Pat Drug Deliv Formul.* 2010 Nov;4(3):245-55.
- Bhagavan HN, Chopra RK, Craft NE, Chitchumroonchokchai C, Failla ML. Assessment of coenzyme Q_{10} absorption using an in vitro digestion-Caco-2 cell model. *Int J Pharm.* 2007 Mar 21;333(1-2):112-7.
- Bhagavan HN, Chopra RK. Plasma coenzyme Q_{10} response to oral ingestion of coenzyme Q_{10} formulations. *Mitochondrion.* 2007 Jun;7 Suppl:S78-88.

Lipoic Acid

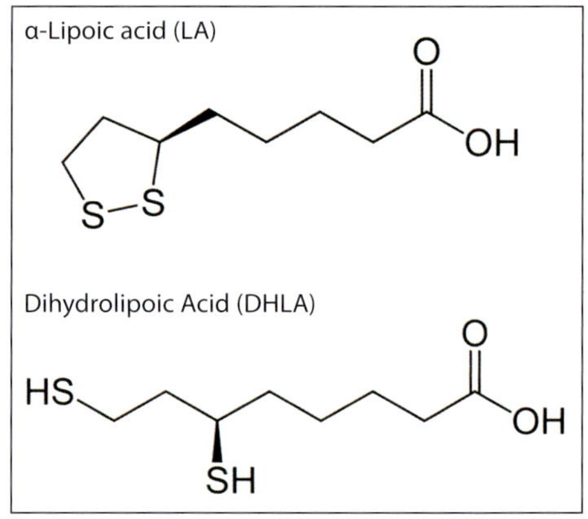

Lipoic acid (alpha-lipoic acid or thioctic acid) is a peculiar molecule synthesized from an eight-carbon fatty acid (octanoic or caprylic acid) within the mitochondria, in very low concentrations. Within the mitochondria lipoic acid is found attached to the lysine residue of several enzyme complexes critical to energy production.

The unique structure of lipoic acid allows for both lipid and water solubility, giving lipoic acid a pleiotropic antioxidant effect, quenching superoxide radicals, hydroxyl radicals, hypochlorous acid, peroxyl radicals, and singlet oxygen. The disulfide feature of lipoic acid also allows for direct reduction of oxidized glutathione (GSH) and, along with recharging vitamin C, lipoic acid may help reduce oxidized vitamin E. Also, lipoic acid has a genomic influence through the NRF2 signaling pathway, allowing for increased production of antioxidant and detoxification proteins regulated through the antioxidant response element (ARE).

Deficiencies of lipoic acid (endogenous or dietary) are not described and are unknown in humans. However, while endogenous biosynthesis of lipoic acid is protein-bound, cells have and use transporter mechanisms for the uptake of free, unbound lipoic acid, both R and S isomers. Decades of basic science, animal studies and human clinical studies suggest increasing free lipoic acid can influence physiology within the cells and organ systems. While these studies use doses that could never be achieved with any known dietary source (usually only a few mcg/gm are found in the highest food sources such as organ meats), these data have led many to postulate insufficient lipoic acid levels from any cause may play a role in diminished mitochondrial energy, increased oxidative burden, diminished glucose sensitivity, the depletion of "metabolic reserve" and the overall aging process. For these and other reasons, lipoic acid supplementation is common for general and therapeutic use in the U.S.

Supplemental lipoic acid is derived from chemical synthesis, starting from modified eight-carbon fatty acids (e.g., 6,8-Dichloro-ethylcaprylate). This process produces a 50:50 (racemic) mixture of the two stereoisomers of alpha-lipoic acid, R and S. Nearly every clinical trial done in humans has been done using this racemic (RAC) lipoic acid—both intravenous and oral dosing. Since about 2001, R-lipoic acid (potassium and sodium salt forms) has become available and sold as a dietary supplement in the U.S. Sometimes touted as the natural form, this ingredient is produced by a complex process that separates the R and S forms after chemical synthesis. While animal and cell culture studies suggest the R-isomer may have benefits over the RAC blend, human clinical studies have yet to suggest this is true.

To date, only small pilot trials have been done to test the pharmacokinetic and clinical differences between R-lipoic acid and RAC-lipoic acid in humans. These studies reveal that there may be large individual differences in R and RAC lipoic acid bioavailability; and also an age-dependent difference in bioavailability. In any event, these studies were performed using high single doses (500 mg), and have not been done with long-term dosing of each ingredient with any meaningful clinical end-points. Since *in vitro* and animal studies suggest many, though not all, of the antioxidant and cell-signaling functions of S-lipoic acid (or RAC) are similar to the R-isomer, it is possible the RAC-form may be clinically similar to R-lipoic acid. Regardless, since there are almost no human clinical studies performed using R-lipoic acid to evaluate, and there are large numbers of studies to help guide clear recommendations for use of RAC alpha-lipoic acid, we believe it is premature to recommend the expensive R-lipoic acid for supplementation or therapeutic intervention at this time. Perhaps further studies, and lower R-lipoic acid cost, may favor the use of R-lipoic acid products in the future.

Alpha-lipoic acid doses of 30 – 100 mg are often found in multivitamins or specialty antioxidant products. Higher doses are usually reserved for various therapeutic protocols. These doses are safe for most subjects. Lipoic acid has been noted in one animal study to inhibit a biotin-dependent carboxylase and shares a transporter with biotin. While lipoic acid has never been shown to hinder biotin metabolism in humans, out of precaution some companies include a small amount of biotin in products containing high amounts of alpha-lipoic acid.

References

- Lipoic Acid Page- Linus Pauling Institute website: http://lpi.oregonstate.edu/infocenter/othernuts/la
- Rochette L, Ghibu S, Richard C, Zeller M, Cottin Y, Vergely C. Direct and indirect antioxidant properties of α-lipoic acid and therapeutic potential. *Mol Nutr Food Res.* 2013 Jan;57(1):114-25.
- Shay KP, Moreau RF, Smith EJ, Smith AR, Hagen TM. Alpha-lipoic acid as a dietary supplement: molecular mechanisms and therapeutic potential. *Biochim Biophys Acta.* 2009 Oct;1790(10):1149-60.
- Suh JH, Shenvi SV, Dixon BM, Liu H, Jaiswal AK, Liu RM, Hagen TM. Decline in transcriptional activity of Nrf2 causes age-related loss of glutathione synthesis, which is reversible with lipoic acid. *Proc Natl Acad Sci U S A.* 2004 Mar 9;101(10):3381-6.
- Teichert J, Hermann R, Ruus P, Preiss R. Plasma kinetics, metabolism, and urinary excretion of alpha-lipoic acid following oral administration in healthy volunteers. *J Clin Pharmacol.* 2003 Nov;43(11):1257-67.
- Keith DJ, Butler JA et al. Age and gender dependent bioavailability of R- and R,S-α-lipoic acid: a pilot study. *Pharmacol Res.* 2012 Sep;66(3):199-206.
- Yamada T, Hashida K, Takarada-Iemata M, Matsugo S, Hori O. Alpha-Lipoic acid (LA) enantiomers protect SH-SY5Y cells against glutathione depletion. *Neurochem Int.* 2011 Dec;59(7):1003-9.
- Zempleni J, Trusty TA, Mock DM. Lipoic acid reduces the activities of biotin-dependent carboxylases in rat liver. *J Nutr.* 1997 Sep;127(9):1776-81.
- For our critique of time-released lipoic acid preparations: see our whitepaper online at http://www.pointinstitute.org/wp-content/uploads/2012/10/Time-release-lipoic-acid-paper.pdf.

Herbals, Botanicals, and Phytonutrients: The Basics

In the United States, botanical or herbal products are sold as dietary supplements; botanical supplement manufacturers are required to follow the same manufacturing and labeling guidelines as those required for vitamin and mineral supplements. It is also very common for dietary supplement formulas to combine botanical ingredients or concentrated phytonutrients with vitamins, minerals, or other nutrients. Since the consumers' intent in using many of these botanical ingredients is generally therapeutic (or health-promoting) in nature, rather than for basic supplementation; this section will explain some of the unique features of herbal products, botanical ingredients and concentrated phytonutrients; while listing references you can use to further your understanding of their therapeutic potential.

Herbal Medicines versus Botanical Ingredients

Before delving into some of the particular aspects of botanical ingredients used in dietary supplements, a distinction should be made between the use of botanicals as medicines (globally and in the U.S.) and the way many botanical ingredients are used in dietary supplements. The historical use of botanicals (or herbals) as therapeutic agents is rooted in nearly every ancient culture. Written evidence of advanced medicinal systems using botanical medicines is found in some of the earliest writings from cultures in the East and West, while numerous oral traditions have been passed on for millennia amongst indigenous peoples in every region of the globe. Some of the most prominent herbal traditions that have persisted and still influence today's use of botanicals are Traditional Chinese Medicine (TCM), Ayurveda (developed in India), and the Eclectic and modern herbalist movements of Europe and the Americas. Each of these traditions (including many adaptations) rely upon different diagnostic philosophies, botanical ingredients, preparations and doses.

In contrast to the more holistic view of botanicals taught in these traditional healing philosophies, the increased amount of research into the chemistry of botanical constituents has had a greater influence on the current use of botanical ingredients in the U.S. In general, botanical ingredients or highly concentrated phytochemical compounds are used for their "active ingredient(s)" and are often formulated in a manner that is quite different from their historical use.[1] Quite often, clinicians or researchers borrow ingredients or isolated constituents from one of the ancient traditions and attempt to test their efficacy using modern Western research methods, with varying degrees of success. Debating the merits of one approach (holistic and traditional) over the other (concentrated constituents) is a complex topic and beyond the scope of this overview.

General Preparations of Botanical Products

When botanical ingredients are used as dietary supplements they may be used in a variety of ways. Products can be sold as dried plants (or plant parts), cut and sifted, dried powders, liquid extracts, powdered extracts, or standardized powdered extracts very often in capsule or tablet dosage forms. Here are some definitions that can be used to help decipher a botanical product.

Infusions and Decoctions

One of the most common ways to deliver herbal ingredients (besides consuming them directly) is using water extracts. An infusion (tea) is simply made by pouring boiling water over a dried herbal preparation, steeping, and then straining. A decoction is similar but

1. There are many licensed healthcare practitioners in the U.S. that have educated themselves in one or more of the ancient healing traditions. These individuals may use (or make) products that are associated with those traditions, even preparing products specific for each patient or teaching the patient to make their own medicines from botanical sources.

requires submerging the plant material in boiling water over a relatively longer period of time before cooling and straining. Infusions are common for leaves and flowers, while decoctions are usually made from denser materials (roots, bark, berries, etc.). Most often, package directions instruct an individual on how to prepare the plant material(s) in loose form or tea bags as needed.

Dried Powders

Botanical ingredients can be delivered merely as dried powders. This is very common for spices used in foods or botanical ingredients used in functional foods and dietary supplements. These powders can be made from virtually any part of a plant (or plant juice) and used in ready-to-mix powders, tablets or capsules.

Tinctures and Liquid Extracts

Liquid extracts can be made by soaking or percolating macerated plant material in ethyl alcohol and water (solvent). The ratio of plant material to solvent, the strength and type of the solvent and the length of time of extraction is usually determined by the traditional use of the plant, the nature of the plant constituents being extracted and desired potency of the final extract. The concentration of the final product is often expressed as a ratio between the plant and the solvent. One part herb to five parts solvent yields a 1:5 extract. Tinctures usually describe more dilute versions of liquid extracts (1:2 or less), although the naming convention that distinguishes tinctures from other liquid extracts is not universal.

The most common solvent is ethanol of various dilutions, but some botanicals are extracted using glycerin, plant oils, or supercritical gases (e.g., liquefied CO_2); some even with industrial solvents like hexane, acetone and ethyl acetate. Where ethanol is the best (and traditional) extraction solvent but undesired in the final product, the ethanol can be slowly evaporated while adding glycerol to provide a similar extract profile without ethanol in the final product (excellent for children's products). Some liquid extract products are also made by reconstituting dried extracts.

Powdered Extracts

Powdered extracts start out as liquid extracts that are made by evaporating the solvent. Depending on the nature of the plant extract, a carrier is often added to the material to allow it to maintain free-flowing characteristics. These carriers (excipients) typically include maltodextrins, cellulose, lactose and/or silicon dioxide. Some liquid extracts are directly spray-dried onto a carrier to form a powdered extract. In some cases, the plant constituents are very oily and form pastes or soft extracts (e.g., Saw Palmetto berry extract), these semi-solid extracts can be delivered in soft gel capsules or diluted with a carrier to produce a powder that can adequately handle the rigors of tablet or capsule preparations.

Powdered extracts are sometimes described by the strength of their extract ratio. These are usually described as a ratio of the weight of the original botanical starting material compared to the weight of the finished extract. These concentrated powders start around 4:1, but some highly concentrated extracts can be 50:1 or greater. These extract ratios can be very helpful when dealing with reputable ingredient manufacturers that use botanicals harvested at their peak (or traditional) season for medicinal activity and that use traditional extraction techniques. However, unscrupulous manufacturers can purchase poor quality herbal materials, use inferior extraction solvents and techniques, and still declare that the final powdered extract meets the starting-to-finished material ratio.

Standardized Extracts

Liquid or powdered extracts that are manufactured to contain a specific amount of one or more constituents (usually described as a percentage) are generally referred to as standardized extracts. The constituent(s) used for standardization are usually those that are either unique to the plant being extracted, are believed to be related to the traditional medicinal use of the plant (i.e., an active ingredient), or simply a measure used to control batch to batch consistency and extract potency. While there are many cases where the use of standardized extracts has proven to be an excellent method to ensure efficacy, there are also many examples where this has not been the case. For example, if a traditional herbal extract is found to generally contain 2% of constituent X; this may be a good marker component for future extracts made using similarly harvested and extracted material. However, it may be possible to harvest the plant at a different time or extract it using a different solvent that would yield a much higher value of constituent X. In this example, if the constituent was only a marker of proper extraction and not the main active medicinal component of the plant, this new extract would appear to be the same on the label, but may have a completely different constituent profile in the other 98% of the extract.

When using standardized extracts, it is important to be able to correlate the type of extract used in successful clinical trials (dose, extraction solvent, standardization) with those found in the product being recommended. In many cases, successful clinical trials will have used a plant powder, a dilute liquid extract, a concentration of the juice, or some other preparation. Most clinical trials using herbal preparations today are very well characterized and will often use standardized extracts of botanicals that have a long history of successful use as non-standardized ingredients in the hands of healers trained to use them. It is important to note that the successful use of a standardized botanical extract does not negate any previous published research or traditional use of the same botanical in an unstandardized form.

How do you know you have the right plant?

Botanical taxonomy is a complex science, made more complicated by the fact that each plant has numerous common names (in more than one language) and the same common name is used in different regions for different botanical species. In 1997 the FDA recognized the standardized common names and corresponding scientific names (Latin binomials) for labeling of botanicals used in dietary supplements as published in the *American Herbal Products Association's Herbs of Commerce, 2nd edition.* This does not guarantee that you will know the exact genus and species used, as some common names refer to more than one taxonomically (and medicinally) related botanical.

More important is the ability of the manufacturer of a dietary supplement to properly identify a botanical ingredient in any preparation (dried herb, powder, extract). This requires expertise in the use of many different laboratory techniques, compendial methods and ingredient specifications. Reputable dietary supplement manufacturers should have the equipment and expertise in-house to ensure the appropriate botanical is being used, although many still rely on outside third-party analytical laboratories for unique or sensitive botanical tests of identity and potency.

The use of very specific chemical fingerprints using high-performance liquid chromatography (HPLC) or high-performance thin-layer chromatography (HPTLC) is becoming more standard for identifying botanicals, and even DNA fingerprinting is being developed for routine quality control procedures where applicable (this would not be useful for extracts which normally retain no DNA).

Adulteration and Contamination of Botanicals

For a general discussion of the quality control measures used to ensure products are free of adulteration and contamination, see our discussion on page 145 and the *HerbalGram* article on DS regulation in the appendix. The issue of adulteration and contamination of herbal products is something that is nearly as complex as the chemistry of the plants themselves and as old as the ancient spice trade. Three leading nonprofit organizations—the American Botanical Council (ABC), the American Herbal Pharmacopoeia (AHP), and the University of Mississippi's National Center for Natural Products Research (NCNPR)— have invested a vast amount of time and resources (underwritten by many forward-thinking and responsible members of the dietary supplement and botanical industry) creating a large-scale program to educate members of the herbal and dietary supplement industry about ingredient and product adulteration. The status of available information for the Botanical Adulterant Program can be found online (www.abc.herbalgram.org). Reputable companies manufacturing dietary supplements using botanical ingredients should be aware of the potential adulterants and contaminants of these ingredients and have methods in place to test for both prior to use in their products.

Concentrated Phytonutrients

Perhaps the most popular current trend for using botanical ingredients in the dietary supplement industry is the use of highly concentrated or isolated phytonutrients. This is primarily due to the growing body of research using isolated plant constituents in mechanistic, cell-culture, and animal studies, as well as human clinical studies; and the ability to screen large numbers of plant constituents for beneficial genomic activity. While different in philosophy from the ancient traditions that delivered these phytonutrients as part of a natural healing system, today's researchers want to decipher the actions of each phytochemical compound, apart from the "noise" of other plant compounds. While this application of botanical medicine can be viewed as merely reducing complex phytotherapy into a drug-like delivery mechanism of only a few compounds, this type of research has done much to explain the healing mechanisms of traditional herbal medicines and has revealed data for compounds that are therapeutically valuable as concentrates/isolates for disease prevention and intervention (e.g., curcumin, quercetin, berberine, etc.).

Few concentrated phytonutrients are considered essential in the same way as vitamins or minerals; although it is now widely-recognized that phytonutrient intake is a major contributor within the disease preventing activities of fruits and vegetables.[2,3] Similar to other nutrient components, phytonutrients can act as cell signaling molecules, redox antioxidants, and enzyme regulators; although many have now been discovered to modulate gene expression (i.e., nutrigenomic and epigenetic activity).[4,5] This explains why many phytonutrients can often act at very low concentrations for some activities (nutrigenomic), but have clear dose-response curves when functioning to directly affect enzyme activities, via receptor interactions (as agonist or antagonist) or as redox antioxidants.[6]

2. Del Rio D, Rodriguez-Mateos A, Spencer JP, Tognolini M, Borges G, Crozier A. Dietary (poly)phenolics in human health: structures, bioavailability, and evidence of protective effects against chronic diseases. *Antioxid Redox Signal.* 2013 May 10;18(14):1818-92.

3. Crozier A, Jaganath IB, Clifford MN Dietary phenolics: chemistry, bioavailability and effects on health. *Nat Prod Rep.* 2009 Aug;26(8):1001-43.

4. Ferguson LR, Schlothauer RC. The potential role of nutritional genomics tools in validating high health foods for cancer control: broccoli as example. *Mol Nutr Food Res.* 2012 Jan;56(1):126-46

5. Shankar S, Kumar D, Srivastava RK. Epigenetic modifications by dietary phytochemicals: implications for personalized nutrition. *Pharmacol Ther.* 2013 Apr;138(1):1-17

6. Kim HS, Quon MJ, Kim JA. New insights into the mechanisms of polyphenols beyond antioxidant properties; lessons from the green tea polyphenol, epigallocatechin 3-gallate. *Redox Biol.* 2014 Jan 10;2:187-195.

Sources of Concentrated Phytonutrients

In many cases, these phytonutrients are simply derived from a highly concentrated extract of the plant for which the constituent is known for having traditional medicinal or dietary use. An example of this would be curcumin, which describes a blend of bright yellow phenolic curcuminoid compounds from the spice turmeric (*Curcuma longa* L.). This highly concentrated extract is typically standardized to contain 95% curcuminoids. This is also true when using concentrates of the catechin polyphenols (e.g., EGCG) from Green tea (*Camellia sinensis* (L.) Kuntze) or the anti-malarial sesquiterpene lactone compound artemisinin from wormwood (*Artemisia annua* L.).

However, not all commercially-available phytonutrients are derived from their traditional medicinal or dietary source. An example of this is resveratrol. While this polyphenol is linked in epidemiological research mostly with the consumption of red wine, nearly all commercially used resveratrol used for dietary supplements is extracted from Japanese knotweed (*Polygonum cuspidatum* Sieb. & Zucc). Likewise, while lutein and zeaxanthin are commonly consumed in the diet through kale, spinach and other green leafy vegetables, supplement forms of these xanthophylls are extracted from yellow petals of Aztec marigold flowers (*Tagetes erecta* L.).

Organic synthesis of chemically-identical phytonutrient compounds is commonly used for research and laboratory standards because they are often nearly 100% pure. The use of chemically-synthesized phytonutrients as dietary supplement ingredients is becoming more common, although their use is being debated within the regulatory framework of DSHEA (Are they "new dietary ingredients"? See page 140 for discussion). Of course, the chemical synthesis of plant compound derivatives is integral to the history of the development of numerous pharmaceutical agents still used today.

Clinicians considering the use of botanical ingredients for basic supplementation or therapeutic intervention should be familiar with the variety of plant parts, preparations, doses and formulas available in today's dietary supplement products. The same plant (but different plant part) may be used in a variety of ways for different conditions (i.e., nettles [*Urtica dioica*

L.] leaf powder for treating allergies, nettles root extract for prostate health). In the hands of a traditional healer, a concentrated phytonutrient would seem out of place, while it may provide great results as a "phytoceutical" when administered by a trained practitioner using it in a similar way as the preparation's positive clinical trial(s) suggests. Conversely, traditional herbal remedies used outside of their diagnostic and historical framework rarely reveal their historical benefits when tested in a clinical setting (or research trial) using Western criteria for diagnostic and clinical end-points. Clinicians should seek products formulated in a manner that fits the intent of their practice philosophy and understand the evidence on which those formulas are based.

Select Botanical References for Healthcare Professionals:

- Blumenthal, M. (2003) *The ABC Clinical Guide to Herbs.* Austin, TX: American Botanical Council.
- Mills, S and Bone, K. (2013) *Principles and Practice of Phytotherapy* 2nd Ed. London: Churchill Livingstone.
- Barrett, M. (2004) *The Handbook of Clinically Tested Herbal Remedies (2 Vol.).* New York, NY: The Haworth Press.
- Mills, S and Bone, K. (2005) *The Essential Guide to Herbal Safety.* St. Louis, MO: Elsevier Churchill Livingstone.
- Brinker, F. (2010) *Herbal Contraindications and Drug Interactions plus Herbal Adjuncts with Medicines, expanded 4th edition.* Sandy, OR: Eclectic Medical Publications.

Supplementing Probiotics: The Basics

While probiotics are not "nutrients" per se, the common use of these products as daily supplements for basic health goals makes them an appropriate topic for this Road map. For a complete discussion of probiotics, prebiotics and the role of the gut microbiota in human health, see our Road map *Functional Strategies for the Management of Gastrointestinal Disorders* (Point Institute 2016).

What are Probiotics?

Within the context of supplementation, probiotics describe micro-organisms intentionally consumed for an intended health benefit, usually to rebalance the natural gut microbiota. These micro-organisms have been part of the food chain for millennia (mostly in fermented foods), although today the vast majority of probiotics are consumed as added ingredients to dairy products (milk, yogurt, kefir) or in capsule, tablet or powder dietary supplements.

Commercial probiotics are not the same thing as commensal (or indigenous) microbiota (see Figure 14) and the use of probiotics should not be viewed as "reinoculating" or "recolonizing" the gut. Instead, probiotics typically survive up to two weeks in the human gastrointestinal tract, where they can perform a host of beneficial effects that are similar to (often indistinguishable from) commensal microbiota.

The human GI tract is host to trillions of micro-organisms from hundreds of different species. These organisms provide a wide range of benefits that can generally be classified as protective functions, structural functions and metabolic functions. Many of these benefits are unrealized when any number of GI disturbances results in microbial imbalance (dysbiosis). A healthy microbiome is important for the production of some vitamins (vitamin K, biotin and folate); improved absorption of many minerals; the fermentation of some dietary fibers into short-chain fatty acids (SCFA), which are nutrient resources for colon cells; and the conversion of certain phytonutrients into their bioactive compounds (e.g., soy isoflavones). While commercially prepared probiotics do not become permanent members of the human GI tract, they often perform some of the same biological functions; but more importantly, they help create a GI environment that favors a healthy

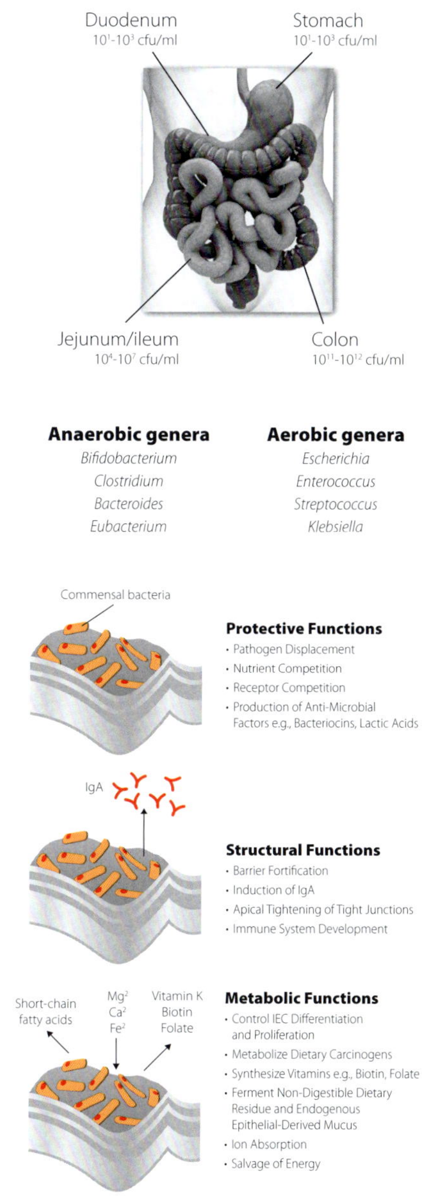

Figure 14: Basic Functions of Commensal Microbiota and some Probiotic strains.

commensal balance. These probiotic-induced changes to the gut micro-environment can have far reaching health consequences that have been noted in numerous clinical trials for a wide range of conditions such as: chronic immune suppression, inflammatory bowel disease, irritable bowel syndrome, atopic conditions, bowel irregularity, *Candida* overgrowth, upper respiratory infections and more.

Where do Probiotics Come From?

Healthy bacteria reach the GI tract from the environment starting at birth, influenced by the mode of delivery and whether or not a child is breast fed (an effect of both breast milk and contact with the mother's breast). After that, organisms in the soil, food and water continue to create an individual's unique population of commensal organisms, detrimentally impacted by the use of antibiotics or GI conditions that greatly alter bowel transit time (chronic constipation or frequent diarrhea).

Like commensal organisms, commercially available probiotic strains also have their *origins* from one of these environmental sources, so that the original isolate used to make the product may have been taken from a variety of sources: plant, soil, dairy or directly from the human GI tract itself. The origin of strain's isolation, however, does not necessarily determine its overall benefit as a probiotic. In order to be a commercially and therapeutically viable strain, these isolates must withstand large-scale fermentation, stability upon freeze-drying, shelf-stability, and the ability to withstand stomach acid, bile and enzyme digestion (i.e., pepsin and pancreatin). Likewise, many probiotic strains are tested for their ability to adhere to intestinal cells, inhibit the growth of pathogenic organisms and resist common antibiotics. Each strain of bacteria differs slightly with respect to all these criteria, depending on their specific genetics, growth conditions and product preparation (see Table 5).

Commercial growth and preparation prevent probiotic strains from becoming permanent residents of the human GI tract. Clinicians should understand this as a good thing, since overgrowth of only a few selected strains (found within the probiotic product) would result in a vastly limited microbiota diversity and lead to major health consequences. Probiotics should be seen as helpful, but temporary, residents within the human GI tract. On the other hand, the use of probiotics on an ongoing (chronic) basis is not necessarily discouraged if the patient's dysbiosis is well established and daily probiotic use proves helpful.

Typical Probiotic Strains

There are a number of micro-organisms that could be defined broadly as a "probiotic." The vast majority fall into the following classifications:

Lactobacilli: By far the most common and well-known probiotics come from this genus of bacteria and have names known to most consumers of probiotics (there are well over 50 commercial strains): *Lactobacillus acidophilus (or L. acidophilus), Lactobacillus bulgaricus, Lactobacillus rhamnosus, Lactobacillus plantarum, Lactobacillus reuteri, Lactobacillus salivarius, Lactobacillus casei, Lactobacillus paracasei,* and *Lactobacillus gasseri.*

Bifidobacteria: The most abundant type of bacteria in the human gut comes from this genus, represented in commercially available strains such as: *Bifodbacterium bifidum, Bifodbacterium lactis, Bifodbacterium longum, Bifodbacterium breve, Bifodbacterium infanti.*

Streptococci: These types of bacteria are usually associated with their negative health outcomes, but two strains in particular are used in some probiotic products due to their positive health benefits: *Streptococcus thermophilus* and *Streptococcus salivarius.*

Spore-forming probiotics: Spores are dormant forms of certain bacteria naturally designed to withstand desiccation and harsh environments. Common types of probiotic spores include: *Bacillus subtilis, Bacillus coagulans* (a.k.a. *Lactobacillus sporogenes)* and other lesser-used *Bacillus* strains.

Yeast probiotics: This category is virtually dominated by a single strain of yeast, similar to brewer's yeast, called *Saccharomyces boulardii*. An extensive amount of research has shown the use of this strain of yeast as an oral probiotic is safe and effective.

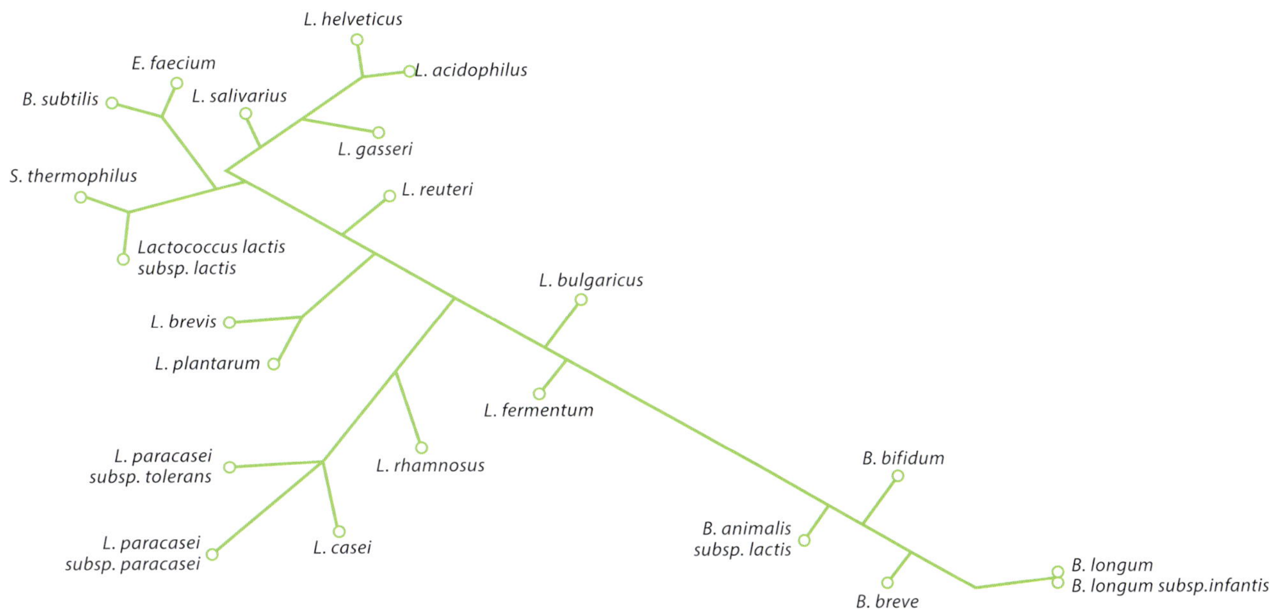

Figure 15 : Phylogenetic relationship between common probiotic strains based on unrooted maximum parsimony clustering of partial 16S rRNA gene sequences (Courtesy of Danisco/DuPont).

Which Strain(s) are the Best?

Since each person's GI tract contains hundreds of different subspecies of bacteria, it is clear biodiversity and balance are key, not the prominence of only a few species. While it is difficult to examine the human GI tract in situ, it appears certain subspecies reside only in particular parts of the GI tract based on pH, nutrient concentrations and their ability to bind different cell surface features. It is for these reasons we believe routine probiotic supplementation should be done not with single organisms, but with products that provide a broad number of probiotic strains. This is how we encounter healthy microbial organisms in the first place.

By using a multi-strain approach, one can take advantage of the fact that each strain has a slightly different range of metabolic and protective functions and may occupy a different micro-environmental niche within the GI tract. The multi-strain approach allows for robust support for more commensal organisms along the entire lower GI tract.[1] Figure 15 shows the genetic similarity (based on 16S rRNA) of the most common subspecies of commercially available probiotic strains. Finding products that contain strains from each of the various branches is one way to increase the potential of this multi-strain approach.

On the other hand, a wide range of clinical trials have been performed using specific strains of probiotics, many as single-strain therapies. How does this information correspond to our recommendation above? Since there are virtually no published "head-to-head" trials using probiotic strains for various clinical outcomes, it is difficult to interpret any of the published data as exclusive to the studied strain(s). For instance, results reported from studies done in subjects using one particular *Lactobacillus acidophilus* strain are likely to be repeatable using nearly all *Lactobacillus acidophilus* strains, assuming the preparation and viability of each strain is similar. This, of course, is not true of different strains, where the clinical outcomes for *Lactobacillus acidophilus* may turn out to be different than *L. rhamnosus* or *Bifidobacterium longum*.

Some interpret the growing published data to suggest different strains or strain combinations should be used for different clinical outcomes (requiring physicians to have a wide range of probiotic products in their formulary). We believe, with the exception of the yeast *Saccharomyces boulardii*, a multi-strain approach

1. Nearly all probiotics are designed to support the commensal organisms in the colon or small intestine. Some strains or strain combinations are designed to support the microbiota within the mouth, stomach, skin or vagina. If these products are intended to be consumed orally, they are still deemed "dietary supplements" in the U.S.

that takes advantage of the genetic diversity of the available commercial strains will have the best overall benefit in the widest number of patients. Obviously, where evidence is strong for a particular strain or strain combination in subjects similar to the patient seeking therapy, the use of these specific products may be warranted.

Formulary Suggestion

- Modest-Dose Multi-Strain Probiotic-Capsule formula and/or powder [15-40 billion CFU]
- *Saccharomyces boulardii*- only capsule: 5 billion CFU/capsule
- High-Dose Multi-Strain Probiotic- sachet or powder [>100 billion CFU]
- Children's Multi-Strain Probiotic- powder or chewable wafer [1-5 billion CFU/dose]

Therapeutic Rotation of Probiotic Strains

Some clinicians recommend patients should rotate (monthly, bi-monthly, etc.) between different probiotic products, believing the use of only one product (or strain) may limit the overall benefit of daily probiotic use. We know of no published study attempting to address this particular question. Based on the principles already mentioned, and our general recommendation to use a multi-strain approach for most patients, this method of rotating probiotics appears unnecessary and adds the potential for patient confusion and noncompliance.

What is the Right Dose for Clinical Probiotic Use?

Probiotic doses are expressed as colony forming units (CFU). Essentially, this means when the product is prepared appropriately (during laboratory enumeration), the dose will yield a given number of live "colony-forming" organisms in the laboratory. Since these organisms are specially prepared by a freeze-drying process, and many organisms could be damaged beyond their ability to become viable, this is the best method we have of enumerating the probiotic potential of a product, though other methods are being explored.

Available products range from as little as one billion CFU/dose to as high as 450 billion CFU/dose. For the purpose of non-disease-specific balancing of the GI microbiota, daily doses of 15 – 40 billion CFU in adults and one to five billion CFU in children are usually sufficient. Much higher doses (some well over one trillion CFU/day) have been reported to benefit patients with specific clinical conditions (like IBD), but are rarely needed to help most patients without specific dysbiotic abnormalities.[2]

Shelf life Issues- Do Probiotics Need to be Refrigerated?

Probiotic organisms in foods or supplements are prone to easy degradation and must be manufactured with great care. Responsible companies understand how the manufacturing process (from the time the frozen raw material reaches their facility to the selection of the appropriate shipping method) affects the eventual shelf life and efficacy of their product. Procedures must be put in place to limit exposure to heat, oxygen and moisture throughout the manufacturing, storage and shipping process. Even when all these factors are considered, companies must still add a significant overage at the time of manufacturing to maintain their stated potency at the time of expiration (do not purchase products that claim potency only at "time of manufacturing").

While it is generally true that all probiotics will have a longer shelf life when kept refrigerated, a significant amount of innovation has been developed to allow manufacturers to make products with significant shelf life at room temperature. This gives the consumer months of shelf life without the need for refrigeration.

Companies are required to have real-time data to show products still meet their label-claim potency at the time of expiration, usually nine to 18 months after the original manufacturing date. Regardless, when receiving product from companies with room temperature shelf life dates, they should be shipped in insulated containers with cold packs (or similar packaging) to prevent high temperatures during shipment.

2. For a review of the use of high-dose probiotics and the therapeutic uses of probiotics at various doses, see our book *Functional Strategies for Supporting Gastrointestinal Disorders*. Point Institute 2016.

Once a probiotic product is opened and exposed to oxygen and moisture, its shelf life greatly diminishes. Product packages should be small enough that a patient will use up the product within a month or two. Once products are opened, refrigeration can contribute moisture, through condensation, and should not be relied upon as a way to extend shelf life. As a rule of thumb, once products have been opened, they should be consumed fairly quickly.

Technologies to Improve Probiotic Stability

As mentioned above, probiotic manufacturers have been developing a number of technologies to improve the stability of probiotics. This includes the initial strain selection, the medium used to grow the bacteria, the harvesting process, and the steps used to put these micro-organisms into a freeze-dried state of suspended animation. These steps are used to protect bacteria from the harsh process of freeze-drying so their cell membranes, DNA and cell metabolites are undamaged, allowing the cells to "re-animate" when reaching the appropriate environment. Without these processes, room temperature stability would be short and impractical. While some of the patented processes used to stabilize probiotics are proprietary, most suppliers will share their basic techniques and processes. With growing interest in probiotic use throughout the world, more technological advances are being introduced on a regular basis.

Do Probiotics Need to be Enteric-coated?

No. Most studies revealing the benefits of commercially prepared probiotics were done using *non-enteric-coated* finished products (capsules, powders, tablets or powders added to foods). This means most of what we know about the effects and the effective dose of various strains of probiotics is related to unmodified products.

Companies are now creating products that deliver probiotics in acid-resistant or enteric-coated capsules and tablets in an attempt to improve cell survival and, hopefully, product efficacy. Since previous studies have confirmed probiotic survival is hindered by stomach acid (some strains more than others), the logic of using acid-resistant doses (or micro-encapsulated powders) to improve product efficacy is not without reason. However, we do not yet believe this justifies using these types of products with lower probiotic potency until specific data measuring survival and clinical efficacy is published.

Should Probiotics be Taken with Food or on an Empty Stomach?

Although many clinical opinions exist, this question is virtually un-researched; many probiotic studies don't even describe the timing of meals respective to probiotic dose. Only one study we know of has attempted to answer this question directly, and because of the lack of validated enumeration of probiotics after human ingestion (see below), this study was performed using an *in vitro* digestive system model, not human subjects. Nonetheless, they used a four-strain, encapsulated, non-enteric-coated product containing *Lactobacillus helveticus, Lactobacillus rhamnosus, Bifidobacterium longum* and *Saccharomyces boulardii.*[3] Two capsules were added to the system 30 minutes before, during or 30 minutes after the addition of a "meal" consisting of oatmeal and 1% milk. Capsules added before the oatmeal also included 250 ml of spring water. Additionally, they tested the differential effect of apple juice, 1% milk or water on the probiotic survival.

In this model system, probiotic survival was slightly better when added to the system before or during the oatmeal, and slightly lower when added 30 minutes after the oatmeal. In most cases these differences were not statistically significant nor, in our opinion, clinically significant. A more noticeable difference was seen when using water or apple juice, both of which significantly decreased probiotic survival compared to the oatmeal or 1% milk alone. The authors believe this was due either to a protective effect of the 1% fat content, a longer buffering of stomach acid by the milk and oatmeal, or a quicker gastric emptying rate (especially water). It should be noted that in each case, the *Bifidobacteria* were more vulnerable to these changes than the *Lactobacillus* strains, while the *Saccharomyces boulardii* had a universally high survival rate, unaffected by beverage selection or meal timing.

3. Tompkins TA, Mainville I, Arcand Y. The impact of meals on a probiotic during transit through a model of the human upper gastrointestinal tract. *Benef Microbes.* 2011 Dec 1; 2(4):295-303.

In general, with the limited data available to answer this question, we believe patients should consume probiotics when it is convenient for them, as the differences noted in this study are insignificant compared to the cumulative benefits of daily supplementation. Since only water, apple juice and 1% milk were compared, it may be suggested that when probiotics are consumed apart from a meal, 1% milk may benefit survival over water or apple juice. Whether milk substitutes with fat (almond, soy or rice) or other fruit juices will behave in the same manner is unknown.

Can Stool Testing Measure Probiotic Effectiveness?

This is still an open question. Some laboratories have the technology (typically requires PCR) to detect or quantify specific subspecies of bacteria in stool samples. Differentiation between commensal strains and similar probiotic strains must be discussed with the provider of the test results. However, changes in overall bacteria ratios, and more importantly other stool functions typical of a balanced gut, may result after probiotic use. Since stool analysis, or bacterial enumeration from stool, is rarely reported in clinical studies where probiotics are used, ask your laboratory for references/studies that relate to their specific test.

Probiotic Therapy During and After the Use of Antibiotics

A common question among clinicians is whether probiotic use is appropriate, effective or contraindicated during antibiotic therapy. These questions stem from the fact that antibiotic use has a well-known detrimental effect on commensal gut microbiota, causing an antibiotic-associated dysbiosis that often leads to bowel symptoms, especially diarrhea. We will address three basic questions related to probiotic use during antibiotic therapy.

- **Does antibiotic therapy render probiotics therapy inert?** While some strains of probiotics are susceptible to certain antibiotics, most strains are resistant or partially resistant to many common antibiotics used today. Broad spectrum antibiotics, such as amoxicillin, ampicillin and penicillin G, are particularly harsh on most commercially produced probiotic strains (see Table 5). The yeast probiotic *Saccharomyces boulardii* is resistant to all antibiotics. Using a multi-strain probiotic that includes *S. boulardii* is recommended during antibiotic therapy to offset potential and harmful dysbiosis caused by the antibiotic.
- **Do probiotics make antibiotics less effective?** There is no evidence to suggest probiotics change the effectiveness of any antibiotic. Since a dose of even 100 billion CFU (if all survived to the gut) would still only represent about 0.1% of the total organisms in the gut, even susceptible strains would offer a small percentage of likely "targets" for any antibiotic, leaving the antibiotic dose undiminished to target other organisms.
- **Are probiotics effective for preventing or treating antibiotic-associated GI side-effects?** The answer is: It depends. A large number of studies have attempted to answer this question, mainly focused on antibiotic-associated diarrhea (AAD), often connected with preferential overgrowth of *Clostridium difficile*. Unfortunately these studies have included a wide range of doses, strains, strain combinations, antibiotics and patient-types, leading to a wide range of reported efficacy.

  In 2012 *JAMA* published a systematic review and meta-analysis of more than 80 studies using probiotics for the prevention or treatment of AAD.[4] Though these studies were generally small, and some of the specific probiotic strains were poorly documented, they concluded the "evidence suggests that probiotics are associated with a reduction in AAD." In fact, in the trials reporting on the number of patients with AAD, the relative risk was reduced by over 40% (RR 0.58). Of the trials used for the analysis, 57 of 82 included *Lactobacillus* alone or in combination (32/82 in combination with a *Bifidobacterium* strain). Sixteen of the studies used *Saccharomyces boulardii* alone, commonly used for AAD and *Clostridium difficile*-related diarrhea.[5]

4. Hempel S et al. Probiotics for the prevention and treatment of antibiotic-associated diarrhea: a systematic review and meta-analysis. *JAMA.* 2012 May 9; 307(18):1959-69.

5. Berni Canani R, Cucchiara S, Cuomo R, Pace F, Papale F. Saccharomyces boulardii: a summary of the evidence for gastroenterology clinical practice in adults and children. *Eur Rev Med Pharmacol Sci.* 2011 Jul; 15(7):809-22.

Probiotic Attribute Chart

	Bif. Bifidum Bb-02	B. animalis subsp. Lactis Bi-04	Lb. acidophilus La-14	Lb. paracasei Lpc-37	Lb. plantarum Lp-115	Lb. rhamnosus Lr-32	Lb. salivarius Ls-33	Lb. casei Lc-11	St. thermophilus St-21
Survival									
Acid Tolerance	★★★★★	★★★★★	★★★★★	★★★★☆	★★★★★	★★★★★	★★★☆☆	★★★★☆	★☆☆☆☆
Bile Tolerance	★★★★☆	★★★★★	★★★★★	★☆☆☆☆	★★★★★	★★★★★	★★★★☆	★★★★☆	★★★★★
Pepsin Resistance	NA	NA	★★★★☆	★☆☆☆☆	★★★☆☆	★☆☆☆☆	★☆☆☆☆	NA	NA
Pancreatin Tolerance	NA	NA	★★★★☆	★★★★☆	★★★★☆	★★★★☆	★★★★☆	NA	NA
Adherence									
Caco-2	★★★★★	★★★☆☆	★★★☆☆	★★★★☆	★★★★☆	★★★★☆	★★★★☆	★★★★☆	★★★★☆
Ht-29	★★★★★	★★★☆☆	★★★★☆	★★★☆☆	★★☆☆☆	★★★★☆	★★★★☆	★★★☆☆	★★★☆☆
Antibiotic Resistance									
Amoxicillin	S	S	S	S	S	S	S	S	S
Ampicillin	I	S	S	S	S	S	S	S	S
Penicillin G	S	S	S	S	R	S	S	S	S
Ciprofloxacin	R	R	R	R	R	R	R	R	R
Clindamycin	S	S	I	S	S	S	S	I	R
Erythromycin	I	S	S	S	I	S	I	I	I
Vancomycin	R	R	S	R	R	R	R	R	S
Polymyxin B (topical, G-only)	R	R	R	R	R	R	R	R	R
Tetracycline	R	R	R	S	R	I	R	R	S
Gentamicin	R	R	R	R	R	R	R	R	R
Kanamycin	R	R	R	R	R	R	R	R	R
Neomycin	R	R	R	R	R	R	R	R	R
Streptomycin	R	R	R	R	R	R	R	R	R
Sulfamethoxazole	R	R	R	R	R	R	R	R	R
Trimethoprim	R	S	R	R	R	R	R	R	R
Pathogen Inhibition									
Pancreatin Tolerance	NA	NA	★★★★☆	★★★★☆	★★★★☆	★★★★☆	★★★★☆	NA	NA
C. difficile	NA	NA	NA	NA	NA	NA	NA	NA	NA
E. coli	★★★★☆	NA	★★★☆☆	★★★★☆	★★☆☆☆	★★★☆☆	★★★☆☆	★★★★☆	NA
Listeria monocytogenes	★★☆☆☆	NA	★☆☆☆☆	★★☆☆☆	★★☆☆☆	★★☆☆☆	★★☆☆☆	★★☆☆☆	NA
Salmonella typhimurim	★★☆☆☆	NA	★☆☆☆☆	★★★★☆	★★☆☆☆	★★☆☆☆	★★☆☆☆	★★☆☆☆	NA
Staphylococcus aureus	★★★★★	NA	★★★★★	★★★★★	★☆☆☆☆	★★☆☆☆	★★★★☆	★★☆☆☆	NA

★★★★★ STRENGTH

S = Susceptible I = Intermediate R = Resistant

Table 5 : Attributes of Commonly Used Probiotics Based on *in vitro* Testing.
Data provided by Danisco/DuPont.

Using Dietary Supplements
What Clinicians Need to Know

In the U.S., nutrient supplementation is primarily accomplished using products regulated as foods: functional foods, dietary supplements or medical foods. As such, these products are available to anyone without a prescription. The additional fact that many of these products are used as therapeutic agents by a large number of Americans (with or without the knowledge and consent of their healthcare providers) has led to confusion about the way in which these products are regulated for safety, quality and efficacy in the United States. This section will provide an overview of relevant issues pertaining to dietary supplement regulation, as well as cover a number of important additional concerns clinicians may have about distributing dietary supplements to their patients as part of their practice/ business.

General Regulatory Framework

A complete history of the regulation of dietary supplements (DS) has recently been covered in "The Regulated Dietary Supplement Industry: Myths of an Unregulated Industry Dispelled," a review published in 2012 by *HerbalGram*. This article describes the history of food regulation in the United States, putting into context the regulatory framework that resulted in the Dietary Supplement Health Education Act (DSHEA) in 1994, and further describes how the FDA has interpreted and implemented DSHEA to create the current regulatory environment. A complete reprint of this article is available in the appendix (Page 160).

Table 6: Overview of FDA's Authorities for Regulating Dietary Supplements

Safety & Quality Authorities
Prohibit any poisonous or deleterious substance injurious to health in a dietary supplement
Prohibit any dietary supplement or dietary ingredient, whether old or new, that presents a "significant or unreasonable risk of illness or injury"
Impose an immediate ban of an imminent hazard
Impose requirements for Good Manufacturing Practices (GMPs)
Inspect facilities
Prohibit any food that is filthy, decomposed, held under insanitary conditions whereby it may have been rendered injurious to health, or otherwise unfit for food
Collect and oversee mandatory reports of serious adverse events associated with dietary supplements and inspect records kept by manufacturers and distributors
Premarketing Notification Authorities
Prohibit (on basis of adulteration) any new dietary ingredient for which there is inadequate information to provide reasonable assurance that it does not present a significant or unreasonable risk of illness or injury
Require FDA approval of food additives (excipients) and color additives used in food, including dietary supplements
Post-Marketing Enforcement Authorities
Issue safety alerts to health professionals and consumers
Initiate enforcement actions (recalls)
Issue warning letters
Seek injunctions through the courts, resulting in civil or criminal penalties
Labeling Authorities
Regulate the content of dietary supplements labels to prohibit misbranding of dietary supplements

Enforce FDCA requirement that all statements in product labeling are truthful and non-misleading, including:
– Statement of identity—product must be identified as a "Dietary Supplement"
– Nutrition information in the form of a Supplement Facts panel
– List of ingredients not listed in the Supplement Facts panel
– Name and address of the manufacturer, packer, or distributor
– Net quantity of contents
– Claims including
    – Health Claims
    – Qualified Health Claims
    – Criteria constituting reliable scientific evidence to substantiate health-related claims
    – Nutrient Content Claims
    – Structure Function Claims

Who Regulates Dietary Supplements?

FDA: Congress has given most of the authorities for regulating laws pertaining to DS to the Food and Drug Administration (FDA), managed through its Center for Food Safety and Applied Nutrition (CFSAN). CFSAN is responsible for all food and cosmetic safety, regulation and labeling. The scope of their responsibilities and authorities related to DS is summarized in Table 6. (see Soller et al. in appendix)

FTC: While the regulation of label-claims is specifically regulated by the FDA (see discussion below), the Federal Trade Commission (in cooperation with the FDA) is tasked with regulating the advertising of DS, with authority to protect consumers from false or misleading claims in print, television, radio or Internet settings.

USDA: Many of the botanical ingredients used in dietary supplements are co-regulated by the U.S. Department of Agriculture, which also regulates a wide range of foods and food labeling (such as the "organic" labeling rules). Importation of agricultural products into the U.S. is partly regulated by the USDA.

Other Federal and State Agencies: The agencies above can, and have been, assisted by other federal and state regulatory agencies to affect the regulation of DS. These might include the Drug Enforcement Agency (DEA), the Department of Homeland Security (DHS), the Centers for Disease Control (CDC), and State Health Agencies. Statutes in some states can also add labeling requirements (e.g., Prop 65 warning in California) or ban certain ingredients, where federal statutes have not been implemented.

Industry Self-Regulation: A number of organizations have emerged within the food and dietary supplement industry to help responsible companies comply with the wide array of federal and state regulatory requirements for DS. These organizations have developed monograph standards for many DS products or herbal products, some created interim Good Manufacturing Practices (GMPs) programs (1997 – 2006) while the FDA was slow in implementing their statutory responsibilities and have hosted hundreds of seminars and training sessions in proper labeling, raw material identification, manufacturing practices and advertising compliance. Even so, a number of companies remain slow in implementing all the regulatory requirements; and the FDA has increased their enforcement actions of DS distributors. Also, rogue manufacturers of non-DS agents (pharmaceuticals, anabolic hormones, etc.) continue to attempt to thwart the FDA by selling products illegally labeled as dietary supplements (usually for weight loss, libido enhancement or sports performance). Purchasing products from companies that have been in the business for many years and have a reputation in the industry is usually one of the best ways to avoid purchasing one of these dubious products.

Industry-Related Organizations

American Botanical Council (ABC)

American Herbal Pharmacopoeia (AHP)

American Herbal Products Association (AHPA)

Consumer Healthcare Products Association (CHPA)

Council for Responsible Nutrition (CRN)

National Center for Natural Products Research (NCNPR)

Natural Products Association (NPA)

NSF International

Global Organization for EPA and DHA (GOED)

United Natural Products Alliance (UNPA)

U.S. Pharmacopeial Convention (USP)

What is a Dietary Supplement?

One of the first things Congress needed to do within DSHEA was to define the meaning of a "dietary supplement" for the purpose of regulation. The statute defines a dietary supplement this way:

A product (other than tobacco) intended to supplement the diet that bears or contains one or more of the following dietary ingredients: a vitamin, a mineral, an herb or other botanical, an amino acid, a dietary substance for use by man to supplement the diet by increasing the total dietary intake; or a concentrate, metabolite, constituent, extract, or combination of any of these ingredients; and is intended for ingestion, is not represented for use as a conventional food or as a sole item of a meal or the diet; and is labeled as a dietary supplement.

Intended for ingestion means products labeled as sublingual, intranasal, intravaginal, topical or intravenous do not qualify as dietary supplements and are considered either drugs, cosmetics, or medical devices. Many dietary supplement companies incorrectly sell products claiming to be "sublingual" (e.g., vitamin B_{12}, hormones, etc.). When these products are labeled or advertised as "sublingual," the products are no longer dietary supplements, becoming drugs from a regulatory perspective. As of 2013, the FDA has not heavily enforced this provision, but warning letters have been issued to some companies making these false claims.

When is an Ingredient Not a Dietary Supplement?

The answer to this question is a bit more complicated than it might, at first, appear. DSHEA declared that products containing dietary ingredients that had been marketed prior to October 15, 1994 could be sold without any "preapproval" by the FDA. This essentially "grandfathered" most of the products sold when DSHEA was signed into law. However, products containing ingredients not marketed in the U.S. as dietary supplements or foods prior to 1994 require the marketer to file a New Dietary Ingredient notification (primarily detailing the ingredient's safety) with the FDA at least 75 days before selling the product in the U.S. Nevertheless, this simple distinction between ingredients generally referred to as "old dietary ingredients" (ODI) or "new dietary ingredients" (NDI), based on their historical use, was fraught with nuance and complications.

First, no official list of "grandfathered," pre-1994 ingredients was created or approved by the FDA, and the definition and requirements for "new" ingredients have yet to be fully resolved between the industry and FDA. In fact, a draft industry guidance document detailing FDA's position on NDIs and the notification process did not appear until 2011 (revised and updated in August of 2016) and has not been finalized as of April, 2017.[1] Numerous and wide-ranging sticking points left unanswered include such matters as:

- Defining a list of ODIs to be agreed upon by both FDA and the industry, if possible
- Considering whether a new "grandfathering" date can be selected (e.g., 2016) to include safe products lacking a known date of introduction into the U.S. dietary supplement market
- Defining when certain new manufacturing processes (e.g., new extraction method/solvent for botanical ingredients) creates a "new" ingredient
- Whether chemically-identical synthetic botanical compounds are eligible as dietary ingredients
- Whether every company selling any formula containing a "new" dietary ingredient must file an additional notification to FDA every time the "new" ingredient is used. [Creating a de facto pre-approval process for all future products containing any ingredient not grandfathered since 1994]

In addition, if ingredients previously sold as dietary supplements are later approved as drugs, the dietary supplement ingredient may still remain eligible for use in dietary supplements unless, according to DSHEA, *"the Secretary [of Health and Human Services] has issued a regulation, after notice and comment, finding that the article, when used as or in a dietary supplement under the conditions of use and dosages set forth in the labeling for such dietary supplement, is unlawful."* For instance, even though certain fish oil products have been approved as drugs (for severe hypertriglyceridemia), similar fish oil products remain available as dietary supplements. However, while nearly identical fish oil products can be sold as dietary supplements, these dietary supplement products cannot make the same triglyceride-lowering claims as the approved drug products. Similarly, niacin sold as a dietary supplement cannot make lipid-lowering claims even if it has the identical ingredient and dose as the approved pharmaceutical version. On the other hand, red yeast rice products (some sold prior to 1994) containing monacolin K (lovastatin) cannot be sold as dietary supplements in the U.S., as FDA has deemed them unapproved drugs.

1. For the latest on the New Dietary Ingredient Notification process, see FDA's website here: https://www.fda.gov/food/dietarysupplements/newdietaryingredientsnotificationprocess/

Understanding Dietary Supplement Labels

Understanding the requirements and nuances of a dietary supplement product label is important in order to evaluate the potential benefit of a product. The following describes the basic features of a dietary supplement label (below) and supplement facts box requirements (page 142).

Basic Components of Dietary Supplement Labels (U.S.)

SUGGESTED USE
Suggested Use information is regulated as a claim. and is often very generic. If a particular dose is "recommended" within the "suggested use" portion of the label, this dose must conform to the serving size within the SFB to prevent confusion by consumers.

PRIMARY DISPLAY PANEL (PDP)
Must have the words "Dietary Supplement" prominently displayed on the front panel of the product label. Must also have a statement of the number of units (capsules, tablets, ounces, etc.) on the front panel of the label.

SUPPLEMENT FACTS BOX (SFB)
Must have a Supplement Facts Box (SFB) to describe ingredient contents. The specific requirements for a Dietary Supplement SFB is detailed on page 142. (Food products will have similar "Nutrition Facts" panels of slightly differing requirements)

SUGGESTED USE: 2 capsules per day or as recommended by your health care professional.

If you are pregnant or nursing, consult your physician before taking this product. As with all dietary supplements, some individuals may not tolerate or may be allergic to the ingredients used. Please read the ingredient panel carefully prior to ingestion. Cease taking this product and consult your physician if you have negative reactions upon ingestion.

KEEP CONTAINER TIGHTLY CLOSED. STORE AT ROOM TEMPERATURE. KEEP OUT OF REACH OF CHILDREN.

This product was sealed for your protection. Do not use if outer neck seal or inner-seal is missing or damaged.

Manufactured for:
Company Name
Address and Phone

Exp. 06/15/2015
Lot #: 123456

PRODUCT NAME

60 Capsules
DIETARY SUPPLEMENT

Supplement Facts
Serving Size 2 Capsules
Servings Per Container 30

2 capsules contain	Amount Per Serving	% Daily Value
Vitamin C (as ascorbic acid)	90 mg	100%
Calcium (as D-Glucarate)	120 mg	9%
Calcium D-Glucarate	1,000 mg	*
Colostrum concentrate (bovine)	2.5 g	*
Immunoglobulin G (IgG)	1 g	*
Lactoferrin	13 mg	*
Papain (6,000 USP Units/mg)	100 mg	*
Rosemary (aerial portion)	100 mg	*

* Daily Value not established

Other Ingredients: Natural Vegetable Capsules. This product may contain one or more of the following: Calcium Silicate, Magnesium Stearate, Microcrystalline Cellulose, Silicon Dioxide, and Stearic Acid.
Contains: Milk.

CONTRAINDICATIONS AND WARNINGS
A variety of other warnings may be included on a product depending on the ingredients, use or type of subjects consuming the product. These may include warnings related to: choking hazards, accessibility to children, storage conditions, contraindications, interactions with other substances, overdose instructions etc.

LOT NUMBER & EXPIRATION DATE
A Lot Number must be printed on the label or bottle of the product so that it can be used for identifying the product for a potential recall. Most companies will also include an expiration date somewhere close to the lot number, though an expiration date is not an absolute requirement for DS products (see page 145 for expiration date issues and DS).

OTHER INGREDIENTS
Ingredients not required to be included in the Supplement Facts Box (SFB) must be listed as "Other Ingredients" below the SFB.

SEAL STATEMENT
All products should have two tamper-evident protections. This is usually accomplished by a neckband (or full-body sleeve) and a seal within the inner cap.

MANUFACTURER INFO
Label must have contact information (made for or made by), of a responsible party in order to report adverse events (see page 147 for requirements related to adverse event reporting).

ALLERGEN STATEMENT
If the product contains one or more of the eight (8) mandatory allergens, a specific statement must be included on the label (see more on allergen statements on page 146).

Reading a Supplement Facts Box

Ingredients with a daily value must be declared using the %DV column. If no subgroup is specified, the %Daily Value column uses values for adults and children above the age of 4. Units for several nutrient DVs have (or will soon) change. See p.19 and individual monographs for more details and conversion factors.

A box must be created with a black line and specifically titled "Supplement Facts" with appropriate (FDA-regulated) size font on the label.

The serving size and number of servings per container must be listed at the top of the SFB. The serving size must conform to the "Amount per Serving" listed below and to the recommended serving in the "Suggested Use" portion of the label, if applicable.

The parent compound used to provide an ingredient claim must be included within a parenthesis after the ingredient claim, such as Vitamin C (as ascorbic acid) or Vitamin B12 (as methylcobalamin).

Minerals with a "percent daily value" are listed above the line, and the amount per serving must correspond to the elemental mineral claim [Calcium (as citrate) 100 mg], rather than the weight of the total compound. This helps individuals compare mineral claims from different compounds equally. Minerals with no DRV can be listed as compounds below the line (such as vanadyl sulfate).

Supplement Facts

Serving Size 2 Capsules
Servings Per Container 30

2 capsules contain	Amount Per Serving	% Daily Value
Vitamin C (as ascorbic acid)	90 mg	100%
Vitamin E (as d-Alpha Tocopherol Succinate)	67 mg	447%
Vitamin D (as cholecalciferol)	20 mcg (800 IU)	100%
Calcium (as D-Glucarate)	120 mg	9%*
Calcium D-Glucarate	1,000 mg	*
Papain (6,000 USP Units/mg)	100 mg	*
Rosemary (aerial portion)	100 mg	*
Mixed Tocopherols	50 mg	*

* Daily Value not established

A thick black line is used to separate those ingredients that have a "percent daily value" (above the line) and those that do not (below the line). The ingredients above the line (vitamins and minerals) must be listed in a particular order irrespective of the amount added, while those ingredients below the line must be listed in the order of prominence.

Ingredients with both elemental and compound-related claims may be listed both above and below the line, as with Calcium D-Glucarate in our example.

Enzyme activity units should be listed in addition to mg amounts as activity rather than mass is more important.

All botanical names must correspond to names listed in the Herbs of Commerce. Botanical ingredients must list specific plant part used and whether or the product is an extract, standardized extract, or merely a dried powder of the plant part.

The FDA has established alternative DVs for the following subpopulations: infants through 12 months of age, children aged 1-3 years, and pregnant and lactating women; designed to be the basis for %DV declared on products marketed to these subpopulations.

The SFB may have multiple columns if a product (such as a chewable multivitamin/mineral product) may be consumed by more than one age group (e.g., infants through 12 months, children 1 through 3 years of age, pregnant and lactating women).

Supplement Facts

Serving Size 2 Capsules
Servings Per Container 30

2 capsules contain	Amount Per Serving	% Daily Value for Children 1 through 3 Years of Age	% Daily Value for Infants through 12 months
Vitamin C (as ascorbic acid)	90 mg	600%	100%
Vitamin E (as d-Alpha Tocopherol Succinate)	67 mg	1,116%	447%
Vitamin D (as cholecalciferol)	20 mcg (800 IU)	133%	100%
Calcium (as D-Glucarate)	120 mg	17%	9%
Calcium D-Glucarate	1,000 mg	*	*
Papain (6,000 USP Units/mg)	100 mg	*	*
Rosemary (aerial portion)	100 mg	*	*
Mixed Tocopherols	50 mg	*	*

* Daily Value not established

Supplement Facts

Serving Size 2 Capsules
Servings Per Container 30

2 capsules contain	Amount Per Serving	% Daily Value for Children 1 through 3 Years of Age	% Daily Value for Adults and Children 4 or more Years of Age
Vitamin C (as ascorbic acid)	50 mg	333%	100%

* Daily Value not established

Controlling the Quality of Dietary Supplements

When one understands the extent of the regulations concerning dietary supplements in the United States, it is absurd that there are those who still claim the industry is "unregulated" or that the FDA has no power to prevent unsafe, adulterated or mislabeled products from reaching consumers. Even so, there are nuances within the methods and language of the regulatory process that can affect the outcome of product quality. Here we discuss, in a Q & A style, some of those issues for you to consider.

Can I trust the label claim on my product?

Good Manufacturing Practices (GMPs), mandated by the FDA for all DS products sold in the U.S., require products meet their label claim up to the date of expiration (see expiration date issues below). Furthermore, GMPs require each raw material added to a product be positively identified to ensure it is the correct raw material. They also detail a long list of procedures to ensure the product is manufactured according to its pre-specified formula, which is linked to the intended label claim. Products that do not meet their label claims, or that are produced without appropriate procedures or documentation, are considered "adulterated" and/or misbranded and would constitute a violation if sold in the U.S.

While it is the role of all DS manufacturers to comply with GMP manufacturing requirements, enforcement of these procedures requires the FDA to do onsite inspections of DS facilities. Such audits have revealed there is a wide range of compliance (or noncompliance) within the industry, requiring the FDA to bring regulatory actions against such companies. While warning letters and other legal actions against companies are made public, the FDA does not publish a list of compliant companies nor does it allow statements such as "FDA-approved" or "GMP-compliant" on company products, literature or websites. A few third-party organizations have created programs to help companies with their quality systems and have included a GMP-style logo for labels or websites; however, these logos and statements are not recognized by FDA and many high-profile companies "approved" under these programs have still received major citations from the FDA based on inadequate compliance with respect to GMPs. Dozens of unscrupulous companies have created "GMP-approved" logos (some even with an FDA logo) that appear on their product label or literature, a practice that is confusing to customers and, in most cases, illegal.

As with any industry, the vast majority of DS companies are honestly attempting to manufacture products according to the strict mandates of the FDA. Some of these companies are finding compliance difficult due to the need for large financial investments or a lack of experience in implementing such complex quality systems. Regrettably, the DS industry still has a small number of rogue manufacturers who do not intend to comply with the GMPs for whatever reason. The FDA has been slow to find, audit and prosecute these companies, leaving some vulnerability for consumers. Like rogue "pharmaceutical" companies attempting to sell counterfeit prescription medications, these companies are on the margins of the industry and do not represent the vast majority of companies producing dietary supplements.

Either way, clinicians should be knowledgeable about the quality-control practices of the companies whose products they are recommending. Most reputable companies will answer straight-forward questions about their quality-control program, share their list of Standard Operating Procedures (SOPs), and even allow clinicians to take a tour of their manufacturing facility.

Does the FDA control the efficacy of dietary supplements?

The basic answer is "No." While the FDA has detailed regulations in place to control the safety and quality of products (i.e., identity, purity and potency), the FDA does not set standards for product efficacy or usage. For instance, the FDA does not mandate an effective dose of a particular ingredient be used in products. As long as the finished product meets the label claim potency, FDA does not regulate whether that dose has any measurable benefit. In addition, for herbal products, the FDA does not mandate the appropriate (or expected) plant part is used, only that the correct name is used for a botanical and that the included plant part is disclosed. So, for instance, while you may think you should be getting the traditionally used root of the *Panax ginseng* plant, it is possible a ginseng product may contain only the leaf and stems. As long as the label correctly declares the plant part(s) used, this product would not run afoul of the GMP requirements (although the FTC may take issue with this practice if the product is represented, in advertising, as containing the root).

Chondroitin sulfate efficacy and GMPs

Good Manufacturing Practices (GMPs) mandate that products contain the amount of each ingredient listed on the label, but do not require that each of those ingredients actually perform clinically. One particular characteristic that affects an ingredient's efficacy is its bioavailability, often determined by a range of physical characteristics. For instance, chondroitin sulfate (CS) is a large polymer with virtually no bioavailability unless it is sufficiently digested into regular, small particles. When various lots and types of commercially available CS were tested, their bioavailability was directly associated with their particle size. In this case, a more expensive process of enzyme digestion (rather than acid hydrolysis) produced consistently small particles with the highest bioavailability (Product A in the table below). Not surprisingly, nearly every positive clinical trial performed with CS has used ingredients prepared in this manner, although a majority of the commercially available CS is still prepared by acid hydrolysis, with lower or very limited bioavailability and efficacy.

Raw Material	Permeability Coefficient ($x 10^{-6}$) (n=3) (cm/sec)
A[1]	10.1 (±0.6)
B	8.73 (±9.07)
C	7.94 (±7.35)
D	0.00 (±0.00)
E	3.63 (±2.07)
F	1.03 (±1.78)

[1]mol Wt + 16.900 dalton (95% Bioiberica)

Permeability coefficient for transport across Caco-2 cells of chondroitin sulfate from different manufacturers.

This table shows both the permeability coefficient and the standard deviation (+x) of different manufacturers' chondroitin sulfate in a Caco-2 cell model of bioavailability. The industry standard for bioavailability (Product A) shows the highest permeability and the lowest standard deviation. This is due to a highly controlled process to maintain a consistent and small molecular weight. Other chondroitin sulfate products have either low or no permeability (Products D, E, F), or have a large standard deviation caused by a range of particle sizes. All of these products, regardless of their bioavailability and efficacy, would meet the FDA's GMP standards for chondroitin sulfate if they met the potency of the label claim.

Source: Adebowale AO et al. Analysis of Glucosamine and Chondroitin Sulfate Content in Marketed Products and the Caco-2 Permeability of Chondroitin Sulfate Raw Materials. *JANA* 2000; 3(1):37-44.

In addition, GMPs do not require products contain ingredients extracted or prepared in a manner ensuring efficacy. If, for instance, published data consistently shows a particular standardized extract of an herb has positive clinical benefits, the use of a different extract with no (or even negative) data is not restricted. The FDA does not evaluate product or ingredient efficacy; only their safety, quality and label claims. Since there is a wide range of ingredients available, and a vast amount of published research to evaluate, clinicians should find trustworthy sources of clinically related dietary supplement information and understand the research that supports the products they recommend.

As part of DSHEA, Congress established the Office of Dietary Supplements (ODS), part of the National Institutes of Health. They have been tasked with gathering and disseminating information about the safety and efficacy of various products sold as dietary supplements. Their website (http://ods.od.nih.gov) has a vast array of information for consumers and healthcare professionals concerning evidence for DS efficacy and safety. In addition, the Linus Pauling Institute is well known for their information on each vitamin and mineral (http://lpi.oregonstate.edu). For monographs and Road maps related to therapeutic uses of dietary supplements and lifestyle therapies, see our other Point

Institute publications where you obtained this Road map (see page 196).

How does the expiration date affect the label claim?
Most dietary supplements have an expiration date printed on the label or the bottle. This date is set by the manufacturer, usually one to three years after the time of manufacturing. Products with short expiration dates (generally less than 18 months) typically contain fatty acids, probiotics, or sensitive food ingredients difficult to maintain over long periods of time. Manufacturers must develop their formulas in such a way that the supplement facts information is still true at the time of expiration, under specified storage conditions. This usually means that an **unopened** bottle of product, kept at room temperature, should meet the potency and purity claims when tested at the expiration date. Products with labels that state a need for refrigeration are likely to have their expiration date based on refrigerated temperatures (4°C or 40°F).

In the case of ingredients that can "break down" over time, manufacturers add specified overages based on the length of the expiration date and the known interaction with other compounds in the formula. Manufacturers use a wealth of historical data, real time and accelerated shelf life testing to determine expiration dates and the proper overages needed to meet these dates. On the other hand, some ingredients are fairly inert (most minerals) or have no specific measurable compound (like a non-standardized powdered herb), in which case overages are not typically added to these products.

While a product doesn't cease to be beneficial the day after the expiration date, few companies will guarantee that a product will meet its intended claims after this time period, and most will dissuade customers form consuming these products. Clinicians who intend to purchase and resell products to their clients should ensure they have sufficient time to distribute products well before the product expires, paying special attention to liquids, softgels, meal-type products and probiotics.

Are ALL ingredients listed on the label?
As we detailed earlier, all ingredients in a finished dietary supplement product must be listed on the label, either within the supplement facts box or outside the supplement facts box in an "Ingredients" or "Other Ingredients" section.

When the FDA finalized labeling rules for foods and supplements, they exempted the need to label ingredients used when manufacturing and processing raw materials, including those excipients added to raw materials *before* reaching the finished product manufacturer. Examples of processing agents not typically listed include the type of extraction solvent used to make an herbal extract and the diluents and flow agents (excipients) used to keep the extract powder free-flowing and of a standard potency. Typically, these excipients include ingredients like microcrystalline cellulose, maltodextrins and various forms of silicon dioxide (see excipient section on page 150 for detailed explanation of these agents). While these ingredients are rarely labeled, manufacturers must notify customers on the label if any of these ingredients introduce one of the eight allergens that require mandatory labeling (see page 146).

What steps are taken to ensure no contaminants are in a product?
As with any product intended for human consumption, manufacturers of dietary supplements are required to ensure their products are safe and free of harmful contaminants. This is usually accomplished by testing each batch of raw materials for the presence of certain chemical contaminants prior to being distributed into the supply chain. Furthermore, finished product manufacturers are also required to validate test results supplied by the raw material supplier to ensure they are accurate and truthful. The most common tests are those for heavy metals, pesticides, herbicides, bacteria, yeast and mold. Additionally, specific potential contaminants known to be associated with a particular raw material should be tested for in those products in which the raw material is used.

As with any product derived from agricultural and manufacturing practices, it is impossible (and cost prohibitive) to test for every possible contaminant, especially for those compounds not historically associated with a particular raw material. For this reason, companies must maintain a robust product-recall strategy able to quickly respond in the event a previously unknown contaminant is discovered in the supply chain.

How are allergens defined for dietary supplement labeling?

As with foods, DS must label the eight required allergens, if they are present within the product, with a statement saying, "This product contains allergens from…" These eight allergens, responsible, according to FDA, for greater than 90% of the reported food allergy cases, are: milk, eggs, fish, crustacean shellfish, tree nuts, peanuts, wheat and soybeans. In addition, regulations require the type of tree nut (e.g., almonds, pecans, walnuts), the type of fish (e.g., bass, flounder, cod); and the type of crustacean shellfish (e.g., crab, lobster, shrimp) to be declared on the label. While wheat must be labeled, other gluten-containing grains need not be labeled as allergens (although their presence should be found in the ingredient list).

One nuance in the allergen labeling law is that ingredients derived from purified oil, which are free of potential protein allergens, need not be labeled as allergens. So for instance, purified fish oil products or vitamin E (derived from purified soybean oil) need not be declared as allergens.

How do I know the organic or GMO status of a product?

Consumers of dietary supplements and functional foods are often interested to know if their products are made with ingredients that are organic or derived from genetically modified organisms (GMO). While these two regulatory categories are related in some cases, the definitions and labeling rules are currently different (as of early 2014).

Organic labeling of dietary supplements

The USDA has specified the parameters of labeling products as "organic" for foods. Since dietary supplements are a subcategory of foods within the regulatory framework, the same organic specifications and labeling rules are in place for dietary supplements. See page 27 for the four ways the USDA permits "organic" to be described on product labels.

Labeling ingredients from genetically modified organisms

While any product with a "USDA Organic" logo on its label is GMO-free, there are currently no regulations mandating the labeling of products containing ingredients derived from genetically modified organisms in the U.S. In fact, there is not even a universal agreement on whether such a disclosure is helpful to consumers, some of whom may assume that ingredients labeled as "GMO-free" are inherently more healthful than those without such a claim.[2] Making the issue more complex is the fact that defining "GMO-free" is not as straightforward as one would like to think. For instance, some governing bodies (i.e., The European Commission) allow ingredients obtained from non-GMO sources to be labeled as non-GMO, even when GMO-derived agents are used in the processing of the ingredient but the processing agent is not part of the finished product. Other groups have disputed the allowance of GMO-containing processing agents to produce supplements labeled non-GMO.

Furthermore, some consumer groups believe any unknown GMO status prevents an ingredient from being labeled as non-GMO. An example of this would be the GMO status of honey made by bees that may have collected pollen from a genetically modified plant, something virtually impossible to rule out, or the GMO-status of vitamin D_3 (derived from the lanolin of sheep wool) being dependent on tracing the GMO-status of all the food the sheep have eaten over their lifetimes.

These issues appear trivial at first, but as third-party groups step in to set up certification programs, the use of different definitions related to what is and what is not GMO-free is certain to be exploited by unscrupulous marketers of products and create more confusion among consumers. Likewise, as producers of raw materials gear up to change agricultural and manufacturing practices, something that could take decades in some cases, they need to have a clear set of guidelines in place. Whether Congress will instruct either the USDA or FDA to create uniform national guidelines for GMO-labeling is still unknown. In the meantime, reputable manufacturers of dietary supplements should be working closely with their vendors to understand the nature of their raw materials in order to provide appropriate information to satisfy their customers' concerns related to ingredients derived from genetically modified organisms.

2. The discussion of the merits and/or harms of ingredients derived from genetically modified organisms and the impact of GMO technology on a wide range of global concerns is beyond the scope and purpose of this Road map; this discussion is designed to outline the definitions and labeling regulations of GMO-derived ingredients in the U.S.

How do I Report Adverse Events?
Since 2008, companies selling over-the-counter drugs or dietary supplements have a mandatory requirement to report (via Medwatch) any severe adverse event within 15 days of notification to the company, and keep on record all reported adverse events (severe or not) for at least six years. While an adverse event is "any health-related event associated with the use of a dietary supplement that is adverse," a serious adverse event is any adverse event that results in: death; a life-threatening experience; inpatient hospitalization; persistent or significant disability or incapacity; a congenital anomaly or birth defect; or requires, based on a reasonable medical judgment, medical or surgical intervention to prevent one of these severe adverse outcomes. The Medwatch report must include an identifiable person (who had the adverse event), an identifiable initial reporter (often this is a clinician), a suspect dietary supplement product, and a describable serious adverse event or outcome.

Manufacturers who receive notification of a severe adverse event must report these to the FDA/Medwatch regardless of evidence (or plausibility) of whether their product actually contributed to the adverse event. Simply put, reporting the event is not an admission that the product in any way contributed to the adverse event.

Clinics that "private-label" or brand their own dietary supplements take notice: *"The manufacturer, packer, or distributor of a dietary supplement marketed in the United States whose name appears on the label of the supplement is required to report serious adverse events."* **You must understand that if your name and contact information is on the label of the supplements you distribute, you are responsible for adverse event reporting (to FDA). You should establish how this responsibility will be handled before distributing these supplements.**

How do I identify a dietary supplement independent of its label?
Unlike pharmaceutical products, dietary supplements are not required to be identifiable when removed from their labeled package. With the exception of a few marketed brands of DS with logos or lettering on the dosage form, many products may be similar in shape, color and size as other (unrelated) products. For this reason, the FDA does not permit the sale of bulk dietary supplements for clinicians to distribute, unless the clinic itself is prepared to hold and package products according to strict GMP guidelines (including FDA inspections). Likewise, clinicians should encourage patients to keep products in their original container or, when using weekly pill containers, keep one dose in the original packaging as a reference.

Dietary Supplement Claims: What is Allowed?

The detailed aspects of all allowable claims for dietary supplements are beyond the scope of this guidebook. There are, however, particular issues related to product claims healthcare professionals should understand, especially those who distribute products as part of their business, and even more so those who private-label or brand their own products.

Any statement made on a product label, or, by extension, any statement linked to a product by inclusion in product literature, advertising, company website or even by proximity on the shelf can be considered a "claim" regulated by the FDA. Any statement that implies a dietary supplement can diagnose, treat or cure a disease, or act in a manner similar to a drug, is considered unlawful and would make the product an "unapproved drug" according to the FDA. Since Congress permitted the use of "structure/function" claims for marketing dietary supplements (within DSHEA), the FDA often uses arbitrary definitions and phrases to determine when a statement is related to a disease and when it is related to healthy function (see below).

Nutrient Content Claims: Like other foods, dietary supplements can make various nutrient content claims if product contents meet specific requirements. Nutrient content claims, more typical of foods, include such claims as: fat-free, low-sodium, rich source of dietary fiber, high in calcium, etc. These types of claims are specific to the type of nutrient, whether those nutrients have a daily value (DV) or not, and a number of other criteria to prevent a truthful claim from becoming a misleading claim. For instance, claiming a particular broccoli product is "fat-free" is only allowable if the claim implies all broccoli products are also fat-free.[3]

Health Claims: These are claims that link a specific nutrient or food ingredient with the risk of a particular

3. For a complete description of all claims allowed for dietary supplements, see the FDA's website: www.fda.gov/Food/IngredientsPackagingLabeling/LabelingNutrition/

disease or health-related condition. For instance, *"Low-fat diets rich in fiber-containing grain products, fruit, and vegetables may reduce the risk of some types of cancer, a disease associated with many factors,"* is an allowable health claim for products that are a good source of fiber (unfortified) and low in fat. A range of health claims and qualified health claims are approved by FDA after undergoing scientific scrutiny (usually after receiving a petition for the claim). Other allowable claims are authorized based on an authoritative statement by federal scientific bodies.

Structure/Function Claims: These claims are unique to dietary supplements, specifically added by Congress under DSHEA. Structure/Function claims are designed to allow manufacturers to describe how a product or ingredient affects normal (non-disease) structure or function, or means by which a product or ingredient acts to maintain such structure or function. These types of claims include statements such as "helps maintain healthy prostate function." When structure/function claims are included on product labels, a standard disclaimer must be used that states: *"This statement has not been evaluated by the Food and Drug Administration. This product is not intended to diagnose, treat, cure, or prevent any disease."* While structure/function claims need not go through pre-approval by FDA, companies making any structure/function claim must notify FDA within 30 days of distributing products with such claims.

Structure/Function vs. Disease Claims: An ongoing issue between industry marketing and FDA regulation is the fuzzy (some would say arbitrary) line drawn between an allowable structure/function claim and a disease or drug claim. In fact, the FDA states the following: *"It may not be possible always to draw a bright line between structure/function and disease claims. You should look at the objective evidence in your labeling to assess whether a claim explicitly or implicitly is a disease claim. For example, a statement may not mention a disease but may refer to identifiable characteristic signs or symptoms of a disease such that the intended use of the product to treat or prevent the disease* **may be inferred***"[emphasis added]. Adding more complexity is the fact that the FDA's definition of a disease includes: *"damage to an organ, part,* ***structure****, or system of the body such that it does not* ***function*** *properly (e.g., cardiovascular disease)"* [emphasis added], a definition also based on both the structure and function of the body.

The difficulty arises when companies, attempting to provide truthful, non-misleading, and substantiatable information related to ingredients within their products, are prevented from doing so because a particular individual within the FDA infers an implicit disease claim is being made about the product. Some believe that the FDA's use of such inferences not only violates the First Amendment right of companies to express truthful information, but also violates the spirit and intent of DSHEA, which states that: *"consumers should be empowered to make choices about preventive health care programs based on data from scientific studies of health benefits related to particular dietary supplements"* and that *"although the Federal Government should take swift action against products that are unsafe or adulterated, the Federal Government should not take any actions to impose unreasonable regulatory barriers limiting or slowing the flow of safe products and accurate information to consumers."*

Clinics that market or distribute products must understand claims made about products, or references to studies in relation to marketing products (even if truthful), are not more permissible because they are being made by a healthcare professional. If you are unfamiliar with the appropriate rules in marketing dietary supplements (in your clinic or on your website), contact a regulatory consultant familiar with the FDA's guidelines for DS or your supplement supplier for more information.

Non-Active Ingredients in Dietary Supplements

In order to control the label claim of any product, it is critical a manufacturer control their processes from raw material vendor selection through expiration date testing. Important in this process is selecting the dosing form (powder, capsule, tablet, chewable, liquid) and, when needed, the use of certain non-active ingredients. Below is a discussion of these issues.

Common Dietary Supplement Dose Forms

Powders: The use of powders (usually provided in large jars with scoops) is common when providing large doses of *palatable* products like protein supplements, fiber supplements, meal replacements or green drinks. The advantage of powders is their ability to provide large doses without the extra manufacturing costs of making tablets or capsules, also eliminating the need for certain excipients. On the other hand, because powders are almost always mixed with water, juice, milk or milk substitutes, these products tend to have added sugars, non-nutritive sweeteners, masking agents, flavors and thickeners. Manufacturers are always attempting to create a balance between the clinician's desire for limited added ingredients and the patient's desire for a good-tasting product.

Tablets: One of the most popular forms of delivering dietary supplements is via tablets. The advantages are convenience, size and shelf stability; and because tablets require compression of ingredients, they are typically capable of delivering more ingredients than a capsule. These advantages are often greatly diminished by the fact that tablets require more modified active ingredients and non-active manufacturing excipients. For instance, since many powders are not capable of holding their shape when compressed in a tablet press, manufacturers must purchase "directly compressible" powders (requiring added ingredients and processing) or add ingredients to the nutrient blend prior to tableting. In some cases, a process of wet-granulation is used, which involves making a wet slurry with water or solvents to prepare (after drying) the powder for tableting. As mentioned above, some of these added processing ingredients may not need to be listed on the label.

Important in the manufacture of tablets is their ability to break apart and dissolve properly when consumed. These properties of disintegration and dissolution are dependent on the formula, but also on processing and tablet pressure for each batch. Manufacturers should test the disintegration properties of each batch of tablets they produce prior to approval (although FDA does not mandate this as a requirement in the GMP regulations). Batches that do not meet the maximum time for disintegration should be reworked or rejected, as they may not break apart appropriately after ingestion.

Finally, the manufacturing of the tablet itself involves a higher percent of lubricants and flowing agents than is typical of encapsulation (see below), and most tablets require additional ingredients for coating. It is for this reason we limit our recommendation of tablets to certain multivitamins (to help reduce dose number), chewable tablets and those that require enteric-coating (although some capsules now are acid-resistant).

Capsules: Two-piece hard capsules are also a popular way to deliver dietary and herbal supplements. While requiring some non-active ingredients, they typically can be made using fewer excipients than tablets. Two main types of capsules are used to make dietary supplements: gelatin capsules and cellulose capsules. For years, gelatin (derived from the hooves of animals) was the only major source for the manufacturing of capsules. Cellulose (sometimes called vegetable) capsules are derived from hydroxyproplymethylcellulose, a hypoallergenic polymer derived from tree cellulose (mostly pine and spruce). While it took years to perfect the cellulose capsules to meet the manufacturing stability and properties compared to gelatin capsules, most companies now have a large portion of their encapsulated products in these vegan-friendly capsules.

Two-piece capsules range in size from a large "000" (~1.3 gm of material) to the very small "5" (~130 mg). Most supplement manufacturers limit their production to three sizes ("00," "0," "1"), as most nutrient doses fit into one of these sizes, and each new size requires a completely different set of parts for their encapsulation machines. New technologies are emerging that have allowed for some liquid- and paste-filled hard-gelatin capsules; some technologies even allow for a powder-filled capsule inside a liquid-filled capsule. Whether these types of technologies will be affordable for delivering nutrients is yet to be seen.

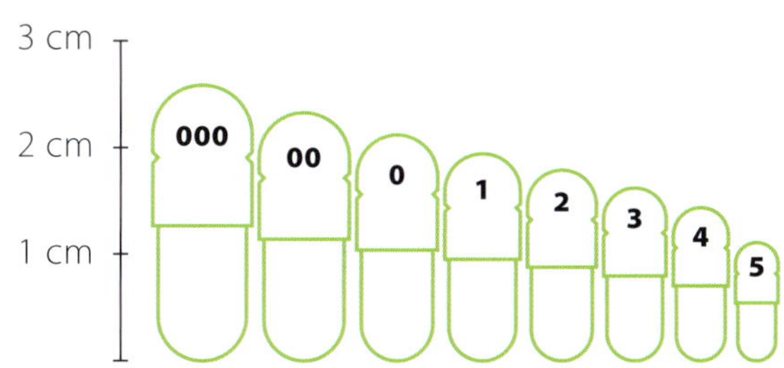

Figure 16: Sizes of two-piece capsules used for DS

Advantages of using capsules

- Available from a non-animal-derived source, allowing suitability for vegetarian, vegan and kosher applications (some gelatin capsules are also kosher).
- Consistent disintegration. Since the thickness and properties of capsules are not changed by the encapsulation process, each batch will have the same (known) disintegration properties when consumed. Unlike tablets, disintegration of capsules is not a batch-to-batch quality control issue.
- Require fewer excipients than tablets while offering similar dose convenience.
- Some capsules can be purchased by the manufacturer with built-in acid-resistant properties. This means ingredients that might be better protected by avoiding the stomach acid (such as probiotics or enzymes) can be delivered in two-piece capsules with greater efficacy.

Soft gelatin capsules: While two-piece capsules and tablets are great for delivering dry powder ingredients, liquid ingredients are often better delivered via soft gelatin capsules (softgels). The specialized equipment designed to make softgels involves melting the gelatin and injecting the liquid material into the gelatin as it forms in a die of various sizes, where it is then cooled and polished. The majority of softgel products use animal-derived gelatin, although fish-source and non-animal source gelatins are being optimized and are now more common. Products typically delivered in softgels might include: fish oil, flax seed oil, evening primrose oil, borage oil, coenzyme Q_{10}, vitamin E, phosphytidylserine, conjugated linolenic acid (CLA), vitamin D and vitamin K.

Liquids: Liquid products (in dropper or pourable bottles) are typically reserved for specific applications. As with drug delivery, some dietary supplements for children are easier to dispense when given in droppers; but as with chewable vitamins for children, taste requirements may force the addition of more sweeteners and flavoring than tablets and capsules intended for swallowing.

Excipients: Due to quality control constraints, powder filling the capsule must have consistent flowing characteristics, and capsules must be mostly full in order to ensure uniformity of the dose. It is necessary to use excipients (flow agents, lubricants, fillers, etc.) to maintain flow and fill characteristics and to ensure friction does not harm the nutrients or the machines. In the case of tablets, these issues are compounded by the need to ensure tablet integrity on the one hand and tablet disintegration and dissolution on the other. This is why tablets also include excipients typically referred to as "binders" and "disintegrants." In many cases, single excipient ingredients perform more than one task in the forming of tablets and capsules. Here we outline basic functions of excipients and give common examples of each (the "other ingredients" portion of a supplement label should disclose all added excipients).

- **Fillers:** As mentioned above, a partially filled capsule or inadequate bulk to compress a tablet can greatly decrease the dose-to-dose precision needed to meet the strict mandates of GMP compliance. In some cases, delivering a small amount of a particular ingredient (without other active ingredients) will not come close to filling the capsule (e.g., 1,000 IU of vitamin D requires only about 10 mg of material). In these cases, various capsule "fillers" are used. The filler most commonly used in the manufacturing of dietary supplements is microcrystalline cellulose, a naturally occurring polymer derived from refined wood-pulp. The need for filler depends on the product formulation and size of capsule/tablet.
- **Flow Agents:** These are excipient ingredients used to help change the flow characteristics of powder (usually to increase flow) for proper tableting and encapsulation. Typical flow agents used in the production of dietary supplements are microcrystalline cellulose (also a filler) and silica derivatives (silicon dioxide, calcium silicate, etc.). Silica helps bind moisture and break apart particles within powders to increase their flowing characteristics. Flow agents typically do not exceed 1 – 2% of the capsule or tablet by weight.
- **Lubricants:** Agents used to coat the powder (after comprehensive mixing) in order to reduce friction, allowing capsules to close and prevent tablets from sticking to punches, are called lubricants. The most commonly used lubricants in tablet and capsule manufacturing are stearic acid and magnesium stearate (the use of which has engendered a wide misinformation campaign, see page 152). These agents are used in formulas from 0.5% – 1.5% by weight.

- **Binders:** Primarily used in tablets, binders are any excipient that helps to hold the powder together to form a finished tablet. Some of these ingredients serve other functions or are even specially prepared "active" ingredients (usually purchased as "directly compressible" ingredients). Binders might be compressible sugars (sucrose, xylitol, sorbitol), hydroxypropyl cellulose and its derivatives or, commonly, dicalcium phosphate (known commercially by the brand Di-Tab®). Some of these agents serve also as fillers or sweeteners in regular and chewable tablets.

- **Disintegrants:** Compounds that help tablets break open faster when reaching an aqueous environment are called disintegrants. Depending on the formula, disintegrants will be used at different levels but are usually limited to less than 5% by weight. The most common disintegrant is croscarmellose sodium, a cross-linked cellulose polymer. Hydroxypropyl cellulose is also sometimes used.

- **Coating Agents:** For coating tablets, there are a number of agents used to seal, protect and color the finished product: Hydroxypropyl cellulose, pharmaceutical lac glaze, chlorophyllin, polyethylene glycol (PEG), titanium dioxide, bees wax, caramel coloring, and a host of natural and artificial colorings. Products that claim to be enteric-coated typically use methyl acrylate-methacrylic acid copolymers or similar agents. Some products that claim to be "naturally" enteric-coated use products described as alginates. These products rarely produce finished products that meet strict USP criteria for enteric-coated products.

Conclusion: In the current GMP environment, manufacturing tablets, capsules and softgels requires judicious use of excipient ingredients. Skilled manufacturers and formulators are capable of producing products that meet these stringent guidelines with minimal use of non-active ingredients. Since the regulatory requirements mandate full disclosure of manufacturing excipients, these agents should be listed on the label below the Supplement Facts panel.

The Use of Magnesium Stearate in Dietary Supplements

For the past several decades, a small but vocal group of individuals, including some well-known clinicians, have raised concerns about the use of magnesium stearate (MagS) and stearic acid. The claims made about the potential harms of MagS use are baseless and unscientific; nonetheless, numerous individuals have believed these claims and some dietary supplement companies actually promote their products based on their refusal to use such ingredients. Let's examine what this is all about.

As mentioned before, MagS and stearic acid are used as lubricants when manufacturing capsules and tablets. For reference, usage of these ingredients is between 1 – 5% for stearic acid and 0.5 – 2% for MagS. Stearic acid is a saturated fatty acid (18:0) found in plants and animals. MagS is the salt formed between one molecule of magnesium and two molecules of stearic acid. Nearly all the stearic acid and MagS used in dietary supplements is plant-source stearic acid (usually palm oil or coconut oil). Once consumed, MagS is separated in the acid environment of the stomach into stearic acid and free (ionic) magnesium. Stearic acid is absorbed along with other fats in the diet and used directly or converted into oleic acid (18:1w9).

Controversy swirls around the unscientific and misapplication of only a few published papers unrelated to the use of stearic acid or MagS in the context of supplements. In 1990 a publication in the journal *Immunology* titled "Molecular basis for the immunosuppressive actions of stearic acid in T-cells" concluded isolated mouse T-cells exposed to stearic acid (as a fatty acid complex with bovine serum albumin and diatomaceous earth) would die due to altered cell membrane function.[1] What most individuals do not realize is this stearic acid phenomenon only occurs in the T-cells of these BALB/c mice, because their T-cells do not properly express the enzyme needed to convert stearic acid to oleic acid (stearoyl-CoA desaturase).[2] These authors later discovered other mice strains have ample expression of this enzyme in T-cells and this response may actually be a strain-specific phenomenon.[3] Perhaps more important, since human T-cells have this enzyme and are rarely bathed in stearic acid-albumin-diatomaceous earth, the relationship between this study and consuming stearates in the diet (e.g., 2,500 mg in 25 gm of chocolate or nearly 4,000 mg in a steak) or through supplements (perhaps a few hundred mg for high supplement users) is unknown. While much has been said about this single study from 1990 (on the Internet and from podiums), this model should never have been considered remotely related to MagS or stearic acid use in supplements.

The other "issues" with MagS use in supplements are more difficult to refute because they simply have no basis in fact. One often repeated is that MagS causes biofilm formation in the gastrointestinal tract, which, according to these detractors, is a sign of something unhealthy. Without delving into the nuances of biofilm (the extracellular matrix produced by mixed colonies of bacteria), it is important to remember biofilm is a normal part of both friendly commensal organisms and potentially harmful organisms. Beyond the basics of biofilm biology, there has never been a referenced study to explain where this MagS-biofilm story originated. Many who have looked into this biofilm issue have even cited a paper that appears to show stearic acid *inhibits* biofilm formation.[4] While this is one way to interpret this study, the result (using a mixture of stearic, palmitic and oleic acids) was isolated to only a few strains of bacteria and not in a biologically relevant (biofilm producing) context. There is no evidence or plausible biology that would lead us to connect MagS in supplements (or drugs) to a change in biofilm formation.

Finally, the issue of whether MagS or stearic acid can inhibit the absorption of the encapsulated or tableted nutrients is often raised. While excessive use of stearic acid or MagS in tablets can increase the disintegration time of tablets, reputable companies should be testing each batch to standard specifications to ensure their formula does not exceed these limits. It is worth pointing out that almost everything we know about supplementing nutrients in tablets and capsules (dosing levels, pharmacokinetics, pharmacodynamics, etc.) have been done with products made with appropriate levels of MagS and/or stearic acid. Nearly every positive (and negative) study performed using an encapsulated or tableted vitamin, mineral, herb or nutraceutical has been performed with products containing these and other excipients.

Supplementing nutrients using the convenience of capsules and tablets has invited a wealth of regulatory and quality guidelines, most of which are focused on the accuracy and consistency of each single dose. Machines currently available to efficiently manufacture capsules and tablets from powdered materials are designed to function properly when lubricants are added directly to the powder (they are not self-lubricating). In an attempt to confuse consumers with baseless claims of harm, manufacturers claiming to exclude MagS and stearic acid as a means to market their products as "better" or "safer" need to provide documented and peer-reviewed evidence for their claims. Until such evidence exists, the use of these excipients should be considered harmless and, in many cases, necessary to produce products of both high quality and sensible economy.

1. Tebbey PW, Buttke TM. Molecular basis for the immunosuppressive action of stearic acid on T cells. *Immunology.* 1990 Jul; 70(3):379-84.
2. Buttke TM, Van Cleave S, Steelman L, McCubrey JA. Absence of unsaturated fatty acid synthesis in murine T lymphocytes *Proc Natl Acad Sci U S A.* 1989 Aug; 86(16):6133-7.
3. Tebbey PW, Buttke TM. Stearoyl-CoA desaturase gene expression in lymphocytes. *Biochem Biophys Res Commun.* 1992 Jul 15; 186(1):531-6.
4. Soni KA, Jesudhasan P et al. Identification of ground beef-derived fatty acid inhibitors of autoinducer-2-based cell signaling. *J Food Prot.* 2008 Jan; 71(1):134-8.

A Suggested Formulary
for Supplemental Nutrients

Macronutrients

Protein-based Supplements (see page 33)

- Multiple Flavors of a mixed vegan protein (e.g., pea, rice, hemp, potato) or whey protein product balanced with healthy fats, fiber and carbohydrates to deliver targeted nutrients or for a caloric meal substitute:
    - Meal Substitute/Replacement: ~20 grams of protein, less than 300 calories
    - Protein Bar: Protein, Fiber and ~250 calories for glycemic control
    - Glycemic Control Product: High in fiber, protein and insulin sensitizing nutrients
    - Inflammation Control/GI products: Hypoallergenic, targeted gut and anti-inflammatory nutrients

Fiber (see page 41)

- Mixture of soluble and insoluble fibers for regularity and glycemic control. Ingredients to look for: Psyllium (husks and seed), pectins, gums, rice bran, glucans, glucomannan, fig or prune powders
    - Powder product to stir into liquid
    - Capsules (remember 12 or more capsules are needed to equal 1 tbs of most fiber)
    - Children's products in liquid: Look for similar ingredients as above in liquid format, may include herbs to settle gas/bloating such as ginger, coriander, caraway or fennel

Fatty Acid Supplements (starting on page 43)

- Evening Primrose Oil: To supply traditional dose of GLA, softgel recommended (see page 47)
- Flaxseed Oil: To supply the plant-based essential omega-3 alpha-linolenic acid, softgel recommended (see page 46)
- Fish oil (TG form of fish oil is recommended- see page 46)
    - High dose multipurpose EPA +DHA (720 mg or more; ratio 2:1-3:2)
    - Children's EPA/DHA- lower dose similar to above (deliver in chew, small capsule, flavored liquid or emulsion)
    - High dose DHA-rich oil (ratio DHA:EPA of ~4:1)
    - High dose EPA-rich oil (ratio of EPA:DHA of ~4:1)

Condition-specific recommendations from the data presented.

Condition	EPA-Rich	EPA/DHA	DHA-Rich
General Health		★★	
Improving w3:w6 ratio		★★	
Low-Risk CVD prevention		★★	★
High CVD Risk/Atherosclerosis		★	★★
Inflammatory Diseases		★★	
Depression	★★	★	
Macular Degeneration			★★
Alzheimer—Dementia		★	★★
Maternal—Childhood Development		★	★★

Notes

Micronutrients

Comprehensive Multivitamins/Minerals (starting on page 49)

- Capsules or tablets providing high doses of most vitamins and minerals in 6 or 8 dose units. Can dose at half (3 or 4) for many patients.
    - o Without Iron: For men and post-menopausal women
    - o With Iron: For pregnant, premenopausal women or those needing daily iron.
- Prenatal Supplement: Use iron version of comprehensive multivitamin or product developed for use in pregnant women. Some packets may contain multivitamins along with DHA softgel. (see page 51)
- Children's Multivitamin/mineral: Chewable wafer large enough to deliver adequate vitamins and minerals for children. (see page 52)

Single Nutrients/Vitamins (starting on page 60)

- Vitamin C: Use with flavonoids or buffering agents (see page 80)
- Vitamin D (multiple doses and forms see page 82)
    - o Capsules: 1,000 IU (25 mcg)
    - o Capsules: 5,000 IU (125 mcg)
    - o Capsules: 50,000 IU (1250 mcg or 1.25 mg) (for once weekly dosing)
    - o Liquid- 1,000 IU (25 mcg) per drop
    - o Children's liquid 400 IU (10 mcg) dropper dose
- Vitamin E:
    - o Softgel (400 IU/268 mg of d-alpha plus mixed tocopherols- measured in mg see page 90)
- Vitamin K2
    - o MK-7 (45-180 mcg) with or without Vitamin D (see page 93)
- Folate
    - o Folic Acid and/or 5MTHF: 800 mcg- 5 mg (depending on intent of use see page 74)

Minerals (starting on page 98)

- Calcium Product (Reacted blend of amino acid chelates and organic salts see page 99)
- Calcium/Magnesium Product (Reacted blend of amino acid chelates and organic salts see page 96)
- Iron Product (Amino Acid Chelate-glycinate see page 105)
- Magnesium Product (Reacted blend of amino acid chelates and organic salts see page 107)
- Magnesium and Potassium (Reacted blend of amino acid chelates and organic salts)
- Zinc Product (Reacted amino acid chelate- glycinate see page 115)
- Multi-mineral Blend containing most minerals with DV

Targeted combinations

- Basic B-complex: A product containing all the B-vitamins along with choline and inositol (see pages 118-119)
- Methylation/Homocysteine product: Combinations of folic acid/5MTHF, vitamin B_{12}, vitamin B_6 and often additional betaine (trimethylglycine) for targeted methylation or homocysteine therapy
- Vitamin C (ascorbic acid) with flavonoids: For targeted use of vitamin C (see page 80)
- Vitamin C with buffering agents (carbonates): for buffered ascorbic acid use at high doses

Notes

Specialty Nutrients

- Co-enzyme Q_{10} (see page 122)
  - o 100 mg softgel of enhanced-absorption CoQ_{10} (ubiquinone)
  - o 300 mg softgel of enhanced-absorption CoQ_{10} (ubiquinone)
  - o Ubiquinol (100 mg or more) for special purposes
- Lipoic Acid (see page 124)
  - o 100-300 mg Lipoic acid capsules
- Carnitine (see page 120)
  - o L-Carnitine (Softgel) or L-carnitine L-tartrate capsules (500-750 mg)
  - o Acetyl-L-carnitine- for specific therapeutic uses (500-750 mg)

Notes

Probiotics (see page 131)

Multi-strain probiotic including 5-7 strains from *Lactobacillus, Bifidobacteria* and *S. boulardii*.

- Versatile mid-range concentration (15-40 billion CFU- capsule, tablet, powder)
- High-dose product (100 billion CFU or more: typically in sachet/packet delivery)
- Children's product (1-5 billion CFU per dose) Strains may differ slightly from products developed for adults.

Notes

Dietary Reference Intakes (DRIs): Recommended Dietary Allowances and Adequate Intakes, Vitamins

Food and Nutrition Board, Institute of Medicine, National Academies

Life Stage Group	Vitamin A (μg/d)[a]	Vitamin C (mg/d)	Vitamin D (μg/d)[b,c]	Vitamin E (mg/d)[d]	Vitamin K (μg/d)	Thiamin (mg/d)	Riboflavin (mg/d)	Niacin (mg/d)[e]	Vitamin B_6 (mg/d)	Folate (μg/d)[f]	Vitamin B_{12} (μg/d)	Pantothenic Acid (mg/d)	Biotin (μg/d)	Choline (mg/d)[g]
Infants														
0 to 6 mo	400*	40*	10	4*	2.0*	0.2*	0.3*	2*	0.1*	65*	0.4*	1.7*	5*	125*
6 to 12 mo	500*	50*	10	5*	2.5*	0.3*	0.4*	4*	0.3*	80*	0.5*	1.8*	6*	150*
Children														
1–3 y	**300**	**15**	**15**	**6**	30*	**0.5**	**0.5**	**6**	**0.5**	**150**	**0.9**	2*	8*	200*
4–8 y	**400**	**25**	**15**	**7**	55*	**0.6**	**0.6**	**8**	**0.6**	**200**	**1.2**	3*	12*	250*
Males														
9–13 y	**600**	**45**	**15**	**11**	60*	**0.9**	**0.9**	**12**	**1.0**	**300**	**1.8**	4*	20*	375*
14–18 y	**900**	**75**	**15**	**15**	75*	**1.2**	**1.3**	**16**	**1.3**	**400**	**2.4**	5*	25*	550*
19–30 y	**900**	**90**	**15**	**15**	120*	**1.2**	**1.3**	**16**	**1.3**	**400**	**2.4**	5*	30*	550*
31–50 y	**900**	**90**	**15**	**15**	120*	**1.2**	**1.3**	**16**	**1.3**	**400**	**2.4**	5*	30*	550*
51–70 y	**900**	**90**	**15**	**15**	120*	**1.2**	**1.3**	**16**	**1.7**	**400**	**2.4**[h]	5*	30*	550*
> 70 y	**900**	**90**	**20**	**15**	120*	**1.2**	**1.3**	**16**	**1.7**	**400**	**2.4**[h]	5*	30*	550*
Females														
9–13 y	**600**	**45**	**15**	**11**	60*	**0.9**	**0.9**	**12**	**1.0**	**300**	**1.8**	4*	20*	375*
14–18 y	**700**	**65**	**15**	**15**	75*	**1.0**	**1.0**	**14**	**1.2**	**400**[i]	**2.4**	5*	25*	400*
19–30 y	**700**	**75**	**15**	**15**	90*	**1.1**	**1.1**	**14**	**1.3**	**400**[i]	**2.4**	5*	30*	425*
31–50 y	**700**	**75**	**15**	**15**	90*	**1.1**	**1.1**	**14**	**1.3**	**400**[i]	**2.4**	5*	30*	425*
51–70 y	**700**	**75**	**15**	**15**	90*	**1.1**	**1.1**	**14**	**1.5**	**400**	**2.4**[h]	5*	30*	425*
> 70 y	**700**	**75**	**20**	**15**	90*	**1.1**	**1.1**	**14**	**1.5**	**400**	**2.4**[h]	5*	30*	425*
Pregnancy														
14–18 y	**750**	**80**	**15**	**15**	75*	**1.4**	**1.4**	**18**	**1.9**	**600**[j]	**2.6**	6*	30*	450*
19–30 y	**770**	**85**	**15**	**15**	90*	**1.4**	**1.4**	**18**	**1.9**	**600**[j]	**2.6**	6*	30*	450*
31–50 y	**770**	**85**	**15**	**15**	90*	**1.4**	**1.4**	**18**	**1.9**	**600**[j]	**2.6**	6*	30*	450*
Lactation														
14–18 y	**1,200**	**115**	**15**	**19**	75*	**1.4**	**1.6**	**17**	**2.0**	**500**	**2.8**	7*	35*	550*
19–30 y	**1,300**	**120**	**15**	**19**	90*	**1.4**	**1.6**	**17**	**2.0**	**500**	**2.8**	7*	35*	550*
31–50 y	**1,300**	**120**	**15**	**19**	90*	**1.4**	**1.6**	**17**	**2.0**	**500**	**2.8**	7*	35*	550*

NOTE: This table (taken from the DRI reports, see www.nap.edu) presents Recommended Dietary Allowances (RDAs) in **bold type** and Adequate Intakes (AIs) in ordinary type followed by an asterisk (*). An RDA is the average daily dietary intake level; sufficient to meet the nutrient requirements of nearly all (97-98 percent) healthy individuals in a group. It is calculated from an Estimated Average Requirement (EAR). If sufficient scientific evidence is not available to establish an EAR, and thus calculate an RDA, an AI is usually developed. For healthy breastfed infants, an AI is the mean intake. The AI for other life stage and gender groups is believed to cover the needs of all healthy individuals in the groups, but lack of data or uncertainty in the data prevent being able to specify with confidence the percentage of individuals covered by this intake.

[a] As retinol activity equivalents (RAEs). 1 RAE = 1 μg retinol, 12 μg β-carotene, 24 μg α-carotene, or 24 μg β-cryptoxanthin. The RAE for dietary provitamin A carotenoids is two-fold greater than retinol equivalents (RE), whereas the RAE for preformed vitamin A is the same as RE.

[b] As cholecalciferol. 1 μg cholecalciferol = 40 IU vitamin D.

[c] Under the assumption of minimal sunlight.

[d] As α-tocopherol. α-Tocopherol includes *RRR*-α-tocopherol, the only form of α-tocopherol that occurs naturally in foods, and the 2*R*-stereoisomeric forms of α-tocopherol (*RRR*-, *RSR*-, *RRS*-, and *RSS*-α-tocopherol) that occur in fortified foods and supplements. It does not include the 2*S*-stereoisomeric forms of α-tocopherol (*SRR*-, *SSR*-, *SRS*-, and *SSS*-α-tocopherol), also found in fortified foods and supplements.

[e] As niacin equivalents (NE). 1 mg of niacin = 60 mg of tryptophan; 0–6 months = preformed niacin (not NE).

[f] As dietary folate equivalents (DFE). 1 DFE = 1 μg food folate = 0.6 μg of folic acid from fortified food or as a supplement consumed with food = 0.5 μg of a supplement taken on an empty stomach.

[g] Although AIs have been set for choline, there are few data to assess whether a dietary supply of choline is needed at all stages of the life cycle, and it may be that the choline requirement can be met by endogenous synthesis at some of these stages.

[h] Because 10 to 30 percent of older people may malabsorb food-bound B_{12}, it is advisable for those older than 50 years to meet their RDA mainly by consuming foods fortified with B_{12} or a supplement containing B_{12}.

[i] In view of evidence linking folate intake with neural tube defects in the fetus, it is recommended that all women capable of becoming pregnant consume 400 μg from supplements or fortified foods in addition to intake of food folate from a varied diet.

[j] It is assumed that women will continue consuming 400 μg from supplements or fortified food until their pregnancy is confirmed and they enter prenatal care, which ordinarily occurs after the end of the periconceptional period—the critical time for formation of the neural tube.

SOURCES: *Dietary Reference Intakes for Calcium, Phosphorous, Magnesium, Vitamin D, and Fluoride* (1997); *Dietary Reference Intakes for Thiamin, Riboflavin, Niacin, Vitamin B_6, Folate, Vitamin B_{12}, Pantothenic Acid, Biotin, and Choline* (1998); *Dietary Reference Intakes for Vitamin C, Vitamin E, Selenium, and Carotenoids* (2000); *Dietary Reference Intakes for Vitamin A, Vitamin K, Arsenic, Boron, Chromium, Copper, Iodine, Iron, Manganese, Molybdenum, Nickel, Silicon, Vanadium, and Zinc* (2001); *Dietary Reference Intakes for Water, Potassium, Sodium, Chloride, and* Sulfate (2005); and *Dietary Reference Intakes for Calcium and Vitamin D* (2011). These reports may be accessed via www.nap.edu.

Dietary Reference Intakes (DRIs): Recommended Dietary Allowances and Adequate Intakes, Elements

Food and Nutrition Board, Institute of Medicine, National Academies

Life Stage Group	Calcium (mg/d)	Chromium (μg/d)	Copper (μg/d)	Fluoride (mg/d)	Iodine (μg/d)	Iron (mg/d)	Magnesium (mg/d)	Manganese (mg/d)	Molybdenum (μg/d)	Phosphorus (mg/d)	Selenium (μg/d)	Zinc (mg/d)	Potass-ium (g/d)	Sodium (g/d)	Chloride (g/d)
Infants															
0 to 6 mo	200*	0.2*	200*	0.01*	110*	0.27*	30*	0.003*	2*	100*	15*	2*	0.4*	0.12*	0.18*
6 to 12 mo	260*	5.5*	220*	0.5*	130*	**11**	75*	0.6*	3*	275*	20*	**3**	0.7*	0.37*	0.57*
Children															
1–3 y	**700**	11*	**340**	0.7*	**90**	**7**	**80**	1.2*	**17**	**460**	**20**	**3**	3.0*	1.0*	1.5*
4–8 y	**1,000**	15*	**440**	1*	**90**	**10**	**130**	1.5*	**22**	**500**	**30**	**5**	3.8*	1.2*	1.9*
Males															
9–13 y	**1,300**	25*	**700**	2*	**120**	**8**	**240**	1.9*	**34**	**1,250**	**40**	**8**	4.5*	1.5*	2.3*
14–18 y	**1,300**	35*	**890**	3*	**150**	**11**	**410**	2.2*	**43**	**1,250**	**55**	**11**	4.7*	1.5*	2.3*
19–30 y	**1,000**	35*	**900**	4*	**150**	**8**	**400**	2.3*	**45**	**700**	**55**	**11**	4.7*	1.5*	2.3*
31–50 y	**1,000**	35*	**900**	4*	**150**	**8**	**420**	2.3*	**45**	**700**	**55**	**11**	4.7*	1.5*	2.3*
51–70 y	**1,000**	30*	**900**	4*	**150**	**8**	**420**	2.3*	**45**	**700**	**55**	**11**	4.7*	1.3*	2.0*
> 70 y	**1,200**	30*	**900**	4*	**150**	**8**	**420**	2.3*	**45**	**700**	**55**	**11**	4.7*	1.2*	1.8*
Females															
9–13 y	**1,300**	21*	**700**	2*	**120**	**8**	**240**	1.6*	**34**	**1,250**	**40**	**8**	4.5*	1.5*	2.3*
14–18 y	**1,300**	24*	**890**	3*	**150**	**15**	**360**	1.6*	**43**	**1,250**	**55**	**9**	4.7*	1.5*	2.3*
19–30 y	**1,000**	25*	**900**	3*	**150**	**18**	**310**	1.8*	**45**	**700**	**55**	**8**	4.7*	1.5*	2.3*
31–50 y	**1,000**	25*	**900**	3*	**150**	**18**	**320**	1.8*	**45**	**700**	**55**	**8**	4.7*	1.5*	2.3*
51–70 y	**1,200**	20*	**900**	3*	**150**	**8**	**320**	1.8*	**45**	**700**	**55**	**8**	4.7*	1.3*	2.0*
> 70 y	**1,200**	20*	**900**	3*	**150**	**8**	**320**	1.8*	**45**	**700**	**55**	**8**	4.7*	1.2*	1.8*
Pregnancy															
14–18 y	**1,300**	29*	**1,000**	3*	**220**	**27**	**400**	2.0*	**50**	**1,250**	**60**	**12**	4.7*	1.5*	2.3*
19–30 y	**1,000**	30*	**1,000**	3*	**220**	**27**	**350**	2.0*	**50**	**700**	**60**	**11**	4.7*	1.5*	2.3*
31–50 y	**1,000**	30*	**1,000**	3*	**220**	**27**	**360**	2.0*	**50**	**700**	**60**	**11**	4.7*	1.5*	2.3*
Lactation															
14–18 y	**1,300**	44*	**1,300**	3*	**290**	**10**	**360**	2.6*	**50**	**1,250**	**70**	**13**	5.1*	1.5*	2.3*
19–30 y	**1,000**	45*	**1,300**	3*	**290**	**9**	**310**	2.6*	**50**	**700**	**70**	**12**	5.1*	1.5*	2.3*
31–50 y	**1,000**	45*	**1,300**	3*	**290**	**9**	**320**	2.6*	**50**	**700**	**70**	**12**	5.1*	1.5*	2.3*

NOTE: This table (taken from the DRI reports, see www.nap.edu) presents Recommended Dietary Allowances (RDAs) in **bold type** and Adequate Intakes (AIs) in ordinary type followed by an asterisk (*). An RDA is the average daily dietary intake level; sufficient to meet the nutrient requirements of nearly all (97-98 percent) healthy individuals in a group. It is calculated from an Estimated Average Requirement (EAR). If sufficient scientific evidence is not available to establish an EAR, and thus calculate an RDA, an AI is usually developed. For healthy breastfed infants, an AI is the mean intake. The AI for other life stage and gender groups is believed to cover the needs of all healthy individuals in the groups, but lack of data or uncertainty in the data prevent being able to specify with confidence the percentage of individuals covered by this intake.

SOURCES: *Dietary Reference Intakes for Calcium, Phosphorous, Magnesium, Vitamin D, and Fluoride* (1997); *Dietary Reference Intakes for Thiamin, Riboflavin, Niacin, Vitamin B_6, Folate, Vitamin B_{12}, Pantothenic Acid, Biotin, and Choline* (1998); *Dietary Reference Intakes for Vitamin C, Vitamin E, Selenium, and Carotenoids* (2000); and *Dietary Reference Intakes for Vitamin A, Vitamin K, Arsenic, Boron, Chromium, Copper, Iodine, Iron, Manganese, Molybdenum, Nickel, Silicon, Vanadium, and Zinc* (2001); *Dietary Reference Intakes for Water, Potassium, Sodium, Chloride, and* Sulfate (2005); and *Dietary Reference Intakes for Calcium and Vitamin D* (2011). These reports may be accessed via www.nap.edu.

Dietary Reference Intakes (DRIs): Tolerable Upper Intake Levels, Vitamins

Food and Nutrition Board, Institute of Medicine, National Academies

Life Stage Group	Vitamin A (μg/d)[a]	Vitamin C (mg/d)	Vitamin D (μg/d)	Vitamin E (mg/d)[b,c]	Vitamin K	Thiamin	Riboflavin	Niacin (mg/d)[c]	Vitamin B_6 (mg/d)	Folate (μg/d)[c]	Vitamin B_{12}	Pantothenic Acid	Biotin	Choline (g/d)	Carotenoids[d]
Infants															
0 to 6 mo	600	ND[e]	25	ND	ND	ND	ND	ND	ND	ND	ND	ND	ND	ND	ND
6 to 12 mo	600	ND	38	ND	ND	ND	ND	ND	ND	ND	ND	ND	ND	ND	ND
Children															
1–3 y	600	400	63	200	ND	ND	ND	10	30	300	ND	ND	ND	1.0	ND
4–8 y	900	650	75	300	ND	ND	ND	15	40	400	ND	ND	ND	1.0	ND
Males															
9–13 y	1,700	1,200	100	600	ND	ND	ND	20	60	600	ND	ND	ND	2.0	ND
14–18 y	2,800	1,800	100	800	ND	ND	ND	30	80	800	ND	ND	ND	3.0	ND
19–30 y	3,000	2,000	100	1,000	ND	ND	ND	35	100	1,000	ND	ND	ND	3.5	ND
31–50 y	3,000	2,000	100	1,000	ND	ND	ND	35	100	1,000	ND	ND	ND	3.5	ND
51–70 y	3,000	2,000	100	1,000	ND	ND	ND	35	100	1,000	ND	ND	ND	3.5	ND
> 70 y	3,000	2,000	100	1,000	ND	ND	ND	35	100	1,000	ND	ND	ND	3.5	ND
Females															
9–13 y	1,700	1,200	100	600	ND	ND	ND	20	60	600	ND	ND	ND	2.0	ND
14–18 y	2,800	1,800	100	800	ND	ND	ND	30	80	800	ND	ND	ND	3.0	ND
19–30 y	3,000	2,000	100	1,000	ND	ND	ND	35	100	1,000	ND	ND	ND	3.5	ND
31–50 y	3,000	2,000	100	1,000	ND	ND	ND	35	100	1,000	ND	ND	ND	3.5	ND
51–70 y	3,000	2,000	100	1,000	ND	ND	ND	35	100	1,000	ND	ND	ND	3.5	ND
> 70 y	3,000	2,000	100	1,000	ND	ND	ND	35	100	1,000	ND	ND	ND	3.5	ND
Pregnancy															
14–18 y	2,800	1,800	100	800	ND	ND	ND	30	80	800	ND	ND	ND	3.0	ND
19–30 y	3,000	2,000	100	1,000	ND	ND	ND	35	100	1,000	ND	ND	ND	3.5	ND
31–50 y	3,000	2,000	100	1,000	ND	ND	ND	35	100	1,000	ND	ND	ND	3.5	ND
Lactation															
14–18 y	2,800	1,800	100	800	ND	ND	ND	30	80	800	ND	ND	ND	3.0	ND
19–30 y	3,000	2,000	100	1,000	ND	ND	ND	35	100	1,000	ND	ND	ND	3.5	ND
31–50 y	3,000	2,000	100	1,000	ND	ND	ND	35	100	1,000	ND	ND	ND	3.5	ND

NOTE: A Tolerable Upper Intake Level (UL) is the highest level of daily nutrient intake that is likely to pose no risk of adverse health effects to almost all individuals in the general population. Unless otherwise specified, the UL represents total intake from food, water, and supplements. Due to a lack of suitable data, ULs could not be established for vitamin K, thiamin, riboflavin, vitamin B_{12}, pantothenic acid, biotin, and carotenoids. In the absence of a UL, extra caution may be warranted in consuming levels above recommended intakes. Members of the general population should be advised not to routinely exceed the UL. The UL is not meant to apply to individuals who are treated with the nutrient under medical supervision or to individuals with predisposing conditions that modify their sensitivity to the nutrient.

[a] As preformed vitamin A only.

[b] As α-tocopherol; applies to any form of supplemental α-tocopherol.

[c] The ULs for vitamin E, niacin, and folate apply to synthetic forms obtained from supplements, fortified foods, or a combination of the two.

[d] β-Carotene supplements are advised only to serve as a provitamin A source for individuals at risk of vitamin A deficiency.

[e] ND = Not determinable due to lack of data of adverse effects in this age group and concern with regard to lack of ability to handle excess amounts. Source of intake should be from food only to prevent high levels of intake.

SOURCES: *Dietary Reference Intakes for Calcium, Phosphorous, Magnesium, Vitamin D, and Fluoride* (1997); *Dietary Reference Intakes for Thiamin, Riboflavin, Niacin, Vitamin B_6, Folate, Vitamin B_{12}, Pantothenic Acid, Biotin, and Choline* (1998); *Dietary Reference Intakes for Vitamin C, Vitamine E, Selenium, and Carotenoids* (2000); *Dietary Reference Intakes for Vitamin A, Vitamin K, Arsenic, Boron, Chromium, Copper, Iodine, Iron, Manganese, Molybdenum, Nickel, Silicon, Vanadium, and Zinc* (2001); and *Dietary Reference Intakes for Calcium and Vitamin D* (2011). These reports may be accessed via www.nap.edu.

Dietary Reference Intakes (DRIs): Tolerable Upper Intake Levels, Elements

Food and Nutrition Board, Institute of Medicine, National Academies

Life Stage Group	Arsenic[a]	Boron (mg/d)	Calcium (mg/d)	Chromium	Copper (μg/d)	Fluoride (mg/d)	Iodine (μg/d)	Iron (mg/d)	Magnesium (mg/d)[b]	Manganese (mg/d)	Molybdenum (μg/d)	Nickel (mg/d)	Phosphorus (g/d)	Selenium (μg/d)	Silicon[c]	Vanadium (mg/d)[d]	Zinc (mg/d)	Sodium (g/d)	Chloride (g/d)
Infants																			
0 to 6 mo	ND[e]	ND	1,000	ND	ND	0.7	ND	40	ND	ND	ND	ND	ND	45	ND	ND	4	ND	ND
6 to 12 mo	ND	ND	1,500	ND	ND	0.9	ND	40	ND	ND	ND	ND	ND	60	ND	ND	5	ND	ND
Children																			
1–3 y	ND	3	2,500	ND	1,000	1.3	200	40	65	2	300	0.2	3	90	ND	ND	7	1.5	2.3
4–8 y	ND	6	2,500	ND	3,000	2.2	300	40	110	3	600	0.3	3	150	ND	ND	12	1.9	2.9
Males																			
9–13 y	ND	11	3,000	ND	5,000	10	600	40	350	6	1,100	0.6	4	280	ND	ND	23	2.2	3.4
14–18 y	ND	17	3,000	ND	8,000	10	900	45	350	9	1,700	1.0	4	400	ND	ND	34	2.3	3.6
19–30 y	ND	20	2,500	ND	10,000	10	1,100	45	350	11	2,000	1.0	4	400	ND	1.8	40	2.3	3.6
31–50 y	ND	20	2,500	ND	10,000	10	1,100	45	350	11	2,000	1.0	4	400	ND	1.8	40	2.3	3.6
51–70 y	ND	20	2,000	ND	10,000	10	1,100	45	350	11	2,000	1.0	4	400	ND	1.8	40	2.3	3.6
> 70 y	ND	20	2,000	ND	10,000	10	1,100	45	350	11	2,000	1.0	3	400	ND	1.8	40	2.3	3.6
Females																			
9–13 y	ND	11	3,000	ND	5,000	10	600	40	350	6	1,100	0.6	4	280	ND	ND	23	2.2	3.4
14–18 y	ND	17	3,000	ND	8,000	10	900	45	350	9	1,700	1.0	4	400	ND	ND	34	2.3	3.6
19–30 y	ND	20	2,500	ND	10,000	10	1,100	45	350	11	2,000	1.0	4	400	ND	1.8	40	2.3	3.6
31–50 y	ND	20	2,500	ND	10,000	10	1,100	45	350	11	2,000	1.0	4	400	ND	1.8	40	2.3	3.6
51–70 y	ND	20	2,000	ND	10,000	10	1,100	45	350	11	2,000	1.0	4	400	ND	1.8	40	2.3	3.6
> 70 y	ND	20	2,000	ND	10,000	10	1,100	45	350	11	2,000	1.0	3	400	ND	1.8	40	2.3	3.6
Pregnancy																			
14–18 y	ND	17	3,000	ND	8,000	10	900	45	350	9	1,700	1.0	3.5	400	ND	ND	34	2.3	3.6
19–30 y	ND	20	2,500	ND	10,000	10	1,100	45	350	11	2,000	1.0	3.5	400	ND	ND	40	2.3	3.6
31–50 y	ND	20	2,500	ND	10,000	10	1,100	45	350	11	2,000	1.0	3.5	400	ND	ND	40	2.3	3.6
Lactation																			
14–18 y	ND	17	3,000	ND	8,000	10	900	45	350	9	1,700	1.0	4	400	ND	ND	34	2.3	3.6
19–30 y	ND	20	2,500	ND	10,000	10	1,100	45	350	11	2,000	1.0	4	400	ND	ND	40	2.3	3.6
31–50 y	ND	20	2,500	ND	10,000	10	1,100	45	350	11	2,000	1.0	4	400	ND	ND	40	2.3	3.6

NOTE: A Tolerable Upper Intake Level (UL) is the highest level of daily nutrient intake that is likely to pose no risk of adverse health effects to almost all individuals in the general population. Unless otherwise specified, the UL represents total intake from food, water, and supplements. Due to a lack of suitable data, ULs could not be established for vitamin K, thiamin, riboflavin, vitamin B_{12}, pantothenic acid, biotin, and carotenoids. In the absence of a UL, extra caution may be warranted in consuming levels above recommended intakes. Members of the general population should be advised not to routinely exceed the UL. The UL is not meant to apply to individuals who are treated with the nutrient under medical supervision or to individuals with predisposing conditions that modify their sensitivity to the nutrient.

[a] Although the UL was not determined for arsenic, there is no justification for adding arsenic to food or supplements.

[b] The ULs for magnesium represent intake from a pharmacological agent only and do not include intake from food and water.

[c] Although silicon has not been shown to cause adverse effects in humans, there is no justification for adding silicon to supplements.

[d] Although vanadium in food has not been shown to cause adverse effects in humans, there is no justification for adding vanadium to food and vanadium supplements should be used with caution. The UL is based on adverse effects in laboratory animals and this data could be used to set a UL for adults but not children and adolescents.

[e] ND = Not determinable due to lack of data of adverse effects in this age group and concern with regard to lack of ability to handle excess amounts. Source of intake should be from food only to prevent high levels of intake.

SOURCES: *Dietary Reference Intakes for Calcium, Phosphorous, Magnesium, Vitamin D, and Fluoride* (1997); *Dietary Reference Intakes for Thiamin, Riboflavin, Niacin, Vitamin* B_6, *Folate, Vitamin* B_{12}, *Pantothenic Acid, Biotin, and Choline* (1998); *Dietary Reference Intakes for Vitamin C, Vitamin E, Selenium, and Carotenoids* (2000); *Dietary Reference Intakes for Vitamin A, Vitamin K, Arsenic, Boron, Chromium, Copper, Iodine, Iron, Manganese, Molybdenum, Nickel, Silicon, Vanadium, and Zinc* (2001); *Dietary Reference Intakes for Water, Potassium, Sodium, Chloride, and Sulfate* (2005); and *Dietary Reference Intakes for Calcium and Vitamin D* (2011). These reports may be accessed via www.nap.edu.

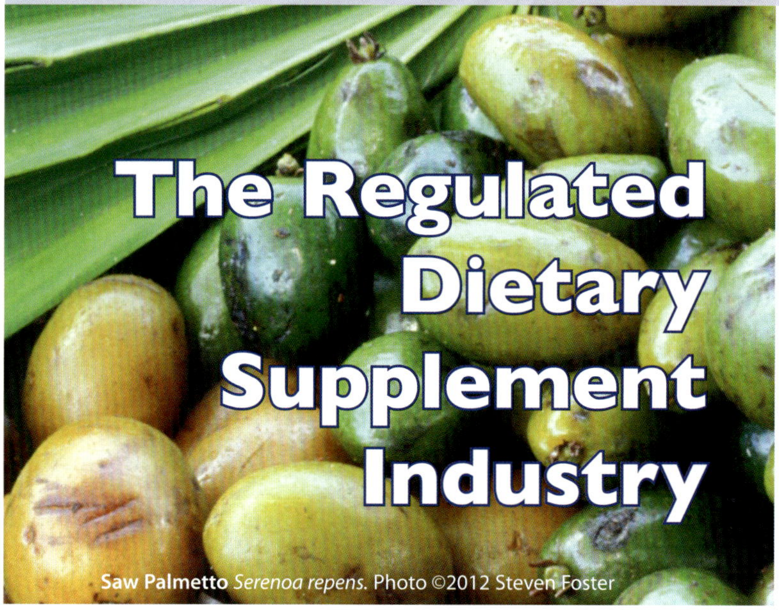

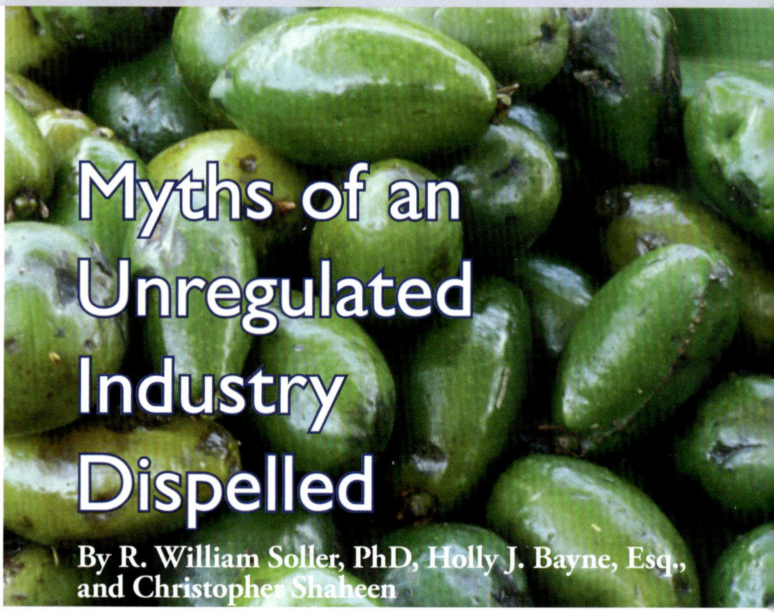

The Regulated Dietary Supplement Industry Myths of an Unregulated Industry Dispelled

Saw Palmetto *Serenoa repens*. Photo ©2012 Steven Foster

By R. William Soller, PhD, Holly J. Bayne, Esq., and Christopher Shaheen

Summary

In 1994, the 103rd US Congress passed the Dietary Supplement Health and Education Act (DSHEA). This legislation, along with previous laws and the 2006 Dietary Supplement and Nonprescription Drug Consumer Protection Act, has provided the US Food and Drug Administration (FDA) with statutory authority to regulate dietary supplements and those who manufacture, distribute, and sell them. It also enabled FDA to take enforcement action against unsafe or mislabeled products and those who sell them—fulfilling the agency's mandate to protect and promote public health and safety. A comprehensive framework of regulations also has evolved through the public notice and comment rulemaking process. These regulations address essential aspects of the safety, labeling, health-related claims, and quality of dietary supplements. Consistent with its legal mandate, FDA has taken a primary role—using interagency collaborations as needed, particularly with the Federal Trade Commission (FTC)—to pursue enforcement actions against non-compliant products and companies. And yet, critics still charge that the dietary supplement industry remains "unregulated" and many members of the media use this word to characterize it. This is a myth. Today, dietary supplements represent a major industry in the national marketplace, the products of which are used widely and safely by millions of Americans under a comprehensive set of statutes of regulations.

Introduction

President Bill Clinton signed DSHEA into law on October 25, 1994.[1] DSHEA amended the federal Food, Drug, and Cosmetic Act (FDCA) in several important ways, thus creating the legal framework for FDA to develop a comprehensive, predictable, and transparent regulatory system for dietary supplements. Importantly, DSHEA confirms that dietary supplements are legally classified as "food," defines a "dietary supplement," and clarifies that "dietary ingredients" in supplements are not "food additives" but have a distinct safety standard.* The law also requires

*Only dietary ingredients are excluded from the food additive provisions of the law; however, other ingredients such as excipients (e.g., preservatives, binders, encapsulation materials, etc.) must be FDA-approved food additives or generally recognized as safe (GRAS) for the intended uses.

FDA's Regulatory Toolbox for Dietary Supplements

The Agency's regulatory toolbox for enforcing the statutory and regulatory requirements for dietary supplements is detailed in a listing of FDA's authorities for monitoring and evaluating product safety, quality, and labeling (Table 2). The major understanding that comes from this table is the following:

a. Congress has established a legal framework for dietary supplements that provides FDA with all of the authority it needs to properly regulate dietary supplements and take enforcement action against unsafe or mislabeled products;

b. The DSHEA amendments to the FDCA expressly define FDA's authority to regulate dietary supplements;

c. From this legal framework, FDA has developed a comprehensive set of rules describing the regulatory expectations of good business practices in the dietary supplement arena;[1]

d. This set of rules, generally developed through participatory public notice and comment rulemaking processes, is able to be applied by FDA to the degree necessary through warning letters, injunctions, seizures, and/or civil penalties, so as to enforce the statutory requirements of the FDCA;

e. Individuals and entities operating outside this framework are on fair notice that they are subject to regulatory action and possibly criminal prosecution for non-compliance with the FDCA and FDA regulatory requirements. As a corollary, FDA makes extensive information available on its website for manufacturers, distributors, and retailers to access regulations and guidance documents that describe a company's responsibilities to ensure compliance with pertinent laws and regulations;

f. FDA regulations concerning the safety, quality, and labeling of dietary supplements, all of which are interrelated, represent an approach that FDA has used successfully under other sections of the Act to regulate, for example, nonprescription drugs and conventional foods.

any manufacturer or distributor of a new dietary ingredient (NDI) that is not present in the food supply prior to the date of DSHEA's passage—and as of the date that the dietary ingredient is offered for sale—to submit to FDA a 75-day premarket notification containing safety data.† DSHEA expressly authorized FDA to prescribe Good Manufacturing Practice (GMP) regulations specific to dietary supplements. In this way, DSHEA became the central building block on which FDA crafted implementing regulations and guidance to ensure the availability of safe and properly labeled dietary supplements meeting technical standards of quality. As with other product categories under FDA's authority, such as conventional foods, prescription and nonprescription drugs, and medical devices, the agency developed regulations and guidance specific to dietary supplements through a public rulemaking process, allowing interested parties the opportunity for input. Since the enactment of DSHEA, FDA has also issued dietary supplement-specific guidance documents addressing a range of issues, such as labeling and claims substantiation. Not unlike the development of regulations for other FDA-regulated product categories, when disagreements have arisen, as might be expected in the implementation of a new law and complex rulemakings by any government agency, stakeholders have sometimes turned to the courts to ask for judicial review of FDA's regulatory policies. While there has been only limited litigation with respect to dietary supplements, the courts have generally upheld FDA's statutory authority to regulate dietary supplements, much to the dismay of some in the industry.‡

A comprehensive review of the available evidence strongly supports the conclusion that FDA has ample authority under current law to remove unsafe dietary supplements from the marketplace and enforce the misbranding (mislabeling) provisions of the law.

Today, under DSHEA and subsequent amendments to the FDCA, FDA has broad statutory authority to regulate dietary supplements appropriately, and those who manufacture, distribute, and sell them, and to take enforcement action against unsafe or mislabeled products and those who sell them to fulfill the Agency's mandate to protect and promote public health and safety. Nevertheless, critics still echo the accusation that dietary supplements are an unregulated industry. This is a myth.[2] In fact, a comprehensive review of the available evidence strongly supports the conclusion that FDA has ample authority under current law to remove unsafe dietary supplements from the marketplace and enforce the misbranding (mislabeling) provisions of the law.[3] Indeed, assessment of the agency's enforcement activities in recent years shows that FDA is applying a risk-management approach using regulatory tools that define dietary supplements as a regulated industry. For example, as high-profile issues have arisen, FDA draws in inter-agency resources by working with groups, such as the FTC, the Drug Enforcement Administration (DEA), and the Centers for Disease Control and Prevention (CDC).

Development of the Regulatory Infrastructure for Dietary Supplements

Since the early part of the 1900s, when vitamins A and D were promoted in fish oil supplements, FDA's predecessor agency (the Department of Agriculture, now the USDA) and what eventually became known as the dietary supplement industry clashed on a number of key issues relating to the sale and marketing of vitamins, minerals, amino acids, botanicals, and other dietary substances (now individually and collectively defined as dietary supplements).§ Their disagreements included the legality of such products, the scope of permissible health-related promotional claims, the appropriateness of marketing practices, and properly balanced federal oversight.

The major events that shaped the development of today's comprehensive regulatory infrastructure for dietary supplements spanned over 100 years, from 1906 to 2011, culminating with the passage of the FDA Food Safety Modernization Act.[4] (see Table 1). The Pure Food and Drugs Act of 1906 was enacted primarily to protect consumers from misbranded and adulterated foods and drugs moving in interstate commerce, motivated by public indignation at dishonesty and fraud in the marketplace. With its principal emphasis on foods, the 1906 Act prohibited any poisonous or deleterious substance that is injurious to health to be used in food.[5] In 1938, Congress passed the FDCA, giving FDA broader authority and enforcement power over foods and drugs.** Significantly, the FDCA specifically recognized that food products may be labeled for and promoted with claims concerning effects on the structure or function of the body and for "special dietary uses."†† FDA was also provided new authority to regulate the labeling of food for "special dietary uses." Under section 403(j) of the FDCA, a food will be deemed misbranded "if it purports to be or is represented for special

†An NDI notification to FDA for an ingredient's being newly introduced for dietary supplement use is not needed if the ingredient is present in the food supply as an article used for food in a form in which the food has not been chemically altered.

‡A noted exception is the Pearson v. Shalala litigation, holding that FDA's regulations and enforcement policies governing the use of health claims (under the Nutrition Labeling and Education Act of 1990) on dietary supplements were more extensive than necessary, thus violating the First Amendment. The litigation paved the way for the use of "qualified health claims" in conventional food and dietary supplement labeling. [Pearson v. Shalala, 164 F. 3d 650 (1999).]

§21 U.S.C. § 321(ff). Under DSHEA, a "dietary supplement" is a product intended for ingestion that contains one or more of the following dietary ingredients: a vitamin; mineral; herb or other botanical; amino acid; a dietary substance for use by man to supplement the diet by increasing the total dietary intake; or a concentrate, metabolite, constituent, extract, or combination of any ingredient listed above.

**Federal Food, Drug, and Cosmetic Act; Pub L. No. 75-717, 52 Stat. 1040 (1938), as amended. The FDCA of 1938 also gave FDA the authority to regulate cosmetics and medical devices.

††The drug definition at section 201(g) of the FDCA, "food" articles (or products) intended to affect the structure or any function of the body are exempt from the drug definition. 21 U.S.C. § 321(g)(1)(C).

Table 1: Summary of Key Developments of the Legal Framework of the Fully Regulated Dietary Supplement Industry	
1906	**Pure Food and Drugs Act:** Adulteration standard that prohibits any added poisonous or deleterious substance injurious to health in food; prohibits filth, decomposed, or putrid animal or vegetable substances; prohibits addition of substances to reduce, lower, or injuriously affect strength or quality of food or to conceal damage; in essence, remains in effect today for both old (pre-1994) and new dietary ingredients. (See also 1994 listing on DSHEA.) *United States Statutes at Large* (59th Cong., Sess. I, Chp. 3915, p. 768-772; cited as 34 U.S. Stats. 768) (June 30, 1906)
1938	**Federal Food, Drug, and Cosmetic Act:** Authorizes foods to bear claims describing effects on [normal] structure or function of the body; establishes a category of foods for special dietary uses; authorizes FDA to specifically regulate such products, which will be deemed misbranded unless the label bears information concerning vitamin, mineral, or other dietary properties as prescribed by FDA regulations as necessary to fully inform purchasers as to the value of the food for such special dietary uses; grants FDA inspectional authority over factories. Pub. L. 75-717 52 Stat. 1040 (June 25, 1938)
1938	The **Wheeler-Lea Act** amended the Federal Trade Commission Act to grant FTC oversight of advertising of FDA-regulated products, except for prescription drugs. Pub. L. 75-447, 52 Stat 111 (1938).
1941	**Federal regulations** published on: (a) labeling of vitamin and mineral supplements (VMS) and other foods for special dietary use containing added vitamins and/or minerals; and (b) minimum daily requirements (MDR) as reference standards for defining the daily need for a vitamin or mineral. No restriction on the amount or variety of nutrients that could be included in a supplement or a fortified food. Fed. Reg. 6:5921-5926.
1958	**Food Additives Amendment of 1958:** Establishes a premarket approval system for "food additives" through FDA petition process; defined a "food additive" as any substance added to food (directly or indirectly), unless the substance is generally recognized as safe for its intended use. Pub L. 85-929, 72 Stat. 1784
1962	**FDA attempts** to: (a) replace the MDR with Recommended Daily Allowance (US RDA); (b) establish a standard of identity restricting the amounts and combinations of vitamins and minerals that could be marketed as dietary supplements; and (c) require a label disclaimer on VMS that in part stated, "there is no scientific basis for recommending routine use of dietary supplements."
1973	**Special dietary use and standards of identity regulations** were published by FDA in 1973 after hearings (1968-70). These regulations omitted the proposed disclaimer but limited quantities of VMS to 150% of US RDA, only permitted a few VMS combinations, and referred products with higher levels to an OTC drug review panel. Fed. Reg. 38:20730-20740.

dietary uses, unless its label bears such information concerning its vitamin, mineral, and other dietary properties as the Secretary determines to be, and by regulations prescribes as, necessary in order to fully inform purchasers as to its value for such uses."[6]

In the years that followed FDCA, until the passage of DSHEA in 1994, the regulatory environment for products later defined by DSHEA as dietary supplements was marked by heightened controversy, especially characterized by FDA's attempts to restrict the sale of high-potency vitamins and minerals and limit the availability of dietary ingredients deemed not essential for human growth and nutrition. In 1976, the industry won a major victory with passage of the Proxmire Amendment, which prevented FDA from classifying vitamins and minerals as (illegal) drug products based on potency, or establishing maximum limits on the potency of vitamins and minerals in foods for special dietary use.[7] Antagonism between FDA and the industry continued during the 1980s and early 1990s, particularly as the use of health claims on food labels proliferated and FDA began issuing proposed regulations implementing the Nutrition Labeling and Education Act of 1990 (NLEA).[8] Industry challenged FDA in the courts and in Congress, resulting in a judicial reining in of FDA's use of its food additive authority, and a congressionally mandated moratorium on regulations that were ultimately withdrawn. In 1994, Congress passed by unanimous consent clarifying legislation (Table 1). DSHEA emerged as viable legislation, promising both a sustainable solution to years of FDA-industry antagonism, as well as the potential to bring the stability, predictably, and transparency expected of a fully regulated industry.

FDA's aggressive enforcement tactics ultimately forced the tipping point that created DSHEA. In the watershed decisions concerning black currant oil (made from seeds of *Ribes nigrum*, Grossulariaceae), then marketed as products by Traco Labs, Inc. and Oakmont Investment Co. Inc., FDA overreached by trying to regulate encapsulated black currant seed oil as a "food additive," earning scathing criticism from the courts for the agency's "Alice in Wonderland" approach that "defenestrates common sense."[9,10,11] There were numerous other instances of what the supplement industry and nutritional advocates considered FDA's overreaching and strong-arm tactics.‡‡ One of America's largest and most successful grassroots efforts ensued.[12,13] An avalanche of activism overwhelmed Congress, and with a leading role played by US Senators Orrin Hatch (R-Utah) and Tom Harkin (D-Iowa), DSHEA was passed in 1994. Although not a part of official legislative history, the Senate Committee on Labor and Human Resources emphasized in its commentary "the need for

‡‡For example, in 1985, FDA issued an Import Alert on Evening Primrose Oil (EPO), instructing FDA officials to detain at the border EPO labeled for food use. FDA's position was that EPO was an unsafe food additive. In 1992, the US Court of Appeals for the Ninth Circuit upheld a lower court's ruling that EPO was an unsafe "food additive," preventing the marketing of what is generally considered a safe herbal ingredient. Also in 1992, FDA agents and armed sheriffs raided a Tahoma, Washington, medical clinic seizing bottles of L-tryptophan and samples of injectable B vitamins from Germany used by Jonathan Wright, MD, in his clinic.

Table 1 Continued

1974	**Dietary use/identity regulations** were overturned and remanded to FDA by the courts.
1975	**Re-proposed dietary use/identity regulations** published by FDA.
1976	**Vitamin/Mineral ("Rogers/Proxmire") Amendment to the FDCA** was passed, which: (a) invalidated FDA's re-proposed regulations; (b) prohibited FDA from classifying VMS as drugs based solely on their combinations or potency (unless drug claims were made), from establishing a standard of identity for these products, and from limiting the quantity or combination of nutrients in them, except for reasons of safety; and (c) incorporated FDA's 1941 definition of special dietary use into FDCA. Late in 1976, FDA **revised and reissued dietary use/identity regulations**. Pub. L. 94-278 (Apr. 22, 1976)
1978	**FDA's regulations, again overturned** by the courts and withdrawn in 1979
1990	**Nutrition Labeling and Education Act (NLEA)** requires all food labels to contain specific information on nutritional content (mandating the "Nutrition Facts" box) and authorizes FDA to consider and permit by regulation claims describing the relationship of specific nutrients to reduced risk of diseases or disorders ("health claims"). In implementing NLEA, FDA proposed regulations to replace the RDAs with new RDIs based on "mean requirements" for vitamins and minerals, which would have had lowered the daily reference amounts for many nutrients. FDA also proposed certain requirements for health claims that appeared to disallow health claims for many dietary supplements. Pub. L. 101-535 (Nov. 8, 1990)
1992	**Dietary Supplement Act** is passed, which (a) prohibited the implementation of NLEA with respect to dietary supplements except for the approved health claims provision, and (b) required regulations pursuant to NLEA regarding dietary supplements to be re-proposed. This created a moratorium on the labeling of dietary supplements to permit Congress and FDA time to consider various related issues. Pub. L. 102-6571 (1992)
1993	**Advance Notice of Proposed Rulemaking (ANPR) on dietary supplements**: proposed *inter alia*: (a) vitamins and minerals be limited to low multiples of the RDIs; (b) some botanicals were inherently drugs and not dietary supplements; (c) many dietary supplements, including amino acids, were unapproved food additives. The ANPR reflected FDA's concepts in prior overturned regulations.
1994	**Dietary Supplement Health and Education Act (DSHEA)**: defines "dietary supplement," exempts dietary ingredients from FDA regulation as "food additives," and establishes a new safety standard, prohibiting any significant or unreasonable risk of illness or injury; it also authorizes FDA to immediately ban any dietary supplement presenting imminent hazard; and authorizes FDA to impose requirements for good manufacturing practices ("GMPs")—none of which apply to conventional food. Pub. L. 103-417, 108 Stat. 4332 (Oct. 25, 1994)
1996	**Food Quality Protection Act:** Amended the Federal Insecticide, Fungicide, and Rodenticide Act and the FDCA to require complete reassessment of all pesticide tolerances; mandates a single, scientifically based standard for all pesticide tolerances in all foods. Pub. L. 104-170 (Aug. 3, 1996)
1997	**FDA Modernization Act:** permits use of health claims and nutrient content claims based on authoritative statements by a scientific body of the US government, such as the National Institutes of Health, provided that premarket notification is submitted to FDA; FDA remains final arbiter on whether claim is permitted. Pub. L. 105-115 (Nov. 21, 1997)
2002	**Public Health Security and Bioterrorism Preparedness Response Act:** requires FDA registration of all food manufacturers and notification in advance of importation of food, including dietary supplements and ingredients (raw materials). Pub. L. 107-188 (June 12, 2002)
2004	**Anabolic Steroid Control Act:** prohibits steroid precursors to be sold as dietary supplements. Pub. L. 108–358(Oct. 22, 2004)
2004	**Food Allergen Labeling and Consumer Protection Act:** requires disclosure on food and dietary supplement labels of 8 major allergens, which account for 90% of food allergies. Pub. L. 108-32, 118 Stat. 905 (Aug. 2, 2004)
2006	**Dietary Supplement and Nonprescription Drug Consumer Protection Act:** requires manufacturers and distributors to maintain records of all adverse event reports (AER) associated with use of a dietary supplement and submit all serious AER data to FDA. Pub. L. 109-462 (Dec. 22, 2006)
2007	**Food and Drug Administration Amendments Act:** prohibits the introduction into interstate commerce of any food to which has been added a drug or biologic, approved respectively under Section 505 of the FDCA or Section 351 of the Public Health Service Act, or a drug or biologic product for which substantial clinical investigations has been instituted and made public. Pub. L. 110-85 (Sept 27, 2007)
2011	**Food Safety Modernization Act:** provides FDA with the authority to order a recall of any food product, including dietary supplements other than infant formula, already subject to FDA recall authority; requires FDA to issue guidance on new dietary ingredients (NDIs) in dietary supplements (issued by FDA in July 2011), and other provisions. Pub. L. 111-353, 124 Stat. 3885 (Jan. 4, 2011)

Congressional action to assure citizens have continued access to dietary supplements and information about their benefits."[14]

FDA Enforcement Policy and Industry Self-Policing in a Post-DSHEA Market

Criticism of dietary supplements did not dissipate after passage of DSHEA.[15,16] One would think that a comprehensive law would calm critics; rather, they continued to charge that dietary supplements were an unregulated industry and that FDA had insufficient enforcement authority to protect the public from unsafe dietary supplements and unsubstantiated health-related claims.[17] For its part, particularly during the immediate years following the passage of DSHEA, FDA arguably abrogated its responsibility to assertively implement DSHEA in a timely fashion. In fact, some in the dietary supplement industry have maintained that, rather than actively collaborating with the responsible majority of the industry, FDA chose a regulatory posture of studied inertia, hoping that wildcat fringe marketers would cause an implosion of the industry as a whole, resulting in a backlash against DSHEA or even its repeal.[12] While there are continued rumblings that DSHEA should be amended or repealed, this has not happened, although occasional legislation proposing to amend DSHEA remains a concern for the industry. Today, there appears to be both strength of purpose from the mainstream industry and its trade associations to defend DSHEA, encourage member compliance with existing FDA regulations and guidances, and engage in more robust self-policing.[§§]

Today, there appears to be both strength of purpose from the mainstream industry and its trade associations to defend DSHEA, encourage member compliance with existing FDA regulations and guidances, and engage in more robust self-policing.

In the 4½ years after the passage of DSHEA, the dietary supplement industry grew exponentially to 100 million daily users and an estimated annual market of $12 billion.[18] In stark contrast to this phenomenal growth in consumer acceptance of dietary supplements, what can be characterized as FDA's non-action in the early years immediately following DSHEA limited progress in publication of comprehensive final regulations needed for a visible, predictable, and balanced regulatory process. Even so, in September of 1997, FDA published the first set of regulations implementing DSHEA, principally addressing statement of identity, ingredient and nutrition labeling of dietary supplements, nutrient content claims, procedures for notifying FDA of "statements of nutritional support" (commonly referred to as structure-function claims) in dietary supplement labeling, and procedures for filing new dietary ingredient notifications. FDA's early period of apparent regulatory neglect began to change with a new commissioner who set the stage for policy changes. In her testimony before Congress, Jane E. Henney, MD,[***] stated in 1999, "Mr. Chairman, notwithstanding our actions to date, I want to acknowledge that FDA still has a long way to go to achieve full implementation of DSHEA. I assure you that as the new Commissioner of Food and Drugs, I am focusing attention on dietary supplements, an issue that is currently a priority for FDA's Center for Food Safety."[19] To be clear, the federal regulatory inactivity immediately post-DSHEA was not a circumstance of Dr. Henney's doing, but rather a legacy of her predecessor, David Kessler, MD, JD,[†††] who remarkably devoted a mere 49 words to DSHEA in a 4,583-word address to the Food, Drug and Law Institute just 2 months after DSHEA's passage.[20]

In January 2000, FDA issued a long-awaited final regulation governing dietary supplement labeling claims, establishing criteria for determining when FDA would object to a statement in dietary supplement labeling because it impermissibly suggests an effect on disease.[21] This rulemaking process began in April 1998, and took almost 2 years to complete, generating significant controversy, the ire of industry, and thousands of public and health professional comments.[22] Significantly, FDA had proposed to expand the regulatory definition of "disease." Under the proposed regulation, certain natural processes such as menopause and aging, for example, would have been considered diseases, prohibiting claims in dietary supplement labeling to affect these conditions. FDA ultimately modified its course and retained the regulatory definition of "disease or health-related condition" established in the health claims rulemaking under NLEA.[23] Thus, claims concerning common conditions associated with natural states or processes that would not cause significant or permanent harm if untreated are not considered as diseases under the final structure-function claims rule.

In other areas, however, FDA took a rigid and limiting approach, curtailing speech that is arguably within the scope of dietary supplement claims authorized by DSHEA (i.e., describing effects in maintaining normal, healthy bodily structure and function). For example, under the final rule, claims in dietary supplement labeling referring to supporting "healthy cholesterol levels" or the maintenance of "normal cholesterol levels" are considered by FDA as impermissible, implied disease claims, *unless* the claim makes it clear that cholesterol levels "are already within the normal range." FDA's enforcement policy in this regard represents a departure from the agency's prior position. Under the proposed rule, a claim such as "helps maintain a healthy cholesterol level" would have been permitted in dietary supplement labeling, if truthful and not misleading. However, according to FDA in the preamble to the final regulation, "references to 'healthy' cholesterol may be misleading to consumers

§§The major industry trade associations: American Herbal Products Association (AHPA), Consumer Healthcare Products Association (CHPA), Council for Responsible Nutrition (CRN), Natural Products Association (NPA, formerly the National Nutritional Foods Association [NNFA]), United Natural Products Alliance (UNPA, formerly Utah Natural Products Alliance).

***Dr. Jane E. Henney, MD, was FDA Commissioner from January 1999 to January 2001. She started as Commissioner in November 1998.

†††Dr. David A. Kessler, MD, JD, was FDA Commissioner from November 8, 1990 to February 28, 1997. Michael A. Friedman, MD, served as lead deputy commissioner while the post of commissioner was vacant from February 28, 1997 to November 30, 1998.

Table 2: Core Elements of the Current Regulatory Infrastructure for Dietary Supplements: FDA Authorities for Monitoring and Evaluating Safety, Quality, and Labeling*
Safety & Quality Authorities
Prohibit any poisonous or deleterious substance injurious to health in a dietary supplement
Prohibit any dietary supplement or dietary ingredient, whether old or new, that presents a "significant or unreasonable risk of illness or injury"
Impose an immediate ban of an imminent hazard
Impose requirements for Good Manufacturing Practices (GMPs)
Inspect facilities
Prohibit any food that is filthy, decomposed, held under insanitary conditions whereby it may have been rendered injurious to health, or otherwise unfit for food
Collect and oversee mandatory reports of serious adverse events associated with dietary supplements and inspect records kept by manufacturers and distributors
Premarketing Notification Authorities
Prohibit (on basis of adulteration) any new dietary ingredient for which there is inadequate information to provide reasonable assurance that it does not present a significant or unreasonable risk of illness or injury
Require FDA approval of food additives (excipients) and color additives used in food, including dietary supplements
Post-Marketing Enforcement Authorities
Issue safety alerts to health professionals and consumers
Initiate enforcement actions (recalls)
Issue warning letters
Seek injunctions through the courts, resulting in civil or criminal penalties
Labeling Authorities
Regulate the content of dietary supplements labels to prohibit misbranding of dietary supplements

Enforce FDCA requirement that all statements in product labeling are truthful and non-misleading, including:
– Statement of identity—product must be identified as a "Dietary Supplement"
– Nutrition information in the form of a Supplement Facts panel
– List of ingredients not listed in the Supplement Facts panel
– Name and address of the manufacturer, packer, or distributor
– Net quantity of contents
– Claims,† including
    – Health Claims
    – Qualified Health Claims
    – Criteria constituting reliable scientific evidence to substantiate health-related claims
    – Nutrient Content Claims
    – Structure Function Claims

*FDA authorities derive from the legislation cited in Table 1, codified into the FDCA.
†See also Federal Trade Commission guidance: Dietary Supplements: An Advertising Guide to Industry (1998).

because the phrase 'healthy cholesterol' is now frequently used to refer to high density lipoproteins (HDL), a specific cholesterol fraction believed to be beneficial."[21]

Also in January 2000, fulfilling Dr. Henney's promise to make dietary supplements a priority, FDA's Center for Food Safety and Applied Nutrition (CFSAN) published the Agency's overall dietary supplement strategic plan, acknowledging that the purpose of DSHEA was to strike the right balance between providing consumers access to dietary supplements and truthful information about them, while preserving FDA's regulatory authority to take action against supplements that presented safety problems or promoted with false or misleading labeling claims.[24,25] In March of 2001, CFSAN Director Joseph A. Levitt, Esq., unveiled to Congress the agency's report on FDA's first comprehensive strategic plan for dietary supplements.[26] The plan gave FDA's vision for a science-based regulatory program to achieve full implementation and enforcement of DSHEA. Notably, however, real progress and finalization of key standards for dietary supplements, namely in the form of GMP regulations, were delayed. Compounded by the agency's limited resources, tangible regulatory advancements were hampered by the necessarily lengthy process needed to obtain stakeholder and public input in developing and finalizing—through notice-and-comment rulemaking—federal standards for the manufacture of finished dietary supplements.[27,28] The slowness in developing these standards was fodder for critics. Yet, high-acuity hindsight must appropriately recognize the complexities of the issues requiring a disciplined and deliberative approach to developing a rational and sustainable regulatory infrastructure for a major industry.

The Effect of the Ephedra Controversy

In February 2004, following years of contentious rulemaking that began in 1997, FDA prevailed in issuing a final rule declaring dietary supplements containing ephedrine alkaloids (mainly from ephedra [*Ephedra sinica,* Ephedraceae]) to be illegal (adulterated) under DSHEA's "significant or unreasonable" risk safety standard.[29] Ephedra-containing dietary supplements—particularly those based on relatively high concentrations of its extracts—promoted for weight loss and athletic performance, rose in popularity during the immediate post-DSHEA years and were characterized as being associated with cardiovascular events and other adverse product experiences. In issuing the regulation, FDA applied a risk/benefit standard, determining that dietary supplements containing ephedrine alkaloids are adulterated under the FDCA because they present an unreasonable risk of illness or injury under the conditions of use recommended in labeling or under ordinary conditions of use, without conferring any benefit.‡‡‡

A legal challenge to the final regulation ensued, with plaintiffs challenging FDA's use of risk/benefit analysis to ban dietary supplements containing low levels of ephedrine alkaloids without any scientific proof of a significant or unreasonable risk of illness or injury at such levels. Although plaintiffs prevailed at the district court level, the Court of Appeals reversed the lower court's decision, essentially upholding FDA's decision to ban dietary supplements containing ephedra, regardless of the level of concentration or directions in product labeling. The court also found that FDA was not arbitrary and capricious in its Final Rule banning ephedrine alkaloids and ephedra, and that FDA had met its evidentiary burden to justify a total ban. The petitioner's subsequent efforts for re-hearing by the Court of Appeals and review by the US Supreme Court were unsuccessful. Notably, the ephedra situation highlighted a safety-related and post-marketing surveillance gap that had yet to be filled by FDA—mandatory reporting of serious adverse product experiences associated with dietary supplements.

In December 2006, the Dietary Supplement and Nonprescription Drug Consumer Protection Act (DSNDCPA) was signed into law, requiring companies engaged in the sale and distribution of dietary supplements and non-prescription over-the-counter (OTC) drugs to maintain records of all adverse event reports received by a company, to report all *serious* adverse events to FDA, and to make such reports available to the agency on request. Several years earlier, the American Herbal Products Association (AHPA), a national trade association consisting of herbal and botanical product companies, filed a Citizen Petition with FDA (March 2003), recommending that the agency impose a mandatory reporting requirement on dietary supplement companies for all "serious adverse event" reports associated with use of a dietary supplement. AHPA's petition requested that FDA establish such requirements through notice and comment rulemaking, modeled on requirements for prescription drug products. The DSNDCPA was not opposed by responsible mainstream components of the dietary supplement and OTC drug product industries.

‡‡‡In the preamble to the final rule, FDA clarified its position as follows: "The Government's burden of proof for 'unreasonable risk' [under Section 402(ff) of the FDCA] is met when a product's risks outweigh its benefits in light of the claims and directions for use in the product's labeling or, if the labeling is silent, under ordinary conditions of use.] Some in the dietary supplement industry have argued that FDA acted improperly in applying the risk/benefit standard, in part, because application of the risk/benefit standard itself was not subject to notice and comment rulemaking and public input.

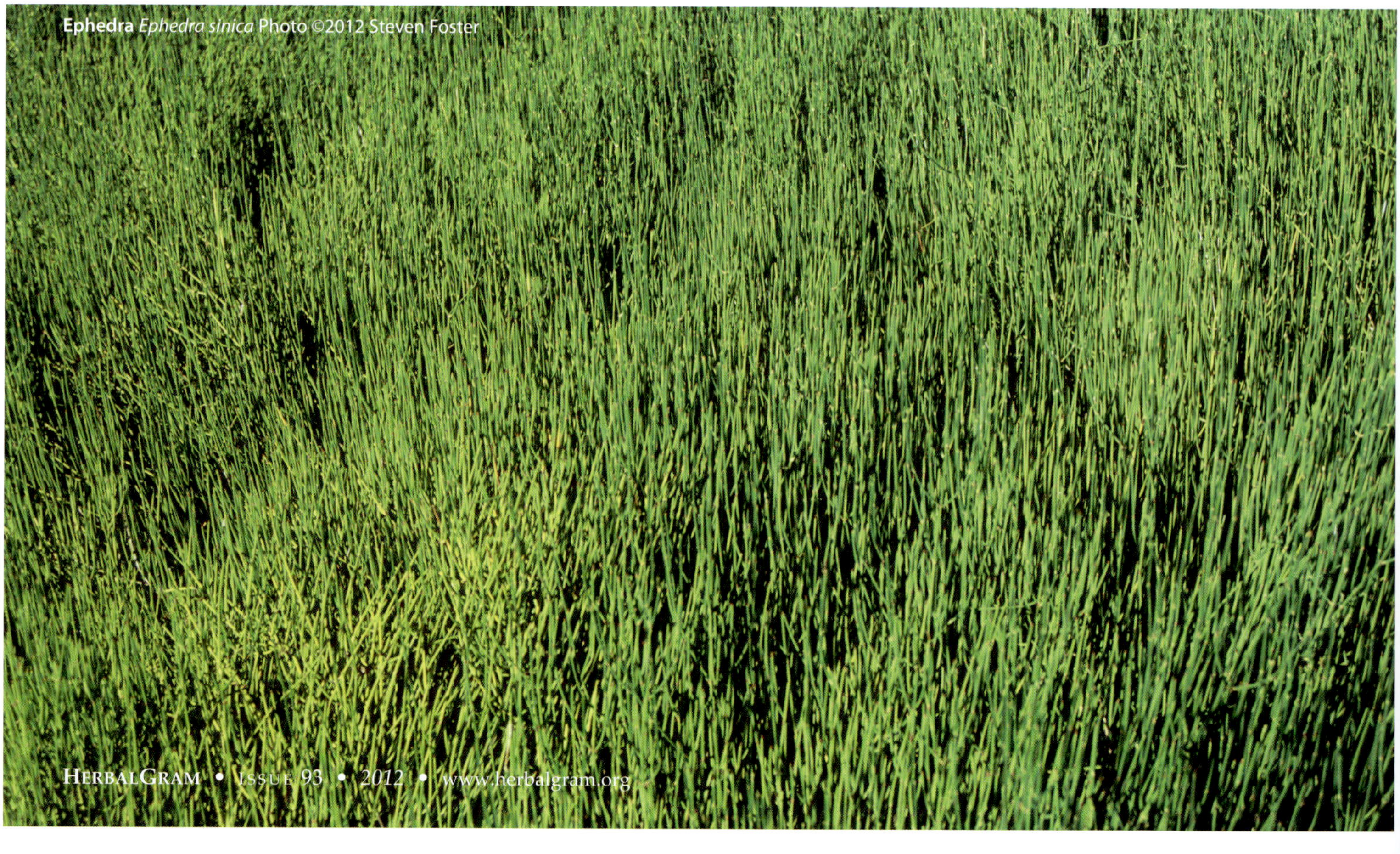

Ephedra *Ephedra sinica* Photo ©2012 Steven Foster

Table 3: Excerpt of FDA Warning Letter to a Dietary Supplement Company Demonstrating Robust Nature of the GMP Regulations for Enforcement [30]
"Failure to conduct at least one appropriate test or examination to verify the identity of a dietary supplement prior to its use" and failure to "specify the identity test or examination the firm would implement in the event that the firm could not successfully identity methodology."
Failure to "to make and keep documentation for why meeting in-process specifications, in combination with meeting component specifications, helps ensure that the dietary supplement meets the specifications for identity, purity, strength, and composition; and for limits on those types of contamination that may adulterate or may lead to adulteration of the finished batch of the dietary supplement, to comply with 21 CFR 111.95(b)(3)."
Failure to "make and keep documentation demonstrating why the results of appropriate tests or examinations for the product specifications selected under 111.75(c)(1) ensure that your dietary supplements meets all product specifications, in accordance with 21 CFR 111.95(b)(4)."
Failure to follow the company's written procedure, "Approval/Rejection of Raw Materials and Packaging Components" for collecting representative samples of each unique shipment of components.
Inadequate quality control program, including: (a) no periodic review of all records for calibration of instruments and controls as required by 21 CFR 111.117(b); (b) inadequate master manufacturing record; (c) lack of documentation that quality control personnel approved, released, or rejected the packaged and labeled dietary supplement to comply with 21 CFR 111.260(1)(4).
Lack of documentation in batch production records to include a statement of percentage of theoretical yield at appropriate phases of processing per 21 CFR 111.260(f).
No specification of corrective actions to use when a specification is not met under 21CFR 111.260(f).

The Senate Report accompanying the bill, introduced in June 2006 by Senator Hatch, stated the legislation "will enhance the Agency's effort to identify potential public health issues associated with the use of these products" and "will give consumers greater assurance that public health officials are on top of emerging, serious safety problems so they can take immediate, appropriate action."[30] The law requires the company whose name appears on the label of a dietary supplement (manufacturer, packer, or distributor) to maintain records of all adverse event reports associated with use of a dietary supplement for a period of 6 years. Reports of "serious adverse events" must be filed with FDA using the mandatory "MedWatch" Form 3500A (the same form used for prescription and OTC drugs and medical devices) within 15 days of their receipt. A "serious adverse event" is defined as an event that results in death, a life-threatening experience, inpatient hospitalization, a persistent or significant disability or incapacity, or a congenital anomaly or birth defect associated with the use of a dietary supplement. Additionally, a serious adverse event includes medical or surgical intervention, based on reasonable medical judgment that is necessary to prevent any of the outcomes listed above.[§§§] Records of all adverse event reports must be made available to FDA upon request, and may be inspected by FDA during a routine GMP inspection.[31] In October 2007, FDA issued draft guidance for industry regarding dietary supplement adverse event reporting and recordkeeping requirements, followed by revised guidance in June 2009, although comments to the guidance may be submitted at any time.[32] The guidance describes the minimum data elements for filing serious adverse event reports to FDA, clarifies the criteria used to determine whether an adverse event report would be considered *serious* by FDA, and addresses a company's recordkeeping obligations.

FDA's implementation of the dietary supplement provisions of the DSNDCPA is consistent with the agency's approach to monitoring the safety of drugs, medical devices, and other FDA-regulated products. Dietary supplement adverse event and serious adverse event reports filed by consumers, health professionals, and industry are maintained by FDA in the CFSAN Adverse Event Reporting System (CAERS), along with adverse event data on foods, medical foods, infant formulas, color additives, and cosmetics. Data are entered by FDA using "MedDRA" medical reporting terminology, the same terminology used to capture adverse event data on drugs, biologics, vaccines, and medical devices.[33] Every entry into the CAERS database is reviewed by an FDA medical officer to evaluate the strength of the evidence suggesting that the dietary supplement caused the adverse event, using categories (e.g., certain, probable, unlikely) described in the World Health Organization's (WHO's) publication *Safety Monitoring of Medicinal Products: Guidelines for Setting Up and Running a Pharmacovigilence Center* (2000).[34] FDA's review process is designed to determine whether a "signal" has been generated by a number of reports (a cluster) in the database suggesting a particular product or ingredient may present a safety problem. If a signal has been identified suggesting a safety problem associated with a dietary supplement, FDA will inspect the manufacturer (or distributor) and inspect the company's adverse event reports to collect additional information about the product. FDA will also convene a "Health Hazard Evaluation Board" consisting of CFSAN's Chief Medical Officer and other FDA medical officers to evaluate all of the data and prepare a written report.[35] FDA effectively used this process in the case of the multi-ingredient dietary supplement "Hydroxycut," which was associated with 23 liver-related adverse effects (idiosyncratic hepatotoxicity) between 2002 and 2009.[36] At FDA's

§§§This is the same definition used for a serious adverse drug experience (or event) (SADE). See: www.fda.gov/newsevents/publichealthfocus/ucm155683.htm. FDA letter to Iovate.

request, Iovate Health Sciences, Inc., initiated a massive recall of Hydroxycut in the United States and Canada, recalling over 21 million units of product. In considering a range of enforcement options available to the Agency, FDA will also conduct a risk-benefit analysis of the product under section 402 (f) of the FDCA to determine whether the dietary supplement presents a significant or unreasonable risk to public health or presents an imminent hazard. FDA's enforcement policy is that dietary supplements generally do not provide significant benefits to outweigh any public health risk and allow for continued marketing, unlike prescription drug products for which greater risk is tolerated based on benefits of treating disease.

Regulation of Current Good Manufacturing Practices

In June 2007, 13 years following DSHEA's enactment, FDA issued final regulations governing dietary supplement GMPs. DSHEA authorized FDA to prescribe GMPs for dietary supplements through notice and comment rulemaking.[37] This was particularly relevant since it is generally accepted by experts and responsible segments of the industry that FDA's food manufacturing, packaging, and hygiene standards that establish GMPs for conventional foods are inadequate for ensuring dietary supplement quality, ingredient identity, and potency as claimed in product labeling. DSHEA required FDA to model dietary supplement GMPs on food GMPs. FDA's progress in issuing the 2007 final regulation was agonizingly slow, spanning about 10 years. Industry proposed a GMP standard to FDA in the fall of 1995, which was essentially published by FDA as an Advanced Notice of Proposed Rulemaking in February 1997. Following industry outreach efforts, FDA published a proposed rule in 2004.[38,39] The final rule in 2007 generally reflects industry's proposed standards, in that they were designed to ensure consumers are provided with dietary supplements that: (1) are safe and not adulterated or misbranded; (2) have the identity and provide the quantity of dietary ingredients declared in labeling; and (3) meet the quality specifications that the supplement is represented to meet.

From 2001 to 2010, FDA issued a total of 314 warning letters relating to dietary supplements, including principally those relating to unapproved new drugs, adulteration, and misbranding.

The dietary supplement GMP regulations mandate that manufacturers of dietary supplements establish a comprehensive system of controls and strictly document each stage of the manufacturing process to help ensure that products have the identity, purity, strength, and composition stated on product labels and that finished dietary supplements meet clearly defined specifications in the manufacturing record and are not adulterated. The final rule establishes the minimum current GMP necessary for activities relating to the manufacturing, packaging, labeling, and holding of dietary supplements to ensure product quality.**** Failure to follow dietary supplement GMP is deemed to adulterate a product under the FDCA, which could subject the product to FDA enforcement action.[40]

Issuance of the final dietary supplement GMP regulations marked a major regulatory achievement for FDA and significantly raised the bar of compliance for dietary supplement manufacturers. Notably, the regulation allowed for a 3-year staggered compliance period, with large companies (500 or more full-time employees) becoming subject to the rule in June 2008, followed by medium companies the following year and small companies (fewer than 20 employees) in June of 2010. FDA has made enforcement of the dietary supplement GMPs a priority. FDA GMP inspections of dietary supplement facilities have risen progressively from 12 in 2008 to 75 in 2010.[41] Of particular note is what appears in one of FDA's first warning letters relating to enforcement of the current GMP regulations for dietary supplements.[42] Table 3 shows a list of FDA's major findings in a recent inspection of a dietary supplement firm, demonstrating the robustness of the GMP regulations in mandating strict quality control procedures from start to finish, to ensure the quality of raw materials and finished products.

Both FDA and industry are supported by non-governmental organizations in meeting their respective twin goals: FDA to ensure that dietary supplements are safe and not adulterated under the law; and industry to ensure compliance and that only properly labeled dietary supplements meeting technical standards of quality reach consumers. The United States Pharmacopeial Convention (USP) is a nonprofit scientific organization that has been setting standards for food and drug ingredients since 1820 as part of its mission to improve the quality and safety of foods and drugs moving in international commerce. Compendial standards established by USP have legal effect under the FDCA and are enforceable by FDA. Under the DSHEA amendments to the FDCA, a dietary supplement will be deemed misbranded if it is falsely represented as conforming to the specifications of an official compendium (such as USP monographs).[43]

In 1995, USP members adopted a resolution to establish standards for botanical and other dietary ingredients (as defined in DSHEA). Since that time, USP has published many botanical, vitamin, mineral, and other dietary ingredient quality monographs. To qualify for development of a monograph, the dietary ingredient must pass a USP safety review, according to defined criteria. USP also develops and publishes both general and specific standards, tests, assays, and other specifications for use in raw ingredient quality control operations and the manufacture of finished dietary supplements. In 2009, USP published the first edition of the *USP Dietary Supplements Compendium* (the "USP Compendium"), a resource of public standards and technical information for dietary supplement manufacturers that includes information developed by the major trade associations and other organizations. For example, the USP Compendium includes materials published by AHPA concerning the use of marker compounds for botanical identification and detection of adulterants and a joint AHPA-American Herbal Pharmacopoeia® (AHP) draft document concerning Good Agricul-

****As defined in the final rule, quality means that the dietary supplement "consistently meets the established specifications for identity, purity, strength, and composition, and has been manufactured, packaged, labeled, and held under conditions to prevent adulteration under section 402(a)(1), (a)(2), (a)(3), and (a)(4) of the Federal Food, Drug and Cosmetic Act."

tural and Collection Practices for herbal raw materials.[††††] The Compendium also includes the "Standardized Information on Dietary Ingredients (SIDI™) Protocol," developed by member companies of national trade associations, including: AHPA, the Council for Responsible Nutrition (CRN), the Natural Products Association (NPA), and the Consumer HealthCare Products Association (CHPA). The SIDI™ Protocol is designed to assist dietary ingredient suppliers in using standardized content and format templates to convey quality-related information about ingredients to downstream manufacturers of finished dietary supplements.

Analytical Methods for Ensuring Dietary Supplement Purity and Quality

In 2001, the USP Dietary Supplement Verification Program (DSVP) was launched. The program was designed to assist dietary supplement manufacturers in ensuring compliance with FDA GMP regulations. Under the program, manufacturers that demonstrate adherence to quality control procedures and undergo an audit may include a USP quality designation mark on dietary supplement labeling. To qualify for use of the USP-DSV mark, the dietary supplement must pass laboratory testing to confirm dietary ingredient identity, potency and purity, and batch-to-batch consistency.

FDA and the industry are also supported by the work of AOAC International, a nonprofit organization founded in 1884, dedicated to the development of analytical methods.[44] AOAC's official analytical methods, published in "Official Methods of Analysis of the Association of Analytical Chemists," are incorporated by reference into FDA regulations, and are used by FDA for compliance and enforcement purposes.[45] FDA's policy is to utilize the AOAC methods of analysis in its enforcement programs when available and applicable, unless another method is prescribed by regulation. The actual work of developing and testing analytical methods for dietary supplements necessary for confirming ingredient identity, purity, and other quality parameters is conducted by AOAC's government and industry stakeholders, with AOAC coordinating the scientific studies, receiving and evaluating the results, sanctioning acceptable and validated methods, and publishing and distributing the methods and performance data. AOAC maintains a committee structure to engage in the prioritization of methods development, based on ingredient market share and public health needs, among other factors. In 2004, under a contract with FDA, AOAC was charged with making recommendations on Best Practices for the validation of Microbiological Methods.

The Office of Dietary Supplements (ODS) within the National Institutes of Health, and the National Institute of Standards and Technology (NIST) within the US Department of Commerce are key governmental stakeholders actively involved in the development of analytical methods for dietary supplements. ODS was created in 1995, as authorized by DSHEA. The purpose and responsibilities of ODS include promoting the scientific study of dietary supplements and serving as a principal advisor to FDA on issues relating to dietary supplements. In 2002, ODS launched its Dietary Supplements Analytical Methods and Reference Materials (AMRM) program, designed to stimulate the development of validated analytical methods and reference materials to support the needs of industry, regulators (namely FDA), contract laboratories, and researchers. The goal of the AMRM program is to develop and validate methods that can be used to reliably identify and quantify ingredients in dietary supplements, including biologically active compounds, markers, and contaminants and other adulterants. To achieve this goal, ODS collaborates with FDA, AOAC, USDA, and NIST, among other organizations.

NIST is a non-regulatory federal agency whose mission is to promote domestic innovation and industrial competitiveness by advancing science, standards, and technology to enhance national security and improve quality of life. While the work of NIST is not widely known, it is nonetheless is making a significant contribution to dietary supplement quality control efforts, particularly in the area of development of botanical Standard Reference Materials (SRMs), which are needed to support adherence to current GMPs and ensure product quality. For example, NIST has developed 2 natural-matrix SRMs for saw palmetto (*Serenoa repens*, Arecaceae) fruit.[46]

Other non-governmental organizations also are engaged in assisting dietary supplement manufacturers and ingredient suppliers in complying with FDA's GMP regulations and ensuring product quality. NSF International—an independent nonprofit organization founded in 1944 to standardize food sanitation and safety requirements, develop public health standards, and certify products—administers its third-party certi-

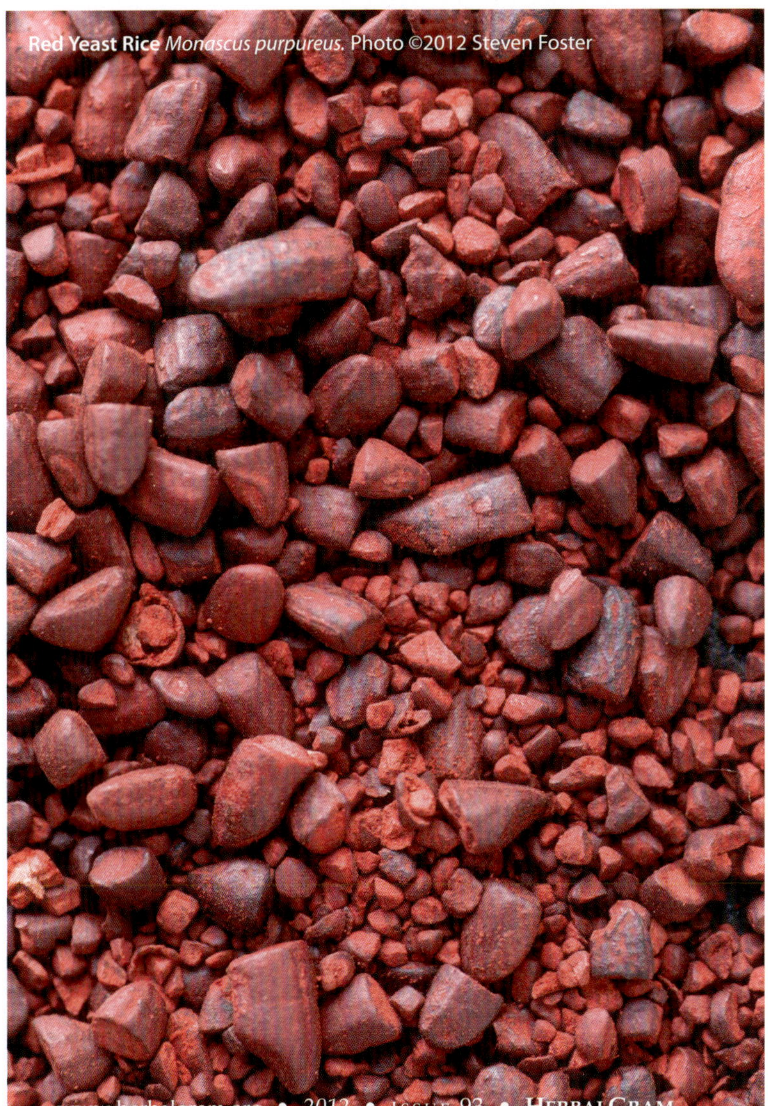
Red Yeast Rice *Monascus purpureus*. Photo ©2012 Steven Foster

††††AHPA has been discussed elsewhere in this article. AHP's mission is to promote the responsible use of safe and effective herbal products through the development of botanical standards of identity, purity, and analytical methods, as well as to critically review traditional and scientific data regarding their efficacy and safety.

fication program for dietary supplements that includes product testing, GMP audit inspections, and—for products that meet NSF's criteria—use of the NSF mark in product labeling and advertising.[47] The NPA, the nation's oldest natural products trade association, primarily consisting of retailers, has instituted a GMP Certification Program using third-party auditors and designed to ensure that products supplied to member companies are produced in accordance with current GMP requirements.[48]

FDA Has Demonstrated DSHEA Works

Public reports from FDA's then Associate Commissioner John Taylor, CFSAN Director Robert Brackett, and then Principal Deputy Commissioner Joshua Sharfstein in 2003, 2004, and 2010, respectively, presented the agency's enforcement report card for dietary supplements, which documented the following actions: successful voluntary destruction of inventories, removal of websites, voluntary recalls, warning letters, cyber letters, consumer alerts, seizures and injunctions, and criminal enforcement proceedings.[49,50,51] These activities show a leveraging of interagency expertise and resources. Some FDA enforcement actions are conducted in collaboration with FTC, a key federal law enforcement agency charged with regulating the advertising of dietary supplements, whose efforts are detailed in the below section on FTC.

FDA's enforcement reports provide evidence of how FDA has exercised enforcement authority to protect public health and safety as envisioned by the agency's strategic plan in 2000. For example, FDA has issued a number of alerts and letters to health professionals on safety issues pertaining to dietary supplement ingredients and/or products, including the following:[52]

- Aristolochic acid: alert on liver toxicity, 2000; as found in *Aristolochia* spp., *Asarum* spp., *Bragantia* spp., *Stephania* spp., *Clematis* spp., *Akebia* spp., *Cocculus* spp., *Diploclisia* spp., *Menispernum* spp., *Sinomenium* spp., *Mu tong, Fang ji, Guang fang ji, Fang chi, Kan-Mokutsu* (Japanese), and *Mokutsu* (Japanese);
- St. John's wort (*Hypericum perforatum*, Clusiaceae): warning about interaction with Indinavir, 2000;
- Tiractricol (or triodothryacetic acid): warning that the product is a thyroid hormone, 2000;
- Comfrey (*Symphytum* spp., Boraginaceae): removal from market, 2001;
- Dietary supplements claiming to prevent or treat Anthrax poisoning, 2001;
- LipoKinetix: warning about liver injury, 2001;
- Kava (or kava kava, *Piper methysticum*, Piperaceae): alert about liver failure, 2002;
- PC-SPES® and SPES®: a multi-herbal combination adulterated with prescription drugs, 2002;
- Certain Chinese diet pills: warning regarding unauthorized ingredient, fenfluramine, 2002;
- ephedrine alkaloids: removal from market, 2004;
- "Better than formula Ultra Infant Immune Booster 117:" warning not to buy, 2004;
- Liqiang 4: warning regrading unauthorized drug, glyburide, 2005;
- Red yeast rice (*Monascus purpureus*, Monascaceae): warning regarding unauthorized drug, lovastatin, 2007;
- Colloidal silver: alert on skin and mucous membrane discoloration, 2009.

Stakeholders and Trade Associations

Stakeholders among the responsible majority of the industry include independent organizations and trade groups. Industry trade associations, including the American Herbal Products Association, Consumer Healthcare Products Association, Council for Responsible Nutrition, and the National Product Association (formerly the National Health Food Association) have developed voluntary programs for labeling, restrictions pertaining to adulterants (e.g., ginseng; goldenseal; kava; lady's slipper; pyrrolizidine alkaloids; St. John's wort; and stimulant laxatives), GMP guidelines, and standards for raw materials, among others.[2,3,4] Compliance with these and other safety and quality-oriented voluntary guidelines by the responsible majority of the industry preceded FDA action in publishing the final GMP regulation by years. In addition, various independent nonprofit research and education groups (e.g., the American Botanical Council and the American Herbal Pharmacopoeia) have published numerous books, peer-reviewed articles, white papers, and monographs that have contributed to the general knowledge base for increased responsible quality control, manufacturing, labeling, and marketing of dietary ingredients and dietary supplement products, as well as increased access to reliable literature on herb quality, safety, and efficacy among various stakeholders in the general public. (American Botanical Council: www.herbalgram.org.; American Herbal Pharmacopoeia: www.herbal-ahp.org.)

In addition, from 2001 to 2010, FDA issued a total of 314 warning letters relating to dietary supplements, including principally those relating to unapproved new drugs, adulteration, and misbranding. The relative percentage of total warning letters seems appropriate to the size of the dietary supplement industry, which is about 1% by sales (2009) of a total $2 trillion in sales represented by all FDA-regulated products for human consumption and other uses (i.e., 1% dietary supplements and herbals, 1% nonprescription medicines, 7% medical devices, 14% prescription medicines, and 77% conventional foods).[53,54,55,56]

FDA's dietary supplement enforcement programs and industry outreach efforts during the past 2 years are attributable to the leadership of Margaret A. Hamburg, MD, who became the 21st Commissioner of Food and Drugs on May 18, 2009, and Joshua M. Sharfstein, MD, principal deputy commissioner under Commissioner Hamburg. Commissioner Hamburg has been charged with FDA's implementation of President Obama's directive for increased transparency and openness in government and in June 2009, launched FDA's Transparency Initiative.[57] A cornerstone of the Initiative is the agency's pledge to more clearly communicate its enforcement policies and requirements to the regulated industries in order to enhance compliance. Indeed, communication to and alignment of non-government stakeholders is an important element for government agencies to use in addressing potentially serious public health issues. In December 2010, Commissioner Hamburg worked with dietary supplement trade organizations to remind companies of their legal obligations and responsibility to prevent tainted products from reaching the US market. As pointed out by the Commissioner in her open letter to the industry, products labeled as dietary supplements that contain "the same active ingredients as FDA-approved drugs, analogs of the active ingredients in FDA-approved drugs, or other compounds, such as novel synthetic steroids … do not qualify as dietary ingredients." These undeclared ingredients may pose a potential of significant risk to consumers due to possible serious side effects and/or food-drug interactions. The letter was prompted by FDA surveillance of the dietary supplement marketplace through laboratory tests that revealed the following drug ingredients as undeclared constituents of products labeled as dietary supplements: anticoagulants (e.g., warfarin), anticonvulsants (e.g., phenytoin), HMG-CoA reductase inhibitors (e.g., lovastatin), phosphodiesterase type 5 inhibitors (e.g., sildenafil), nonsteroidal anti-inflammatory drugs (NSAIDs; e.g., indomethacin), and beta blockers (e.g., propranolol). In addition to recounting how FDA has addressed this problem through warning letters, recalls, and product seizures, the Commissioner announced fair warning that "responsible individuals and companies should be aware that the government may initiate criminal investigations to hold accountable those who violate the Federal Food, Drug, and Cosmetic Act (the Act) and endanger the public health."[58] Five major industry trade associations—CRN, NPA, United Natural Products Alliance (UNPA), CHPA, and AHPA—joined with FDA in calling for media attention to this issue and have agreed to share the letter widely within the dietary supplement industry.

Industry is on notice that, under Commissioner Hamburg, FDA is prepared to initiate criminal misdemeanor prosecutions and felony prosecutions (with a prior offense) working with the Office of Criminal Investigations (OCI), through a rejuvenation of the "Park Doctrine." The Park Doctrine refers to a 1975 US Supreme Court case holding that a corporate official may be prosecuted for introducing misbranded or adulterated foods into interstate commerce, without proof that the official acted with intent or negligence, and even without actual awareness or knowledge of the wrongdoing.[59] The requirements on corporate officials to ensure compliance with the FDCA are "onerous" and "stringent," but as well stated by the court: "They are no more stringent than the public has a right to expect of those who voluntarily assume positions of authority in business enterprises whose services and products affect the health and well-being of the public that supports them."[60]

In these examples and others not addressed here, FDA has demonstrated that under DSHEA and subsequent legislation and FDA's currently implementing regulations, the agency is able to and does address evolving safety, quality, and labeling issues to protect the public from adulterated or mislabeled dietary supplements. Of course, FDA must be adequately supported by Congress with the level of appropriations needed for the agency to achieve its mission.

FTC has extensive investigative and law enforcement authority to prevent companies from engaging in unfair or deceptive acts or practices in dietary supplement advertising.

Federal Trade Commission's Role in Regulating Dietary Supplement Advertising

FDA is supported in its mission to protect the public from false and misleading dietary supplement claims by FTC, which has broad authority to regulate dietary supplement advertising. With overlapping jurisdiction to regulate the labeling and advertising of foods, OTC drugs, medical devices, and cosmetics, FDA and FTC have worked under a liaison agreement (memorandum of understanding [MOU]) since 1954. Under the MOU, FTC has primary responsibility for regulating food advertising and FDA for regulating food labeling.[60] Recently, FDA and FTC have coordinated efforts in removing fraudulent products from the marketplace, particularly those sold on the Internet and promoted with unproven claims for treating or curing a range of diseases, including diabetes and cancer.

To protect consumers from deceptive claims for dietary supplements, FTC works closely with FDA in employing a 3-pronged strategy that consists of: (1) law enforcement, (2) consumer education, and (3) business outreach. FTC's authority stems from Section 5 of the FTC Act, which authorizes FTC to prohibit "unfair methods of competition" and "unfair or deceptive acts or practices" in or affecting commerce.[61] Section 12 of the FTC Act expressly prohibits "false advertisements" for foods, drugs, medical devices, and cosmetics that are likely to induce consumer purchases.[62] Dietary supplement advertising is regulated in a manner consistent with FTC's regulation of advertising generally under Sections 5 and 12 of the FTC Act. Under FTC law, an advertiser must possess "a reasonable basis" of substantiation to support objective advertising claims, both express and implied, at the time the claim is made. Claims concerning health-related benefits of dietary supplements must be supported by "competent and reliable scientific evidence," as interpreted by FTC.‡‡‡‡

FTC has extensive investigative and law enforcement authority to prevent companies from engaging in unfair or deceptive acts or practices in dietary supplement advertising, including the dissemination of false ads and unsubstantiated claims. In exercising its consumer protection enforcement authority, FTC may do the following:

- Request documents and information from a company through the use of voluntary "access letters;"
- Issue subpoenas and "civil investigative demands" requiring production of documentary evidence for any matter under investigation;
- Seek and impose consent orders (through administrative or judicial proceedings in federal court);
- Seek and obtain consumer redress (e.g., disgorgement of profits, refunds);
- Seek and obtain temporary and permanent injunctions, which may include corrective advertising;
- Seek and obtain civil penalties;
- Seek criminal penalties (by referral to the Justice Department).

FTC administrative and judicial proceedings may be directed against companies and individuals. Responsible principals of a company are typically targeted by FTC in its investigation phase. Endorsers, celebrities, and spokespeople engaged in the promotion of dietary supplements may also be held liable for violations of the FTC Act.

‡‡‡‡"Competent and reliable scientific evidence" has been defined through FTC case law as: "tests, analyses, research, studies, or other evidence based on the expertise of professionals in the relevant area, that have been conducted and evaluated in an objective manner by persons qualified to do so, using procedures generally accepted in the profession to yield accurate and reliable results. See FTC Enforcement Policy Statement on Food Advertising (May 1994) at www.ftc.gov/bcp/policystmt/ad-food.shtm.

FTC has been active in its enforcement of legal dietary supplement advertising claims. Two years after DSHEA's passage, in 1996, the Commission issued a resolution authorizing increased FTC investigation of advertisers and marketers of dietary supplements. The resolution provided FTC staff lawyers in any US city the ability to access a company's substantiating data through a "civil investigative demand" without filing a formal complaint. FTC has continued to exercise an active presence in dietary supplement advertising enforcement. In 1998, FTC issued advertising guidance to the dietary supplement industry, clarifying long-standing FTC regulatory policies with respect to the substantiation of advertising claims, including that consumer testimonials alone may not be used to substantiate claims.[63] By that same year, 4 years after passage of DSHEA, FTC had initiated 24 separate dietary supplement enforcement proceedings. In contrast, between 1984 and 1994 (the 10 years preceding DSHEA's enactment), only 35 cases were initiated by FTC. Between December 2002 and early July 2003, as reported by FTC, the Commission filed or settled 17 enforcement actions against parties engaged in deceptive dietary supplement advertising practices, with consumer sales of the targeted products estimated at more than $1 billion.[64] More recently, in May 2010, FTC presented testimony on enforcement activities relating to "Deceptive Marketing of Dietary Supplements" to the Senate's Special Committee on Aging, stating that during the past decade (2000–2010), the Commission "has filed well over 100 law enforcement actions challenging claims about the efficacy or safety of a wide variety of supplements."[65] According to FTC, the Commission's law enforcement actions are focused on national advertising campaigns for products with unproven benefits, products promoted to treat or cure serious diseases, products that may present significant safety concerns to consumers, and products that are deceptively marketed to vulnerable population groups such as children or the elderly.[9]

Indeed, the dietary supplement industry continues to be the focus of increased FTC regulatory scrutiny and enforcement, with significant multi-million dollar civil penalties, redress orders, and other remedies—such as disgorgement of profits—being sought by FTC through federal district courts. A review of recent FTC consent orders provides useful guidance for the general dietary supplement industry. While the substantiation standard continues to be applied on a case-by-case basis, for certain types of health-related claims in dietary supplement advertising, 2 adequate and well-controlled, product-specific clinical trials may be required. Also, when a company relies on third-party ingredient science to substantiate a health-related claim on a finished dietary supplement that has not been clinically tested, the burden will be on the company to demonstrate that the studies were conducted on an "essentially equivalent product."[66] In addition, in a policy shift, FTC has recently made clear that if an advertising claim for a dietary supplement is not permitted under FDA regulations and the governing statute (e.g., the claim indicates disease treatment or prevention, or is not an FDA authorized health claim pursuant to the NLEA), the claim will not be permitted under the FTC Act.[67]

Similar to FDA, FTC has supplemented its law enforcement actions with business outreach and consumer education programs. FTC has communicated to stakeholders that more robust industry self-regulatory efforts are needed to combat the problem of deceptive health-related claims for dietary supplements, particularly claims relating to weight loss. In 2006, CRN announced the launch and funding of a dietary supplement advertising review program, conducted through the National Advertising Division (NAD) of the Better Business Bureau. In 2009, CRN announced that the NAD dietary supplement review program would be extended for an additional 5 years. The NAD's mission is to support effective self-regulation of national advertising claims to ensure truth-in-advertising. While the process is voluntary, companies that refuse to participate do so at their own peril. NAD refers such cases to FTC, which gives NAD referrals priority. CRN's commitment to the self-regulatory process and funding support ($1.5 million over 8 years) has allowed the NAD to hire a dedicated staff attorney to focus solely on dietary supplement advertising claims. During the first 3 years of the program, the NAD opened more than 75 dietary supplement advertising cases, compared to fewer than 10 cases from the year before the CRN/NAD initiative began. At NAD's annual legal conference in 2008, FTC Commissioner J. Thomas Rosch praised the CRN/NAD initiative as "an excellent example of self-regulation that will increase monitoring of advertising for dietary supplements" and encouraged companies to file a competitive challenge with NAD "if they see a supplement ad that's misleading, untruthful, or includes claims that can't be substantiated."[68] [§§§§]

Role of Other Regulatory Agencies

Other regulatory agencies collaborate with FDA to assist the agency in its mission to protect and advance public health, such as the Drug Enforcement Administration (DEA) and US Customs and Border Protection (CBP), among other agencies. While DEA does not have statutory authority to enforce DSHEA (or the FDCA), FDA has statutory authority to investigate the illegal manufacture and distribution of anabolic steroids included in or sold as dietary supplements under the Controlled Substances Act.[69] DEA continues to investigate and uncover products wrongfully labeled as dietary supplements that contain either controlled anabolic steroids or designer steroids that are structurally similar to testosterone. Also, pursuant to the FDA Food Safety Modernization Act of 2011, FDA is required to notify DEA if the agency determines that information submitted in a new dietary ingredient notification is inadequate to establish the safety of the ingredient because it is an anabolic steroid or analogue. The notification to DEA must include the name of the dietary supplement and the name of the person(s) who submitted the notification and/or market the product. [70]

FDA has broad authority to examine, hold, detain, and prevent the importation of dietary supplements (and other FDA-regulated products) under section 801 of the FDCA.[71] FDA is assisted in its mission to prevent the importation of unsafe and improperly labeled dietary supplements by CBP, which is within the Department of Homeland Security. FDA and CBP have had a long history of close cooperation, which was strengthened in 2003 when FDA and CBP signed a MOU. Under the MOU, FDA is allowed to commission thousands of CBP officers in ports and other locations to conduct, on FDA's behalf, investigations and examinations of imported foods. The agreement significantly strengthened FDA's ability to implement the Public Health Security and Bioterrorism Preparedness and Response Act of 2002 (BioTerrorism Act).[72]

§§§§See also a voluntary industry program through the Natural Products Foundation. Truth In Advertising Program. Available at: http://naturalproductsfoundation.org/index.php?src=gendocs&ref=truth_in_advertising&category=FoundationPrograms.

FDA Collaborations with Non-Regulatory Governmental Organizations

As part of the Department of Health and Human Services, the CDC is charged with monitoring, detecting, and investigating health problems and conducting research to enhance the protection of public health. When ephedra was still on the market as a dietary supplement, CDC contributed to identifying adverse event reports by coordinating this effort with numerous state Departments of Health.[73] In addition, CDC manages surveillance studies, such as the National Health and Nutrition Examination Survey (NHANES), which is a program of studies designed to assess the health and nutritional status of adults and children in the United States, including usage patterns of dietary supplements.[74]

Conclusion

The years since the enactment of DSHEA have been marked by a progressive development of regulations and guidance by FDA to help ensure that dietary supplements are safe, of high quality, and appropriately labeled. Not surprisingly, there has not been an absolute consensus in the appropriateness or reasonableness of FDA's approach to regulating dietary supplements. Nonetheless, the core elements of the regulatory infrastructure envisioned by the authors of DSHEA are in place for dietary supplements. These elements are common to every major industry regulated by FDA, and include the following: legal definition for the category; a committed leadership within the agency; a comprehensive claims structure designed to ensure consumers have access to truthful and non-misleading information about a product's health benefits; standardized labeling requirements (e.g., statement of identity, Supplement Facts panel, list of ingredients) for all products in the category; a defined safety standard; a post-marketing surveillance system; strong legal authority for the agency to remove products with unacceptable health/safety risk; health professional and consumer outreach for product safety alerts; and a standard of manufacturing (i.e., GMPs) to help ensure quality products. With these elements, the $27 billion dietary supplements industry clearly represents a major FDA *regulated* industry.[75] With the complex, interrelated infrastructure of regulations now in place to implement DSHEA and subsequent amendments, the myth that dietary supplements are an unregulated industry is definitely dispelled. HG

This article was peer reviewed by numerous food and drug law attorneys with extensive expertise in the dietary supplements industry.

R. William Soller, PhD

Dr. Soller is executive director of the Center for Consumer Self Care Health Sciences and Clinical Professor of Pharmacy in the School of Pharmacy at the University of California, San Francisco (USCF). Dr. Soller has broad-based experience in drug and food law, regulations and health policy, and in consumer and pharmaceutical care research at the national and international levels. He is principal author of numerous drug and dietary supplement-related submissions to the FDA on a wide range of subjects related to self-medication. Dr. Soller received his PhD in Medical Sciences from Cornell University Graduate School of Medical Sciences (Neurobiology & Behavior/Pharmacology), and worked in the pharmaceutical and dietary supplement industries for over 20 years before moving to UCSF in 2002, where currently he teaches health policy, manages a telepharmacy service, conducts research, and consults with industry.

Holly J. Bayne

Holly Bayne is a Washington, DC-based attorney and founder of The Law Office of Holly Bayne, P.C., which specializes in the practice of food and drug law. Ms. Bayne focuses on matters relating to the regulation of functional foods, dietary supplements, and botanicals by the FDA, FTC, and other regulatory agencies. She began her legal career at Hyman, Phelps & McNamara, P.C., the largest law firm in the U.S. exclusively devoted to the practice of food and drug law. Before law school, Ms. Bayne worked as an educator and marketing executive in the dietary supplement and cosmetic industries. She has spoken domestically and internationally on issues concerning the regulation of food, dietary supplement, and botanical products, and has written numerous papers and articles pertaining to these issues. Ms. Bayne is admitted to practice law in the District of Columbia and California, and is also a member of the American Bar Association.

Christopher Shaheen

Christopher Shaheen is a researcher in the Center for Self Care at UCSF School of Pharmacy. Shaheen has a research background in basic and social sciences and experience working in pharmaceutical companies and academic research settings. He is a graduate of the University of California, Santa Cruz, and student of the Class of 2015 at UCSF School of Pharmacy.

References

1. Dietary Supplement Health and Education Act of 1994. Public Law 103-417: 103rd Congress. October 25, 1994. Available at: http://dshedu.com/DSHEA_Legal/dshea.html.
2. Soller RW. Regulation in the herb market: the myth of the "unregulated industry." *HerbalGram*. 2000:49;64-67.
3. 21 U.S.C. § 321
4. Food Safety and Modernization Act. Public Law 111-353. Statute 3885. January 4, 2011. Available at: www.gpo.gov/fdsys/pkg/PLAW-111publ353/content-detail.html. Accessed October 12, 2011.
5. 21 U.S.C. § 342(a)
6. 21 U.S.C. § 343(j).
7. Amendment: Public Health Service Act. Public Law 94-278. Staute 401. April 22, 1976.
8. Nutrition Labeling and Education Act. Public Law 101-533. 104 Statute 2353. 1990.
9. 984 F.2d 814. 61 USLW 2491. US v. Two Plastic Drums, More Or Less Of An Article Of Food, Labeled In Part: Viponte Ltd. Black Currant Oil Batch No. Boosf 039, etc., and Traco Labs, Incorporated. No. 92-1172. United States Court of Appeals, Seventh Circuit. Argued October 21, 1992. Decided January 27, 1993.
10. 987 F. 2d 33. US v. 29 Cartons Of *** An Article of Food, Etc., Defendant Oakmont Investment Co., Inc. Appeal From The United States District Court For The District Of Massachusetts. First Circuit. March 3, 1993.
11. Shelton S. Executive interview: Q&A with Bob Ullman. Engredea News & Analysis. September 8, 2005. Available at http://newhope360.com/executive-interview-qa-bob-ullman. Accessed October 12, 2011.
12. Hutt P. The history & future of the dietary supplement industry. Natural Products Insider. September 21, 2009. Available at: www.naturalproductsinsider.com/articles/2009/09/the-history-future-of-the-dietary-supplement-health-education-act.aspx. Accessed February 24, 2011.
13. McNamara S. Dietary supplements of botanicals and other substances: a new era of regulation. *Food Drug Law J*. 1995;50:341-355.
14. 103rd Congress. Second Session. Senate Report 103-410. Dietary Supplement and Health Education Act 1994. October 8, 1994. Report from the Committee on Labor and Human Resources to accompany S.784: p. 17.
15. Wertheimer L. FDA issues new standards for dietary supplements. NPR News. June 23, 2007. Available at: www.npr.org/templates/story/story.php?storyId=11326842.
16. Landau D. Dietary supplement industry unregulated. Injury Board Blog Network. February 1, 2011. Available at: http://fairfax-loudoun.injuryboard.com/fda-and-prescription-drugs/dietary-supplement-industry-unregulated.aspx?googleid=288118 Accessed February 24, 2011.
17. Green A. Spreading the blame: examining the relationship between DSHEA and the baseball steroid scandal. *Boston Univ Law Rev*. 2010;90:399-430.
18. Henney J. Implementation of the Dietary Supplement Health Education Act. Testimony before the House Committee on Government Reform. March 25, 1999. FDA Speech Archives. Available at: www.fda.gov/NewsEvents/Testimony/ucm115082.htm.
19. Statement by Jane E. Henney, MD, Commissioner Food and Drug Admin-

A Whitepaper Reprint (Updated 2014) from:

POINT INSTITUTE
OF NUTRACEUTICAL RESEARCH

Choosing the Best Marine-Derived Omega-3 Products for Therapeutic Use: An Evaluation of the Evidence

There is overwhelming data to recommend a wide range of therapeutic uses for marine-derived omega-3 fatty acids (primarily EPA and DHA). Likewise, there are also an overwhelming number of different forms, sources and ways to deliver these omega-3 fatty acids; which unfortunately, has led to confusion in product selection for both clinician and patient alike. We will walk through the most common issues discussed in selecting the appropriate omega-3 fatty acid product, with the goal to bring clarity to the decision-making process.

For the most part, the marine omega-3 fatty acid category is dominated by products best described as "fish oil"—that is, while there are products available that deliver omega-3 fatty acids from other marine sources, nearly all the available research has been done with fish oil-derived fatty acids. This fish oil data has become the benchmark for efficacy and safety, and is the standard to which we compare throughout this paper.

The following are the main sources of marine omega-3 fatty acids.

- **Fish Body Oil:** The largest biomass used to create marine-derived omega-3 fatty acids comes from small oily fish caught in the cold waters off the coast of Chile and Peru. The fish species most commonly used are mackerel, anchovies and sardines. Concentrations of these purified oils are the most common therapeutic product used in dietary supplements and pharmaceutical products throughout the world. Other species used to produce fish oil may include salmon, tuna, menhaden, herring and other minor species.[1]
- **Cod Liver:** As a byproduct of the cod meat market, cod liver can be used to provide a blend of fatty acids similar to unconcentrated fish body oil.

1. For detailed information about status and environmental performance of fisheries worldwide (fish species, harvest statistics, regulations and sustainability), see: www.fishsource.com.

- **Krill:** Small crustaceans that feed on plankton and are fed on by many marine mammals, especially whales. Factory ships process krill immediately upon capture off the coast of Antarctica. Krill oil is relatively low in EPA and DHA, but contains small amounts of the carotenoid astaxanthin.

- **Calamari:** A recent, but small, player in the omega-3 fatty acid industry is calamari or squid oil. This oil has a higher ratio of DHA over EPA than is typical of fish. This oil is a byproduct of the calamari food industry.

- **Mussels:** Shellfish are a minor source of commercially available omega-3 fatty acids. Nonetheless, several products are currently available from the fatty acids derived from Green-Lipped Mussels *(Perna canaliculus)*. The diverse fatty acid profile of these mussels includes EPA and DHA in a ratio of about 65:35. Limited research has been done using products derived from mussels for traditional omega-3-related outcomes (mostly arthritis and inflammation studies).

- **Algae:** Various species of algae are commercial sources for omega-3 fatty acids. These products are almost exclusively DHA. Most of the pure DHA raw materials, especially pure DHA used for addition to infant formula, come from these sources.

Additional Considerations on Marine Omega-3 Sourcing

Kosher: Only fish or algae sources are products that can be deemed truly "kosher," however, additional manufacturing processes may influence the ability to officially label a finished product (i.e., soft gelatin capsule) with a particular kosher certificate.

Vegetarian/Vegan: While many vegetarians choose to consume fish oil products even if they avoid consuming fish, strict vegans will avoid all marine lipids with the exception of algae-sourced products. Since EPA can be formed by consuming either DHA from algae or alpha-linolenic acid from flaxseed oil, these may be suitable options for strict vegan individuals. It should be noted that while these vegan omega-3 sources are likely to increase blood levels of EPA and DHA, there are no data yet to suggest these alternatives have the same risk-lowering benefits as EPA and DHA from fish.

Gluten: Marine fatty acids are gluten-free and softgel manufacturing should not introduce gluten to finished products.

GMO Status: None of the biomass—fish, krill, squid or algae—used to produce commercially available fatty acids *today* are known to be genetically modified. Under most global definitions, this would make these products "GMO-Free." Some groups, such as the Non-GMO Project, have proposed strict definitions of GM status whereby the inability to verify the GM status of foods eaten by harvested fish in the wild, or the GM status of the animals that contribute the gelatin for making softgels, would thereby not permit a GMO-Free status. Genetic modification of certain algae, through fermentation, for the production of EPA and DHA is in the works and may soon become commercially available. Also, genetically modified plants (soy, canola, etc.) are also being researched as non-marine sources of EPA and DHA.

Sustainability Issues: One of the concerns with using large quantities of marine omega-3 fatty acids for therapeutic use is long-term sustainability of harvesting the needed biomass. The debate over which source(s) might be in danger of overharvesting or are being harvested ecologically is controversial and made more difficult by the fact that no single final authority defines "sustainability" for the global community. Fisheries that supply both fish meal and fish oil are managed by a number of regulatory bodies around the world where harvest limits are set for fish species, fishing seasons and fishery zones. There is a seasonal variability in biomass, which is controlled by both local and global ocean conditions, affecting the year-to-year availability of EPA and DHA.

Controversy over krill sustainability appears to be more in debate. Most notably, in 2010 the retailer Whole Foods declared they would not sell krill products because of data they believed linked krill harvesting with reduced levels of animals that depend on krill for food. Since that time, the Marine Stewardship Council and other organizations have approved several of the largest krill harvesting companies as being "sustainable." Whole Foods still, as of 2016, does not sell krill products.

The future of the sustainability of marine biomass is influenced by global ocean fluctuations and the growing need for EPA and DHA. Tension between marine-derived EPA and DHA sustainability and the development of more sustainable GMO-produced EPA and DHA from plants will no doubt heighten the controversy.

Allergies to Fish and Shellfish Related to Omega-3 Products

Since the changes required for food allergen labeling went into effect in the U.S. in 2006, there is confusion as to how fish oil products should be labeled and whether individuals allergic to fish can safely consume fish oil. The eight allergens that require mandatory labeling include both fish and shellfish (also soy, wheat, eggs, peanuts, tree nuts and milk). However, the labeling requirements exempt the need to label ingredients that are highly refined oils containing no allergenic proteins specifically as allergens. Highly refined fish oils, like certain soybean oils, therefore do not need to be listed in a separate "contains the following allergens" statement on the label. Some companies using highly refined fish oils still choose to include "fish" in a list of allergens, primarily from a product liability standpoint. Nonetheless, the Supplement Facts box or front panel of a fish oil product must still declare the ingredient itself is concentrated fish oil, thereby notifying users the content contains fish-derived oils, even if no official declaration is made pertaining to fish-derived allergens.

Labeling issues aside, what is the likelihood that individuals who have known allergies to finned fish might also have an allergic reaction to a fish oil product? The answer appears to be: extremely unlikely. First, allergic reactions to fish are well understood and identified to specific proteins. Highly refined fish oil products are virtually absent from any detectable protein and there are no known allergens to fish-derived fatty acids or fish-derived gelatin used in some capsules. This notion was actually tested in a small-scale study where individuals with known allergies to finned fish were given fish oil supplements to see their reaction.[2] Two different fish oil supplements were tested in six subjects with known fish allergies by both skin and oral challenges. None of the subjects reacted in any way to either product.

These data, while limited, agree with the notion that highly refined fish oil products contain no reactive allergens and should be safe to consume by individuals with mild-to-moderate fish allergies. Highly sensitive individuals or those with life-threatening fish allergies should probably avoid the use of fish oil products out of the abundance of caution and look to get omega-3 fatty acids from plant sources such as algae (DHA) and flax (ALA). We are not aware of any published articles that similarly test krill or mussel-derived fatty acid products for shellfish allergies.

2. Mark BJ, Beaty AD, Slavin RG. Are fish oil supplements safe in finned fish-allergic patients? *Allergy Asthma Proc.* 2008 Sep-Oct;29(5):528-9.

Fatty Acid Forms and Structures

When fatty acids are harvested from their source, they are typically in the form of triglycerides (TG), phospholipids (PL) or free fatty acids (FFA). When these fatty acids are delivered as dietary supplements or pharmaceutical products, they can be delivered as triglycerides (in a purified but unconcentrated form or a concentrated re-esterified form [rTG]), ethyl esters (EE), free fatty acids (FFA) or phospholipids. These differences may alter the bioavailability and, perhaps, the efficacy of the fatty acids used (discussed below).

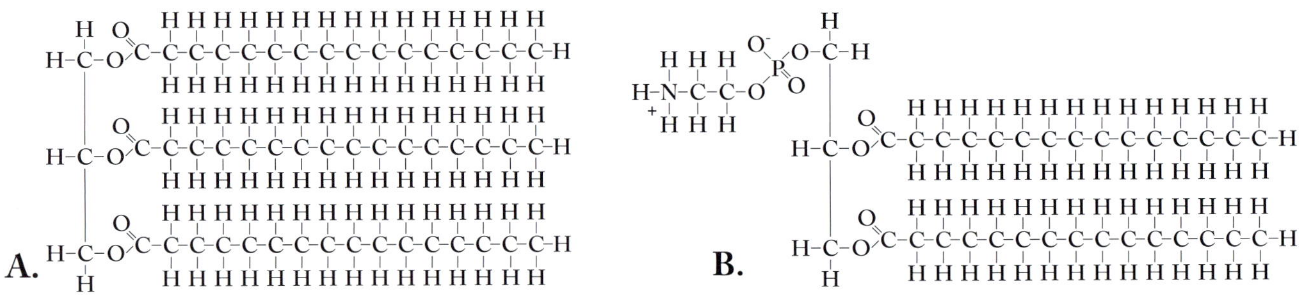

Figure 1: (A) Structure of triglyceride molecule (B) Structure of phospholipid: A phospholipid contains only two fatty acids connected to the glycerol backbone, substituting one of a variety of groups (choline, serine, or ethanolamine as shown here) for the third fatty acid chain.

The processes that transform "crude oil" harvested from fish into the three main fish oil products for therapeutic use involves a number of specific steps.[3] We will briefly describe each:

Deodorization: This process takes crude oil from the fish and, by use of an evaporator, removes the free fatty acids and many of the organic pollutants that may be in the oil. This process is sometimes referred to as "molecular distillation," since heating and cooling is used in this process. Some steam deodorization is still used by some companies.

Ethylation: This process removes the fatty acids from the glycerol backbone and, after neutralizing with a dilute acid, forms ethyl ester fatty acids, essentially a free fatty acid with an ethanol attached to the carboxyl end.

Distillation/Concentration: Under low vacuum and heat, this molecular distillation removes shorter chain ethyl esters and saturated fatty acids and can be continued until the desired EPA and DHA content is achieved (within limits; see CO_2 concentration below[4]).

Cold Filtration: This process precipitates solids that cloud the oil. These precipitates are filtered and removed. This step is sometimes called winterization.

Glycerolysis: This process allows for the enzymatic, or acid/base-catalyzed, reattachment or re-esterification of the concentrated fatty acids (mostly EPA and DHA) molecules to a glycerol molecule creating triglyceride and diglyceride molecules. These molecules might be deemed "bioidentical," as they are chemically the same as the original TG compounds, only with two or three times the number of EPA or DHA molecules attached to the glycerol backbone. This process is obviously not performed when products will be sold as ethyl esters.

3. Krill biomass requires a multistep process involving solvent extraction and various filtration steps that differ from fish oil production.

4. CO_2 "Super-critical" distillation: Some companies add an additional step using a special system that allows for super critical distillation using CO_2. The oils used for such processes have usually gone through most or all of the steps above. The additional distillation process allows for a higher concentration of EPA and DHA, especially when using EE forms.

Molecular Distillation: Similar to the deodorization/distillation, this process removes excess glycerol or fatty acids not reacted in the previous step.

Clay Filtering (Bleaching): This is a step to remove small contaminants that can be bound and removed by a special clay mixture.

Blending: The resultant oil is mixed with agents to protect oxidation (e.g., vitamin E, antioxidant oils, etc.) and blended with other similar oils as necessary to meet specific total omega-3 fatty acid or EPA/DHA specifications before being put in drums for shipping.

Bioavailability Studies

The efficacy of omega-3 fatty acid therapy is affected by their bioavailability.[5] Therefore, numerous studies have been performed to compare short- and long-term bioavailability in human subjects using omega-3 fatty acids from different sources and in different molecular forms. We will first discuss studies using fish oil preparations, and then address the question of krill versus fish oil.[6]

Ethyl Esters vs. Triglycerides

Since the creation of the ethyl ester (EE) forms of omega-3 fatty acids, many people have questioned the potential change in bioavailability of these forms compared to the natural triglyceride forms. The early studies were small, but already these data revealed either a slightly reduced bioavailability of the EE forms (compared to TG forms) in the absence of additional dietary fat or a statistically similar bioavailability between EE and TG forms. However, several larger and better-designed studies have shown a superior bioavailability of rTG forms over EE forms.

In fact, one of the largest studies performed to date compared similar doses of EPA and DHA using five different forms: unconcentrated triglycerides (what they called fish body oil-FBO), cod liver oil (similar TG form as FBO), rTG, EE or FFA, along with a "placebo"

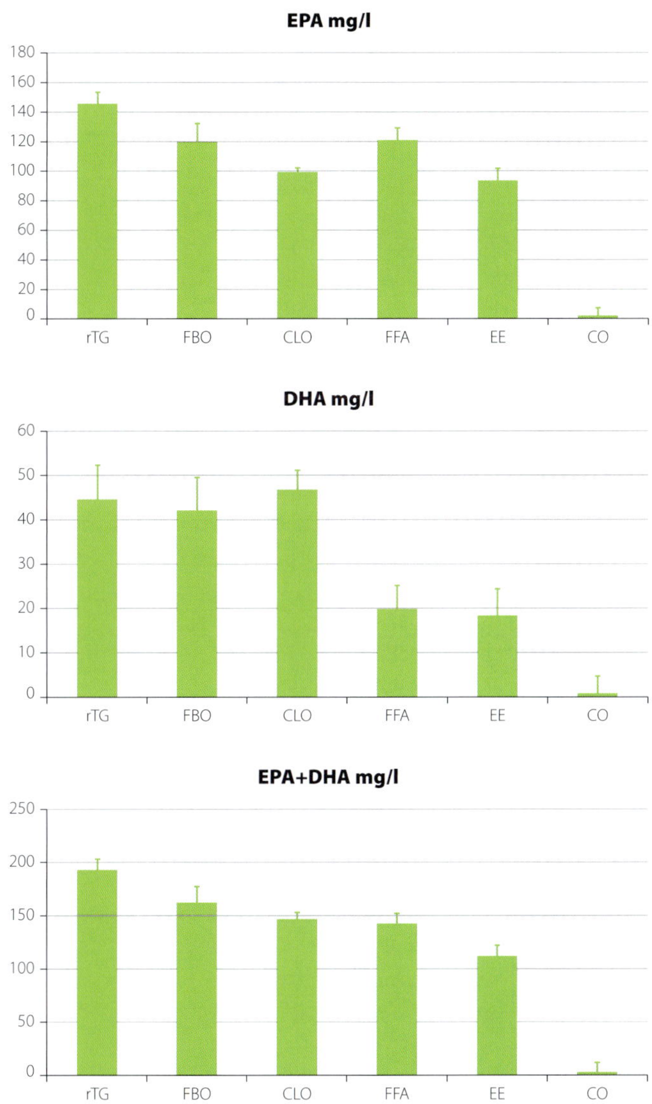

Figure 2: Bioavailability of Omega-3 Preparations from Dyerberg et al. See text for more details.

of corn oil (CO). In this study, 72 subjects were randomly assigned 3.3 gms per day of an EPA+DHA blend as capsules for two weeks.[7] Serum fatty acids (combined serum TG, PL and cholesterol esters) were analyzed at baseline and after two weeks. Figure 2 shows the changes from baseline to two weeks in EPA, DHA, and EPA+DHA in subjects consuming these different forms. In these subjects, the bioavailability of EPA+DHA from re-esterified triglycerides (rTG) was superior (+24%) when compared with natural fish oil (FBO +CLO), whereas the bioavailability from ethyl

5. Several studies suggest fatty acids may act within the intestinal lumen prior to becoming available in the bloodstream, in which case efficacy would not require absorption. In addition, individuals with limitations for fat absorption will clearly show differences in their ability to benefit from omega-3 fatty acid therapy. These nuances are beyond the scope of this particular overview.

6. For a recent review of EPA and DHA bioavailability studies, see: Schuchardt JP and Hahn A. Bioavailability of long-chain omega-3 fatty acids. *Prostaglandins Leukot Essent Fatty Acids.* 2013 Jul;89(1):1-8.

7. Dyerberg J, Madsen P, Møller JM, Aardestrup I, Schmidt EB. Bioavailability of marine n-3 fatty acid formulations. *Prostaglandins Leukot Essent Fatty Acids.* 2010 Sep;83(3):137-41.

esters (EE) was inferior (-27%) to natural TG and nearly 70% less bioavailable than rTG in these subjects. The authors suggest increased bioavailability of rTG over the unconcentrated TG form may be due to the fact that rTG products also contain diglycerides, along with a small amount of monoglycerides, which act as "partially digested forms" of the natural triglyceride, potentially enhancing bioavailability over the natural fish body oil. Concerning the EE form, numerous studies have shown a decreased lipase enzymatic activity when ethyl ester substrates are used, perhaps accounting for their decreased absorption when consumed away from a meal containing fat.

Ultimately, what we would like to know is whether any differences in bioavailability over two weeks might translate into long-term differences in fatty acid incorporation into important tissues and whether these differences can be measured in a clinically meaningful outcome. These sorts of studies have been carried out by researchers in Germany, where they looked at the incorporation of EPA and DHA into red blood cell membranes, commonly referred to as the omega-3 index, when individuals consumed either EE or rTG forms of fish oil.

This study looked at 150 hyperlipidemic subjects who were also taking statin drugs.[8] Subjects were given soft gelatin capsules containing EPA (1,008 mg) and DHA (672 mg) daily in either rTG or EE forms (corn oil used in placebo group). They were followed for six months. Figure 3 shows the change in omega-3 index (%EPA+DHA in RBC plasma membrane). Subjects consuming the rTG form had, on average, a statistically higher omega-3 index than those consuming the EE form after three months, which was maintained after six months of daily intake.

In a separate publication, the lipid-lowering effects of these two therapies were discussed.[9] What they found was that while both the EE and rTG reduced serum TG levels in these patients compared to placebo, rTG changes were nearly double that of the EE form. The only therapy to reach statistical significance was rTG therapy (Figure 4).

8. Neubronner J, Schuchardt JP, Kressel G, Merkel M, von Schacky C, Hahn A. Enhanced increase of omega-3 index in response to long-term n-3 fatty acid supplementation from triacylglycerides versus ethyl esters. *Eur J Clin Nutr*. 2011 Feb;65(2):247-54.

9. Schuchardt JP, Newbronner J, Kressel G, Merkel M, von Schacky C, Hahn A. Moderate doses of EPA and DHA from re-esterified triacylglycerols but not from ethyl-esters lower fasting serum triacylglycerols in statin-treated dyslipidemic subjects: Results from a six month randomized controlled trial. *Prostaglandins Leukot Essent Fatty Acids*. 2011 Dec;85(6):381-6.

Hypertriglyceridemia is prevalent across a wide range of subjects in the U.S., especially in those prescribed statin drugs. The use of a similar dose of concentrated omega-3 fatty acids as rTG provided as a dietary supplement (all current pharmaceutical products are EE fatty acids) can easily be obtained in two softgel capsules. It is our view that, when available, "bioidentical" rTG concentrates are preferable to EE forms for clinical therapy and provide much more "payload" of EPA and DHA when compared to unconcentrated fish oil triglycerides.

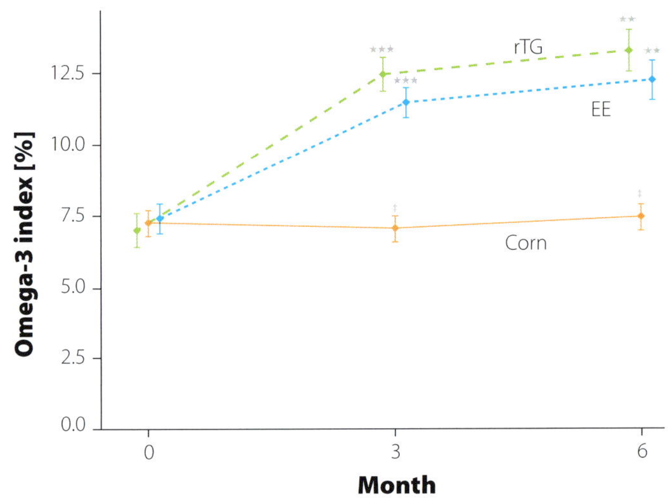

Figure 3: Change in Omega-3 Index consuming rTG, EE or placebo (Corn oil). *- P<0.001; **- P<0.01.**

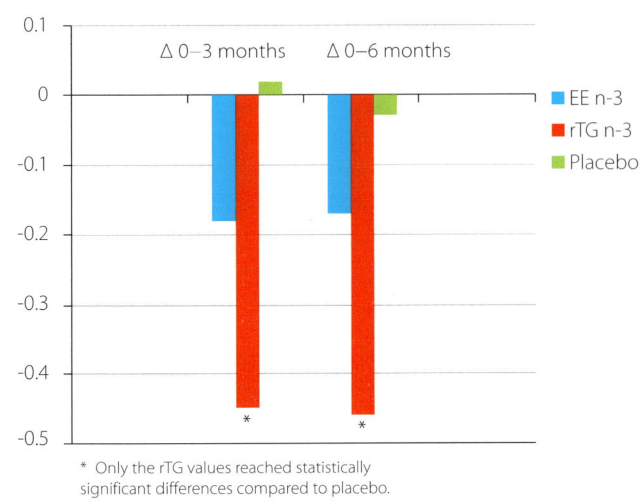

Figure 4: Change in serum TG at 3 and 6 months using rTG vs EE fish Oil (mmol/l).

Omega-3 Index: Risk Assessment, Dose Effects and Goal Setting

The omega-3 index is a measure of the quantity of EPA and DHA within red blood cell phospholipid fatty acids (as a percent). It was discovered that the omega-3 index correlated not only with the fatty acid profile of important cardiac tissues, but is highly correlated with cardiovascular risk, as well as other chronic disease outcomes. A number of laboratories now provide clinicians a variety of ways to easily measure omega-3 index in their patients.

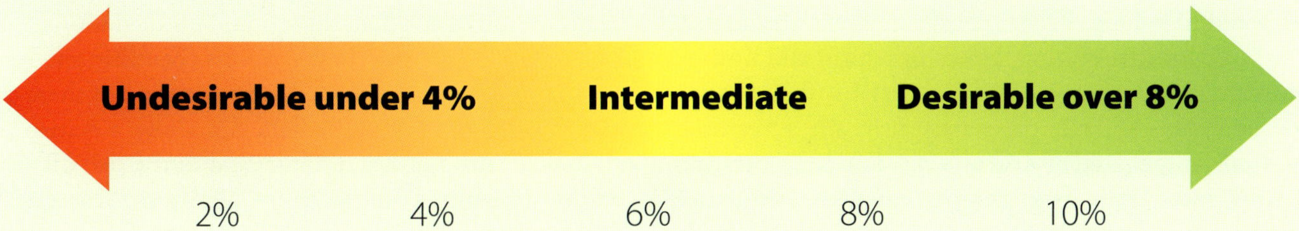

Likewise, many studies use the change in omega-3 index over time to assess the relative long-term bioavailability of a particular omega-3 fatty acid product (see main text). Flock et al. have recently shown the treatment dose of EPA and DHA from fish oil has a predictable effect on the change in omega-3 index; but they also discovered that individual differences, especially body weight, account for a high degree of variability in omega-3 index changes after consuming EPA and DHA. What is essential for the clinician to understand is that without testing a person's omega-3 index, it may not be possible to predict their current, or change in, omega-3 index even when using a clinically-effective dose of EPA and DHA.

Change in Omega-3 Index after 5 months of Different Doses of EPA +DHA in Healthy Subjects

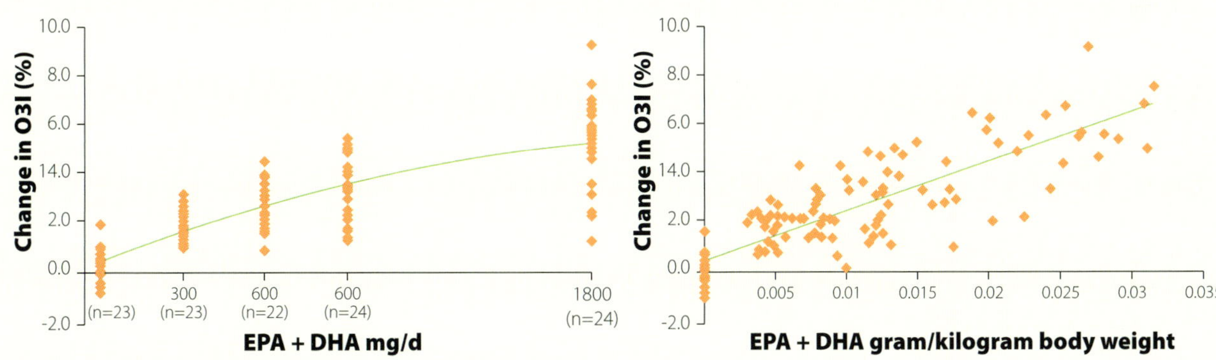

Adapted from Flock et al.

References:

- Harris WS. The omega-3 index: clinical utility for therapeutic intervention. *Curr Cardiol Rep*. 2010 Nov;12(6):503-8.
- Pottala JV, Yaffe K, Robinson JG, Espeland MA, Wallace R, Harris WS. Higher RBC EPA + DHA corresponds with larger total brain and hippocampal volumes: WHIMS-MRI Study. *Neurology*. 2014 Feb 4;82(5):435-42.
- Grenon SM, Conte MS, et al. Association between n-3 polyunsaturated fatty acid content of red blood cells and inflammatory biomarkers in patients with peripheral artery disease. *J Vasc Surg*. 2013 Nov;58(5):1283-90.
- Flock MR, Skulas-Ray AC, Harris WS, Etherton TD, Fleming JA, Kris-Etherton PM. Determinants of erythrocyte omega-3 fatty acid content in response to fish oil supplementation: a dose-response randomized controlled trial. *J Am Heart Assoc*. 2013 Nov 19;2(6):e000513.

Bioavailability: Krill Oil vs. Fish Oil

In the past decade, the market has been flooded with information about the use of, and purported superiority of, omega-3 fatty acids from krill. These claims have primarily come from two properties of krill oil: that it is derived mostly of phospholipids (PL, as opposed to TG) and that it contains trace levels of astaxanthin, a bioactive carotenoid. Additionally, some studies have suggested these properties, particularly the PL nature of the fatty acids, account for superior bioavailability compared to fish oil. We will examine this claim first.

As of this writing, only short-term and limited comparisons are available to ascertain the relative bioavailability of krill oil versus fish oil, a research question complicated by krill oil's very low concentration of EPA and DHA. One group studied the difference between the use of krill oil and menhaden oil (fish body oil, natural TG) or placebo (olive oil) in their ability to alter plasma fatty acids when consumed by overweight and obese subjects (n=76).[10] Each subject was to consume two gm/day of each oil for four weeks before being tested for changes in plasma fatty acid levels. It is important to note that the two gm of menhaden oil contained 212 mg of EPA and 178 mg of DHA (390 mg total), while the krill oil preparation contained 216 mg EPA and 90 mg of DHA (306 mg total). Compared to olive oil, both the krill and menhaden oil significantly increased the EPA and DHA levels of the subjects; Krill EPA (+ 89%), DHA (+23 %); Menhaden EPA (+ 81%), DHA (+ 45%). These data suggest bioavailability of EPA and DHA from krill and unconcentrated menhaden oil are statistically similar. In this study, the systolic blood pressure response in the control group differed significantly from that in the menhaden group (P = .032), but no significant differences were present for krill. This is likely due to the fact that menhaden oil provides higher DHA content (much of fish oil's antihypertensive activity seems to be due to DHA levels).

The second study often cited was a seven-week study comparing the change in plasma fatty acids in subjects with "normal or slightly elevated" lipids when given either krill or fish oil.[11] This study compared six capsules of krill oil, providing 543 mg of EPA+DHA and three capsules of fish oil (unspecified form) providing 864 mg of EPA+DHA. Compared to control subjects (unsupplemented subjects), both krill and fish oil were able to statistically increase EPA and DHA in those consuming each. However, while the average increase in EPA and DHA was slightly higher in the fish oil group, the difference between the groups was not statistically significant. This led the authors, and many krill advocates, to suggest this data is proof a lower dose of krill is equivalent to a higher dose of fish oil. A closer examination of the data show standard deviations of the fatty acid levels at both time-points (baseline and seven weeks) is so large that no real interpretation of these data is possible. Even so, their data did show a statistically significant drop in arachidonic acid in the fish oil group while showing a statistically significant increase in AA in the krill group. The clinical significance of this change in arachidonic acid, generally favoring the fish oil group, is unknown. Regardless, we find it curious the authors designed the study with such a discrepancy in EPA+DHA, since they could have easily given two, instead of three, fish oil capsules to get a near-equivalent dosing comparison to study.

Trials using equal amounts of EPA/DHA from fish and krill are limited or severely flawed. One recent study compared equivalent doses of EPA+DHA from krill, rTG and EE fish oils.[12] Unfortunately this was a single-dose, 72-hour study that measured changes in plasma phospholipids only, unlike the previous krill studies (plasma fatty acids) or the long-term fish oil study (omega-3 index/RBC FA). Twelve healthy males were recruited to consume each of the three omega-3 preparations (crossover design, 14 days apart) containing a total of 1,680 mg of EPA+DHA. The particular products used required four capsules of fish oil (rTG or EE) or 14 krill oil capsules to obtain the necessary EPA+DHA. Blood samples were taken before dosing (7 a.m.) and at two, four, six, eight, 24, 48 and 72 hours after capsule intake.

Like the previous study, due to high standard deviation values, there were no significant differences for EPA, DHA, or the sum of EPA+DHA levels between the three treatments. The authors did note nonstatistical "trends" in higher levels of plasma PL-EPA when subjects consumed krill. When one examines the data closely it does appear this trend may

10. Maki KC and Reeves MS et al. Krill oil supplementation increases plasma concentrations of eicosapentaenoic and docosahexaenoic acids in overweight and obese men and women. *Nutr Res.* 2009 Sep;29(9):609-15.

11. Ulven SM, Kirkhus B, Lamglait A, Basu S, Elind E, Haider T, Berge K, Vik H, Pedersen JI. Metabolic effects of krill oil are essentially similar to those of fish oil but at lower dose of EPA and DHA, in healthy volunteers. *Lipids.* 2011 Jan;46(1):37-46.

12. Schuchardt JP, Schneider I, Meyer H, Neubronner J, von Schacky C, Hahn A. Incorporation of EPA and DHA into plasma phospholipids in response to different omega-3 fatty acid formulations--a comparative bioavailability study of fish oil vs. krill oil. *Lipids Health Dis.* 2011 Aug 22;10:145.

indeed indicate a higher plasma phospholipid level in individuals consuming equal levels of EPA+DHA from krill versus fish. The conclusion, however, that krill is a "better" source of EPA+DHA is complicated by at least three issues. The first is that these nonstatistical trends were performed with a single dose in only 12 male subjects; this was a pilot study at best. Secondly, this study measured plasma phospholipids, not omega-3 index or total plasma fatty acids. This is important because it is postulated that PL can be incorporated into chylomicrons directly and, since krill provides most of its fatty acids as PL (they reported that about 22% of krill oil was actually FFA), the fish oil fatty acids may have been incorporated in TG, cholesterol esters or FFA. In fact, the "trend" in the increase of plasma PL could have been a 72-hour artifact of consuming krill PL over fish rTG. EE forms performed worse than both.

Lastly, and perhaps most important for practical clinical consideration, it took 14 krill oil capsules to provide 1,680 mg of EPA+DHA; something now provided easily in two concentrated fish oil capsules (they used four). The most widely commercially available krill oil products typically contain only 90 – 120 mg of EPA+DHA per capsule; while even unconcentrated fish oil products contain 300 mg of EPA+DHA per capsule. In fact, a recent study attempting to compare the omega-3 index effects of equal amounts of EPA/DHA from krill oil or fish oil using the same number of capsules had to admit (after publishing their article), that the fish oil was actually diluted with corn oil.[13] In the author's rebuttal, they described their reasons this way:

"Our primary objective was to compare effects of consumption of same amount of n-3 fatty acids from krill or fish oil. When designing a double blinded placebo controlled randomised cross over trial, it was felt that the amounts of treatment products as well as the bioactives of interest be maintained consistent across different interventions. However, the n-3 PUFA content of the krill oil fell below that of fish oil. In order to match the concentrations of n-3 PUFA and volumes between krill and fish oil, the fish oil was diluted with the placebo, corn oil at a ratio of 1.3:1.0."

Even so, while providing only one-third of the amounts of EPA+DHA as the lowest concentrations of fish oil, krill oil products are typically five to 10 times more expensive. Economic comparisons between krill oil and the concentrated rTG products recommended here, which can provide seven to eight times more EPA+DHA per capsule, are similar. Unless a higher amount of EPA+DHA can be delivered by krill for an economical price, fatty acids from krill would need to be seven to 10 times more bioavailable than fish TG to be considered either therapeutically or economically equivalent. That said, there is limited evidence to suggest that similar doses of EPA+DHA from krill, if delivered to a patient, would have an inferior biological effect than those proven in studies using fish oil-derived EPA+DHA. A recent study, however, casts some doubts on the reliability of krill oil EPA/DHA to lower triglycerides; one of the most studied benefits of fish oil.

The title of this article (written by scientists employed by the manufacturer of the krill product used) was deceptively hopeful: *Krill oil supplementation lowers serum triglycerides without increasing low-density lipoprotein cholesterol in adults with borderline high or high triglyceride levels.*[14] Unfortunately, the data proved to be anything but a straight-forward TG-lowering effect from krill oil.

The study was designed much like TG-lowering studies of fish oil. Three-hundred patients with high triglycerides were recruited and given placebo or 0.5, 1, 2 or 4 grams of krill oil providing 0, 100, 200, 400 or 800 mg of EPA/DHA over 12 weeks. Blood lipids and omega-3 index were measured at baseline, six weeks and 12-weeks after consuming the krill products. After 12-weeks of krill oil consumption the change in TG levels in these individuals (with a mean baseline TG of 231) was as follows: Placebo (+3.9%), 100 mg (-10%), 200 mg (-3.8%), 400 mg (-6.7%), 800 mg (+0.9%); none of the 12-week changes reached statistical significance. The authors claim that the lack of efficacy and dose-response was due to the overwhelming intra-individual TG measurements and high standard deviation- making it impossible to measure fasting TG as an outcome. How then, with these numbers (even showing an increase in TG using 800 mg of EPA and DHA) were they able to

13. The original article, commentary and rebuttal (all open access) are needed to follow this story.
- Ramprasath VR, Eyal I, Zchut S, Jones PJ. Enhanced increase of omega-3 index in healthy individuals with response to 4-week n-3 fatty acid supplementation from krill oil versus fish oil. *Lipids Health Dis.* 2013 Dec 5;12:178.
- Nichols PD, Kitessa SM, Abeywardena M. Commentary on a trial comparing krill oil versus fish oil. *Lipids Health Dis.* 2014 Jan 2;13:2.
- Ramprasath VR, Eyal I, Zchut S, Jones PJ. Response to commentary on a trial comparing krill oil versus fish oil. *Lipids Health Dis.* 2014 Jan 22;13:17.

14. Berge K, Musa-Veloso K, Harwood M, Hoem N, Burri L. Krill oil supplementation lowers serum triglycerides without increasing low-density lipoprotein cholesterol in adults with borderline high or high triglyceride levels. *Nutr Res.* 2014 Feb;34(2):126-33

declare a TG-lowering effect in the title?

The reviewers of the paper allowed these authors to circumvent the "limitations" of the study and use *"an explorative data analysis approach to increase the statistical power of the study."* In essence what they did was pool together all the doses, including the 6-week data points which happened to be better for nearly all the doses, and analyzed the data as if a theoretical average EPA/DHA content of 385 mg was given to all the subjects. The authors then boldly declare that *"Relative to subjects in the placebo group, those administered krill oil had a statistically significant calculated reduction in serum TG levels of 10.2%."* Even if we accepted this flawed explorative data analysis, this data showed only a 6.3% reduction from baseline TG levels- a level that even if achieved in this study, represents a small clinical difference. In contrast, fish oil studies routinely see drops in TG (from baseline) of >25%, show clear dose-response and are maintained or even continue to improve between 6 and 12 weeks.

Astaxanthin from Krill

Astaxanthin is a reddish-colored xanthophyll (carotenoid, similar to the compound zeaxanthin) found in a variety of marine organisms, from algae to salmon. Krill biomass contains about 120 ppm astaxanthin and most krill oil preparations claim a small amount of it on their label. To date, no studies have been done using krill oil-derived astaxanthin, making the various marketing claims difficult to evaluate. Microalgae sources, and some synthetic sources, are the commercially available forms used in the limited clinical studies using astaxanthin. For context, the few studies available using astaxanthin in humans used doses ranging from four mg to 20 mg per day; the average krill oil capsule claims to have 0.5-0.8 mg of astaxanthin per capsule.[15] Perhaps additional studies will be performed attempting to understand the role and benefits of delivering astaxanthin from krill oil, but currently there are no such studies.

15. Earnest CP, Lupo M, White KM, Church TS. Effect of astaxanthin on cycling time trial performance. *Int J Sports Med.* 2011 Nov;32(11):882-8.

Differential uses of EPA and DHA

We have previously reviewed the differential uses of EPA and DHA in a paper available at www.pointinstitute.org. Table 1 summarizes the evidence-based usage of EPA and/or DHA below.

Quality Control Issues of Fish Oil and Related Products

We are several decades into the regular use of fish oil-derived omega-3 fatty acids as dietary supplements and pharmaceutical products worldwide. Nearly all of the quality control issues that plagued the first few years of fish oil availability, such as heavy metal contamination, pesticide residues and oxidation, are rare instances in today's products. A number of highly reputable organizations (e.g., GOED-Global Organization for EPA and DHA; CRN, The Council of Responsible Nutrition) have developed standards for fish oil products that set specific limits for heavy metal contamination, a wide variety of organic pollutants and oxidation limits. Most global fish oil providers maintain all their products to these high standards. This is especially true of the concentrated products (rTG and EE forms); and since heavy metal and pesticide residue are virtually impossible to add during the manufacturing process, monitoring oxidation of the fatty acids is one of the critical steps in producing a high-quality product.

Condition	EPA-Rich	EPA/DHA	DHA-Rich
General Health		★★	
Improving w3:w6 ratio		★★	
Low-Risk CVD prevention		★★	★
High CVD Risk/Atherosclerosis		★	★★
Inflammatory Diseases		★★	
Depression	★★	★	
Macular Degeneration			★★
Alzheimer—Dementia		★	★★
Maternal—Childhood Development		★	★★

Table 1 : Condition-specific recommendations for EPA and DHA use. General recommendations for the differential uses of EPA and DHA. An "★★" recommendation is used when clinical trial and/or mechanistic data suggest better outcomes using a product rich (although not exclusively) in EPA or DHA. The data used to make these suggestions can be found in a whitepaper on our website http://www.pointinstitute.org/white-papers/.

Fish oil oxidation is measured using two methods. The first measures oxidized fatty acids directly as a peroxide value (PV or POV). Since these peroxides are transient and can form secondary oxidized molecules, like aldehydes, a second test is used to detect these oxidized compounds: the anisidine (or p-anisidine) test. When we combine these values by adding the aniside value to twice the peroxide value (AV+2PV), we get the TOTOX value.[16] To control the oxidation of the fish oil raw material and finished product, most manufacturers add a variety of antioxidant compounds. The most popular are vitamin E, vitamin A, flavonoids, and rosemary extracts or other spice extracts; synthetic antioxidants are rarely used. Most commercially available products will contain one or more of these antioxidants, at very low doses, in the finished product. Manufacturers of liquid-filled bottles or softgel capsules also utilize nitrogen (to purge available oxygen), low light and cold temperatures in the manufacturing process to reduce oxidation and extend shelf life. Products should not be used after their expiration date and should be thrown away, as oxidized fish oil can act as a pro-oxidant and limit the benefits realized if consumed.

Enteric-Coated Capsules and Flavored Oils

In the early days of fish oil therapy it was common to experience unpleasant GI side effects when consuming fish oil, including upset stomach, changes in bowel consistency and the dreaded fish oil burp. Obviously, some people are more prone to these issues than others, and the data from an overwhelming number of clinical trials show fish oil to be extremely well tolerated in a variety of subjects. Even so, to combat some of the unpleasant side effects of consuming fish oil, some manufacturers have taken to adding flavors in fish oil products or have enteric-coated the softgel delivering the fish oil. Are these measures necessary and do they alter the efficacy or safety of the products?

For the most part, the small amount of flavoring used to give the oil a hint of citrus or other flavors have no real measurable impact on the quality or efficacy of the oil, and they can be made from natural sources. It should be noted that once most flavors are added to the oil, they very often interfere with the anisidine test in the final product, which relies on colorimetric analysis. In these cases, oxidative analysis needs to be done before flavoring is added, while any changes in the peroxide value can be used to monitor the oxidation that may have been introduced between flavoring and bottling or encapsulation. Since many people experience burping independent of the fish oil quality, flavoring the oil may prevent this issue from causing them to discontinue the product, creating a better clinical outcome. Fish oil provided in a liquid form is often flavored to provide a pleasant aroma and flavor at the point of consumption.

Over the past several years, some fish oil soft gelatin capsules have been provided with various forms of enteric coating, preventing the release of the fish oil in the stomach, which virtually eliminates the ability to burp up any fishy taste. There are two potential issues with this approach clinicians should be aware of before considering the use of enteric-coated fish oil products: potential for reduced bioavailability and synthetic compounds used to make enteric coating. The second issue is more straightforward, so we will address it first.

A true "enteric-coated" product must meet specific criteria for disintegration, allowing it to remain intact in the stomach while still releasing the active ingredients in the small intestines. To do this, capsules must be coated with a series of chemicals to allow for pH-specific performance. The problem is the chemicals needed to make soft gelatin capsules truly enteric-coated are typically not the sort that healthy consumers and their clinicians want to consume unless enteric-coated delivery is absolutely necessary —chemicals like methyl acrylate-methacrylic acid copolymers, cellulose acetate succinate, hydroxypropyl methylcellulose phthalate and polyvinyl acetate phthalate (PVAP) to name a few. While these chemicals are capable of creating the ideal gastric/enteric release profile, it is no wonder most companies are reluctant to label these additional ingredients. In fact, companies that choose to label these ingredients as merely "enteric coating" are not in compliance with the labeling requirements for food or dietary supplements in the U.S.

There are numerous products that claim to have more natural forms of enteric coating. While these coatings do avoid most of the chemicals listed above, the precision of their enteric coating does not meet the same standards as studied products using the synthetic chemical coatings. Either way, additional handling and coating increases the cost of the final product and increases the chance for exposure to oxidation. It also adds the potential to diminish bioavailability.

It is well-known that marine fatty acids need to be partially digested with pancreatic lipases with

16. For a more detailed explanation of this, a helpful summary can be found online at http://www.oilsfats.org.nz/Oxidation%20101.pdf.

the help of bile salts in the small intestine prior to absorption. These free fatty acids and monoglycerides form mixed micelles and move into enterocytes, where they are then packaged into chylomicrons to be carried into the bloodstream. The concentration of bile salts and lipase enzymes in the duodenum is intended to interact with fatty acids immediately after they leave the stomach allowing for absorption within the upper jejunum. However, in the case of enteric-coated products, this may not occur for 30 minutes or more after arriving in the small intestine (USP analysis allows for up to an hour in simulated intestinal fluid).[17] This delay may act to reduce the interaction of the ingested contents of the enteric-coated capsule with the bile salts and enzymes, thereby reducing bioavailability.[18]

There is, on the other hand, data that suggest certain coated fish oil capsules have adequate bioavailability. One particular study compared EPA and DHA (rTG form) from either an uncoated soft gelatin capsule or a gastric acid-resistant coated capsule in 12 subjects following a crossover design.[19] After subjects consumed a single dose of four capsules containing 1,680 mg of EPA+DHA, their plasma PL changes in EPA and DHA were followed for 72 hours. There were no statistical differences between the area under the curve (AUC), the timing (Tmax) or peak concentrations (Cmax) between ingesting the coated and uncoated products. Dissolution information was described for these gastric-coated capsules, showing they complied with the European Phamacopeia for gastric-coated soft gelatin capsules. It should be noted that European Pharmacopeia specifications for this type of coating requires softgels to dissolve (once past the gastric resistance portion) in less than 30 minutes, though this study claims these particular capsules released in less than 15 minutes.

Nearly all other studies using standard enteric-coated capsules use EPA and DHA delivered as free fatty acids (FFA), which do not require digestion by lipase and bile to prepare them for absorption. In this form, EPA and DHA appear to be bioavailable, at least compared to the poor absorption of the EE form (Lovaza) consumed during a low-fat meal.[20] It is interesting to note the overwhelming published data for enteric-coated fish oils has been for direct gastrointestinal use in patients with inflammatory bowel disease[21], particularly Crohn's disease and colon polyps[22], where delayed absorption may be helpful. Dietary supplement companies selling enteric-coated TG, rTG, EE or PL forms of EPA and DHA should be asked to provide lot-specific pharmacokinetic/bioavailability results from their own products and about the quality-control procedures they use to ensure batch-to-batch consistency for capsule dissolution. Without this information, it is difficult to ensure the product will have the same properties as those described in the limited studies described here.

Dietary Supplements vs. Pharmaceutical Products

Currently there are only two approved pharmaceutical products on the market in the U.S. Lovaza (formerly Omacor: GlaxoSmithKline), an EE fish oil product providing 465 mg of EPA and 375 mg of DHA (840 total) in a single softgel; and Vascepa (Amarin), a one-gm capsule of an EE form of EPA only; both indicated for severe hypertriglyceridemia (TG>500mg/dl). The rationale for the newer EPA-only Vascepa, according to Amarin's marketing perspective, is that EPA does not raise LDL-C like DHA does. Neglected in this perspective is that DHA also raises HDL-C and dramatically increases LDL particle size, which is both cardio-protective and the very reason LDL-C is increased when DHA is administered. This "anomaly" of DHA (slight increase in LDL-C) is actually a signal of a beneficial shift in lipid metabolism. Unfortunately, since the lipid-lowering guidelines are fixated on reducing LDL-C as a primary goal, the marketing of

17. USP Disintegration and Dissolution of Dietary Supplements-June 2011 http://www.usp.org/sites/default/files/usp_pdf/EN/USPNF/revisions/2040disintegration dissolution.pdf.

18. Lack of proper enteric-coating was a major culprit in the failure of numerous clinical trials involving enteric-coated garlic tablets- used to avoid the taste of garlic. Lawson LD et al. Allicin release under simulated gastrointestinal conditions from garlic powder tablets employed in clinical trials on serum cholesterol. *Planta Med.* 2001; 67(1):13-8.

19. Schneider I, Schuchardt JP, Meyer H and Hahn A. Effect of gastric acid resistant coating of fish oil capsules on intestinal uptake of eicosapentaenoic acid and docosahexainoic acid. *J. Functional Foods* 2011 3:129-133.

20. Davidson MH, Johnson J, Rooney MW, Kyle ML, Kling DF. A novel omega-3 free fatty acid formulation has dramatically improved bioavailability during a low-fat diet compared with omega-3-acid ethyl esters: the ECLIPSE (Epanova(®) compared to Lovaza(®) in a pharmacokinetic single-dose evaluation) study. *J Clin Lipidol.* 2012 Nov-Dec;6(6):573-84.

21. Turner D, Zlotkin SH, Shah PS, Griffiths AM. Omega 3 fatty acids (fish oil) for maintenance of remission in Crohn's disease. *Cochrane Database Syst Rev.* 2007 Apr 18;(2):CD006320.

22. West NJ and Clark SK, et.al. Eicosapentaenoic acid reduces rectal polyp number and size in familial adenomatous polyposis. *Gut.* 2010 Jul;59(7):918-25. doi: 10.1136/gut.2009.200642.

an EPA-only product for cardiovascular health will no doubt mislead many who target LDL-C alone.

Some dietary supplement companies refer to their fish oil products as "Pharmaceutical Grade." While this term is misleading in that no such designation exists for products not approved as pharmaceuticals in the U.S., reputable suppliers of highly concentrated fish oil dietary supplements provide products that are just as pure and effective as those approved as pharmaceuticals. In fact, the rTG form that proves to be the best choice for clinicians is currently only available as a dietary supplement. Additionally, the United States Pharmacopeia (USP) has created a verification program that includes specifications for both fish oil raw materials and finished products. While "USP Verified" products are not technically "Pharmaceutical Grade," these products are usually of the highest quality possible.

Recommendations for Selecting Therapeutic Marine Omega-3 Fatty Acid for Supplementation

- The best therapeutic option for delivering marine omega-3 fatty acids is a concentrated "bio-identical" rTG form of fish oil. A single softgel containing rTG fish oil can easily provide well over 700 mg of EPA and DHA; rTG forms outperform the EE version of fish oil in terms of bioavailability and raising omega-3 index.
- Prescription pharmaceutical omega-3 fatty acids are only available in an EE form. However, in the event a patient's insurance is willing to pay for these products upon the diagnosis of severe hypertriglyceridemia (TG>500), these products have been shown to be safe and effective; albeit slightly less so than rTG forms available as dietary supplements. EE products should be consumed with a high-fat meal for best absorption, though it is important to instruct patients to add only healthy fats.
- Clinicians should consider having, or recommending, various blends of omega-3 products—some high in EPA, high in DHA, or a blend of EPA and DHA—to address different therapeutic targets. (see our paper addressing different therapeutic uses of EPA and DHA at www.pointinstitute.org.)
- Clinicians can use blood testing, such as the omega-3 index, to determine the EPA and DHA status of patients and monitor dose accordingly.
- While krill products appear to be adequate alternative sources of EPA and DHA, their low potency and high relative cost make them poor therapeutic substitutes for rTG fish oil, even if the suggested benefits of PL bioavailability can be proven in future clinical trials.
- Low-dose fish oil products, while reliable sources of EPA and DHA are like krill oil in that they provide too low a payload of EPA/DHA to be a viable therapeutic product. They are, however, a cost-effective way to increase omega-3 fatty acids in low-risk individuals desiring to augment a healthy diet.
- Enteric-coated capsules increase the potential for ingesting unwanted chemical compounds and increasing the lot-to-lot variability in omega-3 absorption. Clinicians should ask their supplier for enteric-coating ingredients and lot-specific dissolution information before relying on these products. The additional cost of enteric coating is usually not warranted when using highly purified and concentrated oils.

24 Hour Diet and GI Diary

Patient Name: ______________________________ Date: ______________

Food & Beverage (Please include as much detail as possible including serving sizes.):	**Time of Meal**	**Where Meal Was Consumed***	**How Meal Was Consumed****
Breakfast	A.M./P.M.		
	A.M./P.M.		
	A.M./P.M.		
	A.M./P.M.		
	A.M./P.M.		
Lunch	A.M./P.M.		
	A.M./P.M.		
	A.M./P.M.		
	A.M./P.M.		
	A.M./P.M.		
Dinner	A.M./P.M.		
	A.M./P.M.		
	A.M./P.M.		
	A.M./P.M.		
	A.M./P.M.		

* Please indicate if the meal was consumed at Home (H), Work Cafeteria (WC), Car (C), Restaurant (R) or Other (Please Specify).
** Please indicate how the meal was consumed. Alone (A), With Others (WO), Sit-down meal (S), On-the-go (OG), or Other (Please Specify)

Snacks (Include coffee, soda, candy, gum, etc.)

______________________ Time: __________ A.M./P.M.
______________________ Time: __________ A.M./P.M.
______________________ Time: __________ A.M./P.M.
______________________ Time: __________ A.M./P.M.
______________________ Time: __________ A.M./P.M.
______________________ Time: __________ A.M./P.M.

Food Groups:

As you write down the foods you eat at each meal, check the boxes for the corresponding food group per serving.

Dairy.................................☐☐☐☐☐☐☐☐☐☐☐☐☐☐☐
Meats................................☐☐☐☐☐☐☐☐☐☐☐☐☐☐☐
Grains (including rice and corn).....☐☐☐☐☐☐☐☐☐☐☐☐☐☐☐
Fruits................................☐☐☐☐☐☐☐☐☐☐☐☐☐☐☐
Vegetables.......................☐☐☐☐☐☐☐☐☐☐☐☐☐☐☐
Sugar (Soda, Candy, Etc.)...☐☐☐☐☐☐☐☐☐☐☐☐☐☐☐
Chips and Junk Food....☐☐☐☐☐☐☐☐☐☐☐☐☐☐☐

Water Intake:

Mark off each eight-ounce serving of water you drink today.

☐☐
☐☐
☐☐
☐☐
☐☐
☐☐

Bowel Movements:

1. Time: __________ A.M./P.M.
2. Time: __________ A.M./P.M.
3. Time: __________ A.M./P.M.
4. Time: __________ A.M./P.M.
5. Time: __________ A.M./P.M.
6. Time: __________ A.M./P.M.

Notes:

Food Frequency and Dietary Habits

Patient Name: ________________________________ Date: ____________

This questionnaire will give us information about your eating habits. There are no "right" or "wrong" answers. Accurate and thoughtful responses will allow us to pinpoint your good habits as well as the habits that you should consider changing.

- Use the **past month** as your standard for how you eat.
- Recall the times during the day when you ate, and what you had.
- Include snacks and "nibbles" as well as meals and beverages.
- If you ate out regularly or traveled, remember to include those foods, too.
- Be sure to answer every item on this form. If you did not eat a food listed below — or ate it less than once a week—write a "0" in the space provided. Please do not leave blanks.

Part I. We want to know how often you ate certain foods. For each of the foods listed, please indicate how many servings per week you **usually** ate in the past month. Where indicated, check whether your servings are large, small or about average in size.

Food Item	Average Weekly Servings	Serving Size: Lg.	Av.	Sm.	Size of Average Serving
Red Meat (beef, pork and ham, veal, lamb)	____	____	____	____	4 ounces*
Meat Dishes (casseroles, tacos, pizza, meat sauce)	____	____	____	____	1 cup casserole, 1 taco or pizza slice
Chicken or Turkey	____	____	____	____	1 lg or 2 sm pieces
Fish (including canned in water)	____	____	____	____	4 ounces,* ½ can
Shellfish (including canned in water)	____	____	____	____	4 ounces,* ½ can
Bacon, Sausage	____	____	____	____	2 pieces
Luncheon Meats (salami, bologna, hot dogs, etc. including turkey and chicken varieties)	____	____	____	____	1 piece
Low-Fat Luncheon Meats (at least 95% fat-free)	____	____	____	____	1 piece
How many of the above servings are from fast food outlets? (McDonald's, Taco Bell, etc.)					____________
Soy-Meat Substitute (protein drink)	____	____	____	____	Varies according to package
Whey Protein (meal replacement)	____	____	____	____	8 ounces

* 4 ounces of meat or fish is roughly the size of a deck of cards.

Food Item	Average Weekly Servings	Size of Average Serving
Whole eggs or egg yolks	____	1 egg or yolk
Milk, yogurt or cottage cheese	____	1 cup (8 ounces)
Cheese or cream cheese	____	1 ounce/slice
Ice cream	____	½ cup (1 scoop)
Fruits, fresh or dried	____	1 whole piece or 1 cup cut-up fruit
Fruit juice	____	½ cup (4 ounces)
Vegetable salads or raw vegetables	____	1 cup
Corn	____	½ cup
Cooked vegetables (fresh, frozen, or canned)	____	½ cup
Spaghetti, noodles or other pastas	____	1 cup
Dried beans, split peas or lentils	____	¾ cup (cooked)
Potatoes	____	¾ cup or 1 potato
Rice	____	¾ cup
Bread, bagels, rolls, tortillas, English muffins	____	1 piece
Biscuits, bakery muffins, croissants, flaky rolls	____	1 piece or slice
Sugared cereal	____	1 med. bowl
"Healthy" cereals (whole grain, oatmeal, etc)	____	1 med. bowl
Salad dressing	____	2 Tbsp.
Mayonnaise	____	1 Tbsp.
Nuts, nut butters (like peanut butter)	____	2 Tbsp.
Chips or French fries	____	1 cup
Baked desserts and pastries (cake, cookies, etc.)	____	1 slice or 2 cookies
Donuts or sweet rolls	____	1 piece
Chocolate or candy bars	____	1 candy bar
Alcoholic drinks	____	1 drink, 1 can beer, 1 glass wine
Sweetened beverages, not including diet drinks (soft drinks, fruit drinks, etc.)	____	1 large glass, 1 can
Coffee Beverages and Tea	____	1 cup

Part II. For each of the following items, check the **one** answer that best describes you. Use your eating habits of the past month as your standard.

How many meals do you eat out per week? ________________

How many glasses of water do you consume each week? ________________

How often do you choose organic foods?

____ Always
____ Sometimes
____ Never

Are there any foods that you avoid because you have a reaction to them?

____

On average, how often do you eat breakfast in a week? ________________

When I eat meat, fish or poultry,

____ 1. I almost always have it fried or cooked with oil or another fat, or with gravy.
____ 2. I almost always have it broiled, baked or stewed, and without any gravy or fat.
____ 3. I do both.
____ 4. I don't eat meat, fish or poultry.

When I eat cooked vegetables,

____ 1. I almost always have them with butter, margarine or sauce; or cooked with butter, margarine, oil or another fat.
____ 2. I almost always have them without any of the fats listed above.
____ 3. I do both.
____ 4. I don't eat cooked vegetables.

Validated 14-item Questionnaire of Mediterranean Diet Adherence: Used in The PREDIMED Trial

Questions	Criteria for 1 point	Check if True
1. Do you use olive oil as main culinary fat?	Yes	☐
2. How much olive oil do you consume in a given day (including oil used for frying, salads, out-of-house meals, etc.)?	≥4 tbsp	☐
3. How many vegetable servings do you consume per day? (1 serving : 200 g [consider side dishes as half a serving])	≥2 (≥1 portion raw or as a salad)	☐
4. How many fruit units [servings] (include natural fruit juices) do you consume per day?	≥3	☐
5. How many servings of red meat, hamburger, or meat products (ham, sausage, etc.) do you consume per day? (1 serving: 100–150 g)	<1	☐
6. How many servings of butter, margarine, or cream do you consume per day? (1 serving: 12 g)	<1	☐
7. How many sweet or carbonated beverages do you drink per day?	<1	☐
8. How much wine do you drink per week?	≥7 glasses	☐
9. How many servings of legumes do you consume per week? (1 serving : 150 g)	≥3	☐
10. How many servings of fish or shellfish do you consume per week? (1 serving 100–150 g of fish or 4–5 units or 200 g of shellfish)	≥3	☐
11. How many times per week do you consume commercial sweets or pastries (not homemade), such as cakes, cookies, biscuits, or custard?	<3	☐
12. How many servings of nuts (including peanuts) do you consume per week? (1 serving 30 g)	≥3	☐
13. Do you preferentially consume chicken, turkey, or rabbit meat instead of veal, pork, hamburger, or sausage?	Yes	☐
14. How many times per week do you consume vegetables, pasta, rice, or other dishes seasoned with sofrito (sauce made with tomato and onion, leek, or garlic and simmered with olive oil)?	≥2	☐

Total: ____________

Relative risk for nearly every chronic disease is lower as the MedDiet Adherence score increases. Scores below 7 are associated with higher risk. Risk continues to decrease as the score gets higher.

A Quick Guide to Implementing a Low-Glycemic Mediterranean Diet

In a low glycemic impact, Mediterranean diet, carbohydrates should comprise about 40 percent of the diet (with a focus on non-starchy vegetables); the remaining 60 percent of the diet is split equally into healthy fats and proteins. In this pattern, meals are typically eaten five times a day, as three main meals and two snacks. The following is a detailed explanation of the main components of a modified Mediterranean diet and the specific foods to emphasize. Aim to choose foods that are local and in season, and remember to implement the principles of enjoyment and pleasure by savoring your food, drinks and meals with others whenever possible.

Whole grains: Though the traditional Mediterranean diet allows wheat-based grain products such as pasta, bulgur and couscous, as well as white rice; gluten-free grains such as quinoa, wild rice, millet and amaranth may be used as nutritious alternatives. **Begin by reducing refined carbohydrates** (i.e., white bread, white pasta, white rice and muffins) and focus, instead, on the listed whole grains that are rich in vitamins, minerals, fiber and other phytonutrients. Whole grains can be toasted, then cooked, and drizzled with olive oil for main meals, or served as a hot breakfast cereal with fruit, nuts and seeds.

Legumes, nuts and seeds: Legumes are an excellent source of protein and fiber. Commonly consumed legumes include lentils, chickpeas and white beans that can be found in salads, as dips (like hummus) and in soups. Nuts, preferably raw, are also used throughout the Mediterranean diet as snacks and to add flavor and texture to main dishes. Almonds, cashews, peanuts, pumpkin seeds, sesame seeds, sunflower seeds and walnuts are all included; and all are good sources of healthy fats, protein and fiber. Choose organic almonds for a great snack; pumpkin seeds make a great addition to salads, and toasted sesame seeds make healthy additions to grain dishes alone or served as tahini dressing or spread. Peanuts and cashews should be consumed more sparingly.

Olive oil: Perhaps the most famous component of the traditional Mediterranean diet, olive oil is used liberally in this diet. It is rich in phytonutrients and monounsaturated fatty acids, which are known to increase good HDL cholesterol levels. Olives can be served as appetizers or incorporated into main dishes, and olive oil is used both as a salad dressing and low temperature cooking oil. Look for a high-quality, fresh, extra-virgin olive oil (EVOO). When using EVOO in cooking, reserve it for quick sautéing in order to prevent burning and oxidation, which destroys monounsaturated fatty acids.

Vegetables: The consumption of a variety of local and seasonal vegetables is central to the Mediterranean diet. Vegetables offer phytonutrients and fiber as well as an array of vitamins and minerals. Choose mineral-rich, green leafy vegetables and brightly colored vegetables, which improve insulin sensitivity and reduce inflammation. The Mediterranean diet also highlights the use of garlic, which is rich in cardiovascular benefits and has potent anti-inflammatory and anti-bacterial properties. Vegetables can be cooked in a variety of ways or eaten raw, drizzled with olive oil. Vegetable salads can be enjoyed at all meals, including breakfast.

Herbs and spices: Fresh herbs are included in almost all meals as a salad staple as well as in cooked dishes, and their presence reduces the need for added salt in dishes. Herbs offer great antioxidant value, reduce inflammation and assist in the digestive process. Commonly used herbs include oregano, thyme, basil, cilantro, parsley and mint, in fresh and dry forms, and brewed into herbal tea.

Fruits: Fruits are virtually omnipresent in the Mediterranean lifestyle and diet. Commonly consumed fruits include plums, dates and figs, although fruits should be eaten based on what is local and in season if possible. Fruits are commonly offered after meals as dessert in place of sugary pastries. Berries are especially rich in vitamins and polyphenols and have anti-inflammatory properties. They are also an excellent source of insoluble fiber, key for glycemic control and a healthy gut.

Fish and meats: Fish is an excellent source of protein and the fatty varieties are rich in omega-3 polyunsaturated fatty acids, including tuna, herring, sardines, salmon and bream. Shellfish and crustaceans such as mussels, clams and shrimp have similar benefits and are commonly consumed in the Mediterranean diet, as are a variety of lean white fish, often grilled and baked, and drizzled with olive oil, herbs and garlic.

Dairy and eggs: Although many adults are lactose intolerant, fermented dairy products can often be eaten in moderation. The Mediterranean diet emphasizes cultured dairy products such as strained and Greek yogurt and soft cheeses, which are good sources of calcium and protein. Eggs are typically eaten in moderation, up to four times a week. Also excellent sources of protein, eggs are most often used in baking or as omelets with veggies.

Polyphenol-rich drinks: The traditional Mediterrenan diet is known to include moderate intake of wine, an excellent source of polyphenols. However, the benefits of polyphenols can also be attained by drinking the juices of pomegranates and dark grapes. For those who would like to include wine during meals, moderate consumption means up to one five-ounce glass of wine per day for women, and up to two five-ounce glasses for men.

Sample daily snacks

Choose higher protein or higher fiber etc. depending on personal needs.

- 2–3 tbsp. mixed almonds and walnuts (preferably unroasted)
- 1 handful assorted dried fruits such as dates, figs or apricots
- 12–15 low-fat blue corn chips with ¼ c. salsa or guacamole
- ¼ c. hummus and ½ c. vegetable sticks
- 1 medium, sliced apple with 1 tbsp. almond butter
- 1 low-fat cheese stick with whole-grain crackers
- 3 turkey and lettuce roll-ups with mustard
- 2 brown rice cakes with tahini and jam spread
- 1 c. vegetable juice plus 4–6 whole grain crackers
- ½ c. celery sticks plus 1 tbsp. peanut butter
- 1 cup steamed soybeans in pods (edamame) with sea salt
- 1 hard-boiled egg and ¼ c. carrot sticks
- 2–3 oz. salmon jerky
- ½ c. mixed berries and cherries
- 3 mini whole-wheat pita pizzas made with low-fat mozzarella, tomato sauce and oregano
- 1 handful of spiced, dried green peas and chickpeas
- 4–6 rye crackers and roasted vegetable dip
- 1 small whole-grain bran muffin
- 1 berry smoothie made with 6 oz. of nut milk and ½ c. fruit and flax seeds

Sample low-glycemic, Mediterranean meal options

Meals are typically eaten five times a day, as three main meals plus two snacks.

Breakfast options:

> Low-fat yogurt with sliced bananas and strawberries, handful chopped walnuts or muesli, drizzled with honey

> High-fiber cereal with low-fat milk (soy or nut milk may be substituted), topped with berries

> Soft-boiled egg with slice of whole-grain toast, and sliced tomatoes and cucumbers drizzled with olive oil, small glass of pomegranate juice

> Whole-grain (preferably steel-cut) oatmeal topped with slivered almonds, chopped dates or berries and one cup low-fat milk (soy optional)

> Protein smoothie made with frozen fruit, scoop of rice protein, and rice or almond milk

Lunch options:

> Chicken strips over a Greek salad with walnuts and whole-wheat pita wedges, and a sliced orange

> Tuna wrapped in whole-wheat tortilla with lettuce, carrots and alfalfa sprouts, and side of mixed bean salad or cup of Mediterranean vegetable soup

> Grilled tilapia or local fish over a greens salad with olive oil dressing, a side of brown or wild rice and sautéed cauliflower, small bowl of dark grapes

> Rice bowl with black beans, sautéed vegetables, topped with guacamole and fresh salsa

Dinner options:

> Herbed chicken with sautéed broccoli (in olive oil) and sweet potato fries

> Grilled shrimp kebabs, lentils with herbs and olive oil, tomato and cucumber salad

> Sesame ginger tofu with sautéed greens and roasted vegetables over buckwheat groats or other whole grain

> Grilled salmon filet over spinach with a side of wild rice

> 3-Bean dish topped with chopped herbs, served with crusty, whole-grain bread

No Mediterranean-style diet is complete without integrating the principles of the Mediterranean lifestyle. Here are some of the key aspects to implement:

- Slow cook whenever possible.
- Set aside enough time to eat in a relaxing atmosphere.
- Take the time to savor each bite of food.
- Enjoy meals with friends and family.
- Lead an active lifestyle and walk whenever possible.
- Take some time to soak in the sun's rays every day.
- Set aside some time each afternoon to relax, even 15 minutes to enjoy a cup of tea in the fresh air.
- Remember to give thanks for the food on your plate.

THE STANDARD
ROAD MAP SERIES

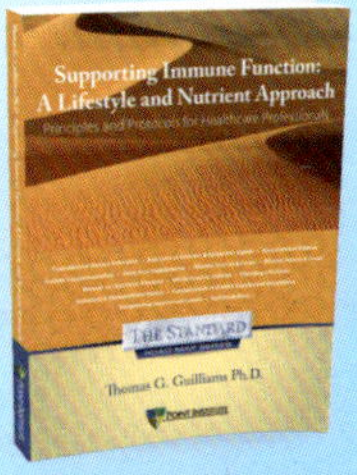

Supporting Immune Function: A Lifestyle and Nutrient Approach
Principles and Protocols for Healthcare Professionals

This Road map summarizes the latest knowledge concerning clinically-relevant immune system function (including autoimmune dysfunctions). Evidence for lifestyle and nutrient interventions affecting immune functions are discussed in detail; along with suggested protocols for improving immune function related to both acute and chronic immune challenges.

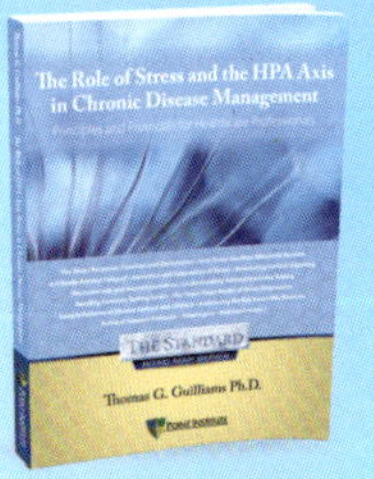

The Role of Stress and the HPA Axis in Chronic Disease Management
Principles and Protocols for Healthcare Professionals

This Road map outlines the evidence connecting HPA-axis and stress-related dysfunction with a wide-range of chronic diseases. Different testing and protocol strategies are reviewed, allowing the clinician to design a diagnostic and treatment strategy that suits their practice and patients. Intervention strategies emphasize lifestyle, nutritional and nutraceutical therapies.

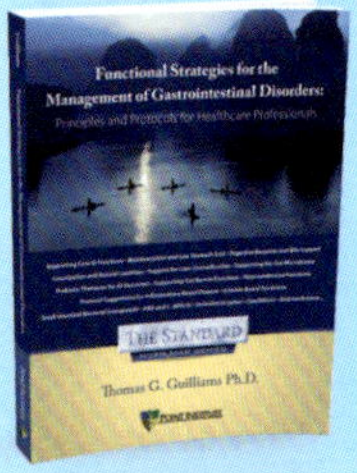

Functional Strategies for the Management of Gastrointestinal Disorders
Principles and Protocols for Healthcare Professionals

This Road map outlines the basic functions and dysfunctions of the GI-system, as viewed through the lens of functional medicine. Protocols are based upon rebuilding each of the functions of the GI tract; focusing on evidence-based therapies using lifestyle and nutraceutical interventions.

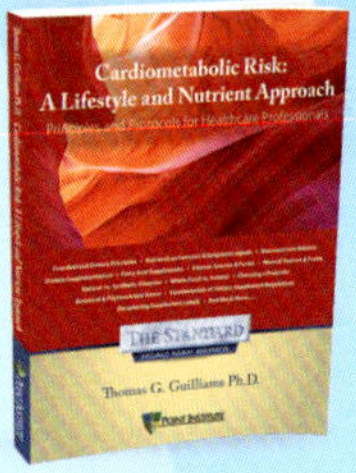

Cardiometabolic Risk: A Lifestyle and Nutrient Approach
Principles and Protocols for Healthcare Professionals

This Road map discusses the relationship between lifestyle inputs and the mechanisms that drive both type 2 diabetes and cardiovascular events. Strategies to help assess patient's insulin resistance, inflammatory status and lipid metabolism will be coupled with evidence-based implementation strategies that include diet, exercise, stress-control and nutraceutical interventions.

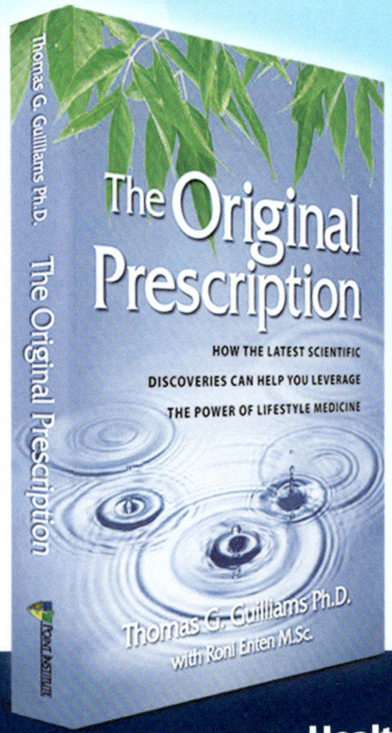

The Original Prescription

Thomas G. Guilliams, Ph.D.
with Roni Enten, M.S.

Includes 48 timeless and fundamental principles from all of the seven spheres of lifestyle signals- empowering patients to leverage their own health decisions.

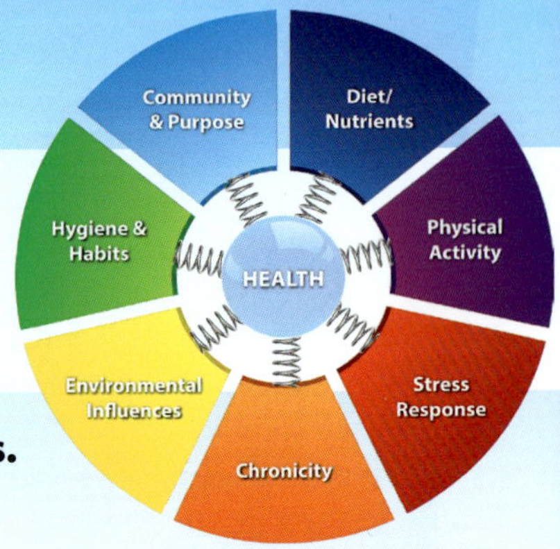

Copies available at volume discounts for use with patients.
Contact the Point Institute (info@pointinstitute.org) or the retailer of this handbook for more information.

Health Solutions should work with our body, not impose an outcome upon it.
***The Original Prescription* is that solution, one that our bodies are waiting for us to fulfill.**